A Contemporary Manual of Left Atrial Appendage Closure

Steven J. Filby • Luis Augusto Palma Dallan
Mauricio Arruda
Editors

A Contemporary Manual of Left Atrial Appendage Closure

Springer

Editors
Steven J. Filby
Division of Cardiology, Harrington Heart & Vascular Institute, University Hospitals Cleveland Medical Center
Cleveland, OH, USA

Luis Augusto Palma Dallan
Division of Cardiology, Harrington Heart & Vascular Institute, University Hospitals Cleveland Medical Center
Cleveland, OH, USA

Mauricio Arruda
Division of Cardiology, Harrington Heart & Vascular Institute, University Hospitals Cleveland Medical Center
Cleveland, OH, USA

ISBN 978-3-031-68443-2 ISBN 978-3-031-68441-8 (eBook)
https://doi.org/10.1007/978-3-031-68441-8

This Springer imprint is published by the registered company Springer Nature Switzerland AG
The registered company address is: Gewerbestrasse 11, 6330 Cham, Switzerland

We dedicate this book to all of our fellows, residents, nurses, and staff, without whom we would not be able to provide the excellent care to our patients and most of all to our families, who make it possible and worthwhile to do so.

Preface

It is with great pleasure and profound gratitude that we introduce this comprehensive volume on left atrial appendage closure. There has been tremendous growth in this space over the last decade, and with several randomized clinical trials on the horizon and future devices in development, there will certainly be more interest in this therapy in the years to come.

This book represents a collaborative effort among many esteemed authors from both interventional cardiology and electrophysiology and is intended to serve as a resource for clinicians performing this procedure. The manual is divided into three sections, spanning pre-procedural assessment, procedural approach, and post-procedure management. At every opportunity, we have attempted to provide the most clinically useful teaching points to benefit operators of all experience levels and to highlight the most contemporary approaches for this procedure.

In acknowledging the efforts of the authors, we extend our heartfelt appreciation for their diligence, enthusiasm, and perseverance throughout the creation of this book. Their collaborative spirit has not only enriched the content within but has also elevated the discourse surrounding this important therapy.

We hope that this book will serve as a valuable resource, fostering continued dialogue and advancements in the field.

Cleveland, OH, USA

Steven J. Filby
Luis Augusto Palma Dallan
Mauricio Arruda

Contents

Part II Procedural Approach

Part I
Pre-procedural Assessment

Chapter 1
Epidemiology: Atrial Fibrillation, Stroke, and Anticoagulation

Richard Pham and Ivan Cakulev

Highlights
- From 1990 to 2019, the worldwide prevalence of atrial fibrillation/atrial flutter has risen from 19.1 million to 59.7 million people.
- In the United States, it is projected that 16 million Americans will suffer from AF by 2050.
- Anticoagulation is remarkably underutilized despite its importance in the prevention of stroke.
- Future directions in the treatment of AF include novel anticoagulation strategies, refining patient treatment options, and clarifying the mechanism of stroke in AF.

Epidemiology

Atrial fibrillation (AF) is the most common arrhythmia worldwide and is a leading cause of morbidity, mortality, and healthcare costs. Defined as uncoordinated irregular activity of the atrium, AF is associated with increased risk of stroke, heart failure, dementia, hospitalizations, death, and disability [20, 47]. The Global Burden of Disease (GBD) study has noted that between 1990 and 2019, the prevalence of AF and atrial flutter (AFL) has risen from 19.1 million to 59.7 million people worldwide. When adjusting for age and population, the United States leads in prevalence with 1331.4/100,000 people. Internationally, AF/AFL incidence peaks between 75 and 80 years. The burden of disability-adjusted life years (DALYs) attributable to AF/AFL has also risen from 3.78 million to 8.39 million between 1990 and 2019, representing a substantial loss and burden to human health globally. Notably there

R. Pham · I. Cakulev (✉)
Division of Cardiology, Harrington Heart & Vascular Institute, University Hospitals Cleveland Medical Center, Cleveland, OH, USA
e-mail: Richard.pham@uhhospitals.org; Ivan.cakulev@uhhospitals.org

S. J. Filby et al. (eds.), *A Contemporary Manual of Left Atrial Appendage Closure*, https://doi.org/10.1007/978-3-031-68441-8_1

has been a rapid increase in the prevalence growth rate of AF/AFL that coincides with rapid economic development in Middle Eastern countries between 1990 and 2019. This may be due to the westernization of the Middle Eastern diet with resultant development of western metabolic and cardiovascular risk factors [27].

In the United States, the lifetime risk of developing atrial fibrillation after the age of 40 has been estimated to be 1 in 3 to 1 in 5. These estimates are based on population cohort studies including the well-known ARIC (Atherosclerosis Risk in Communities) and Framingham Heart Study (FHS) cohorts. Although prevalence continues to rise in the United States, incidence rates have been generally stagnant when examined in the more diverse cohort in ARIC. In ARIC, Black individuals had a 1 in 5 lifetime risk of developing AF, whereas White individuals had a 1 in 3 lifetime risk. The incidence rate of AF was 45% higher in men when compared to women and 32% higher in White compared with Black individuals [12, 43]. Prevalence will continue to grow, and by 2050 it is projected that there may be up to 16 million Americans suffering from atrial fibrillation [34].

The growth in prevalence is concerning, as AF is indicative of substantial mortality, with age-adjusted mortality rates attributable to AF as 6.5% per 100,000 people in 2019 in the United States. According to the findings from the Framingham study, AF is associated with an increase in all-cause mortality with a hazard ratio of 1.9 compared to those without AF. The consequences of AF are numerous, with strokes accounting for 7% of deaths, sudden cardiac death in 22% of cases, and progressive heart failure in 15% of cases [47].

Risk Factors for Developing AF

A significant portion of DALYs associated with AF globally are attributed to several associated risk factors including age, elevated systolic blood pressure, increased sodium intake, obesity, and smoking in the GBD study [27]. In ARIC, the population attributable fraction for AF in order was hypertension, obesity, smoking, cardiac disease, and diabetes [47].

Age

Advancing age is a prominent risk factor for the development of AF as well as increasing incidence [42]. In a Scottish study, the incidence rates per 1000 persons were 0.5 for age 45–54, 1.1 for age 55–64, 3.2 for age 65–74, 6.2 for age 75–84, and 7.7 for age $\geq$ 85 years [36]. The FHS examined temporal trends in AF risk factors. During the most recent time-period studied (1998–2007), participant age of 60–69, 70–79, and 80–89 years was associated with 4.98, 7.35, and 9.33 fold risk of AF, respectively, compared with individuals aged 50–59 years [42]. Accordingly, a stepwise increment in age has been incorporated in AF risk prediction scores.

Sex Differences

It is now recognized that the epidemiology of atrial fibrillation differs between men and women, with a higher incidence overall in men [25]. In the FHS, the AF incidence (per 1000 person-years) was 3.8 in men and 1.6 in women [42]. The Olmsted County Minnesota, Study [34] and the Rotterdam Study [5] reported the AF incidence (per 1000 person-years) in men to be 4.7 and 11.5, respectively, compared to 2.7 and 8.9 in women. Gender differences however do differ at different age groups. In the GBD study, females have a greater overall incidence than males after age 65 with postulated estrogen having a protective effect on AF earlier in life.

High Blood Pressure

Hypertension is the most significant risk factor in those with AF/AFL. In the FHS, the risk factor-adjusted odds ratio for AF was 1.5 and 1.4 in men and women with hypertension, respectively [23]. Some studies have found that the pulse pressure rather than mean blood pressure is more predictive of developing atrial fibrillation [33]. However in the CHARGE-AF study, both systolic and diastolic blood pressures were predictive of AF [2]. Furthermore, while the rate of treated hypertension increased and severe hypertension is less prevalent, the population attributed risk for developing atrial fibrillation is unaffected suggesting that the antihypertensive therapy does not completely eliminate the AF risk associated with hypertension [42].

Obesity

Obesity independently increases the risk for AF [11, 35, 50]. A meta-analyses of 5 studies found that obesity confers a 49% increased risk of developing AF [49]. Notably, weight loss does result in significantly reduced incidence of atrial fibrillation [1] and improved outcomes after atrial fibrillation ablation [37].

Diabetes Mellitus

Diabetes confers an increased risk of AF. In meta-analysis of prospective studies, there is a relative risk increase of 1.1 for the development of AF in diabetics [38]. In observational studies, the relative risk was 1.28 for diabetes and 1.20 for patients with prediabetes [4]. In machine-learning models, when comparing patients with type 1 and type 2 diabetes, there is a similar risk of incident AF, but with female diabetics conferring a higher risk of incident AF as compared to males [53].

Sleep Disorders

Obstructive sleep-disorder breathing (SDB) is associated with an overall increased odds ratio of 1.4 in a meta-analysis of 8 studies [55] for AF. The treatment of sleep apnea has been shown to decrease the risk of progression to permanent AF [17] as well as maintain sinus rhythm after ablation and cardioversions [7, 45]. Smaller trials however do not demonstrate differences in AF burden or recurrence when treating SDB in either primary or secondary prevention [46].

Heart Disease

Sharing many antecedent risk factors, AF and cardiovascular disease are closely related. Among those with either AF or heart failure, 40% will develop the other condition. Pooled data from multiple population studies show that a history of MI and HF were associated with a risk of AF with hazard ratios of 1.64 and 2.02, respectively [2]. An outcome among those with AF in the Olmstead County cohort, incidence of HFpEF (HF with preserved ejection fraction) was 3.3 per 100 person-years as compared to 2.1 for HFrEF [41]. Another important risk factor for AF is congenital heart disease, with a large Swedish study demonstrating a 22 times higher risk of developing AF [29].

Other Risk Factors

AF is often secondary to reversible conditions and triggers. Cardiothoracic surgery, infection, and acute myocardial infarction are among the most common. Coronary bypass surgery is associated with a 33.1% risk-adjusted incidence of AF [9] and 10.9% in those undergoing noncardiac surgery [8]. Among a Medicare sample of patients with sepsis, 25.5% of patients had AF [48]. Other areas of interest include air pollution where meta-analysis has shown incremental increases of AF in areas with worsening particulate pollution concentrations. Psychosocial factors are also an area of interest with demonstration of an increased risk of AF after adjusting for confounders in patients with post-traumatic stress disorder, depression, and job strain [47].

Stroke

Notably, 795,000 patients will have a new or recurrent stroke each year, and among first-time patients, 24% exhibit AF upon monitor detection which is likely underestimated [47]. In a randomized control trial, long-term monitoring of patients with cryptogenic stroke detected a cumulative incidence of AF of 30% by 3 years, and approximately 80% of first-time AF episodes were asymptomatic [6, 40]. Since the early 1970s, an increased incidence of stroke and transient ischemic attacks in patients with atrial fibrillation has been observed [30, 51]. In the Framingham Health Study, the attributable risk of AF for stroke was 1.5% among 50–59-year-olds, whereas among 80–89-year-olds, it was 23.5% [51]. Strokes in AF patients are associated with increased morbidity and mortality, with larger infarcts and involving the cerebral cortex in patients with AF [22].

Anticoagulation and Considerations

Anticoagulation is a cornerstone in AF treatment in the prevention of embolic stroke. Compared to control or placebo, VKA reduces stroke by 64% and all-cause mortality by 26% [14]. The introduction of direct oral anticoagulants (DOACs) has changed the current landscape of stroke prevention in AF patients worldwide, offering relatively improved efficacy, safety, and convenience compared with the traditional vitamin K antagonists. All DOACs have demonstrated reduced bleeding incidence when compared to warfarin especially with intracranial hemorrhage and GI bleeding [19, 26].

The decision to offer oral anticoagulation therapy (OAT) to prevent thromboembolic complications must be balanced against the risk of bleeding. Scores have been designed to help with decision-making, but some patients may fall outside the usual calculated risk scores when considering other important factors. For instance, current risk scores do not consider AF subtypes (i.e., paroxysmal AF, persistent AF, permanent AF) as prior studies show that stroke risk is dependent on underlying risk factors rather than the arrhythmia subtype [13, 16, 28]. It does appear that persistent AF contributes to more strokes when compared with paroxysmal AF [44]. In the non-anticoagulated AF patients, persistent atrial fibrillation was the second strongest predictor after prior stroke or TIA (transient ischemic attack) with 83% and 44% increased risk for permanent and persistent AF compared to paroxysmal AF [3]. Furthermore, subclinical AF is associated with an increased stroke risk in patients with cardiac implantable electronic devices (CIED). In the Asymptomatic Atrial Fibrillation and Stroke Evaluation in Pacemaker Patients and the Atrial Fibrillation Reduction Atrial Pacing Trial (ASSERT) (n = 2580), subclinical AF duration of 24 h was associated with a significant increased risk of subsequent stroke or systemic embolism (hazard ratio [HR] 3.24, [1.51–6.95]) [39].

To this day it is unclear what duration of AF should warrant initiation of OAT. Two recent trials illustrate the need to incorporate duration of the AF, risk factors for stroke, and bleeding when deciding when to offer OAT to patients with subclinical AF. The Non–vitamin K antagonist Oral anticoagulants in patients with Atrial High rate episodes (NOAH-AFNET 6) trial (n = 2536) randomized participants to edoxaban or comparator (acetylsalicylic acid (ASA) or placebo according to clinical indication). NOAH-AFNET 6 was stopped prematurely due to safety concerns and trend towards futility despite that there were numerically fewer thrombotic events in patients randomized to edoxaban [24]. The incidence of stroke was approximately 1% per patient-year in both groups, and the mean duration of AF was 2.8 h. The ARTESiA study of 4012 patients were randomized to apixaban or aspirin and reported that apixaban significantly reduced the risk of the primary efficacy of ischemic stroke or systemic embolism. Both trials showed higher rates of bleeding [15]. A meta-analysis of the two trials provided insights from a broader population with greater power to detect differences in efficacy and/or harm [31] confirming key findings that anticoagulation therapy reduced ischemic stroke risk in device-detected AF, but increased the risk of major bleeding. Notably, there was no reduction in all-cause mortality or CV death with anticoagulation therapy. It is also notable that the overall rate of stroke was lower than anticipated in both trials, suggesting that this may not be a particularly high-risk group (average duration of AF was 1.5–2.8 h). As such, most patients with device-detected subclinical AF should not be treated with anticoagulation therapy, and it remains unclear what duration of atrial fibrillation matched for the specific patient risks warrants OAT.

Importantly, there are other clinical scenarios where OAT is warranted irrespective of the calculated risk score. Patients with hypertrophic cardiomyopathy and amyloidosis who have significantly higher risk for thromboembolic phenomena should be anticoagulated irrespective of the CHA2DS2-Vasc score. Furthermore, patients post-ablation involving the left atrium, or those cardioverted, should be anticoagulated. In patients who have had electrical isolation of the LAA, the incidence of left atrial appendage thrombus despite OAT is close to 20% [10]. These patients would best be served with consideration for a staged or concomitant left atrial appendage closure or removal.

Despite the importance of anticoagulation, studies have consistently demonstrated significant underuse. Important factors for underuse include substance use disorders, noncompliance, dementia, falls, renal impairment, female gender, non-commercial insurance, and bleeding diatheses. Black patients are less likely to receive direct oral anticoagulants after adjusting for socioeconomic factors in the United States. The Get With The Guidelines Stroke program performed a retrospective analysis of 94,474 patients with stroke who had known previous AF, and nearly 84% of patients were not receiving therapeutic anticoagulation therapy prior to their stroke. Data from the NCDR PINNACLE (National Cardiovascular Data Registry's Practice Innovation and Clinical Excellence) registry of patients with AF demonstrated that less than half of patients with a CHA2DS2-VASc score of ≥4 received oral anticoagulation [18, 47, 52].

The underutilization of anticoagulation underscores an unmet need for alternative treatments for stroke prevention. In 1996, Blackshear et al. conducted a review of studies which suggested that in nonrheumatic atrial fibrillation, 91% of thrombi formation could be localized to the left atrial appendage (LAA). Early surgical ablation procedures were often followed by surgical excision of the LAA, and often surgical LAA exclusion coincided with other cardiac surgeries. Data in this area are mixed and limited, often with retrospective studies clouded by concurrent use of anticoagulation. Although surgical LAA exclusion has been demonstrated to potentially reduce stroke and all-cause mortality, the benefit may not be apparent in those already on anticoagulation. There remains benefit of oral anticoagulation after LAA exclusion [21, 32, 54]. Endovascular, catheter-based solutions have been introduced in modern times as an additional alternative to stroke prevention, demonstrating non-inferiority to warfarin in the PROTECT-AF and PREVAIL trials. The evolution of catheter-based LAA occlusion strategies has introduced a new frontier and will be further explored in this book.

Future Directions and Research

There remains a great need to better define patient selection for which OAT is needed to reduce thromboembolic risk while reducing bleeding complications and cost. As the field advances with LAAO technologies, cardiac ablation, and more consumer monitoring devices that quantify AF burden, decision-making has become more complex beyond the CHA2DS2-Vasc score. Ongoing trials OCEAN, ODIn-AF, and REACT AF will attempt to answer some of these questions. Novel anticoagulation strategies are also at the forefront of AF treatment. Factor XI inhibitors, the latest focus of interest in this field, are potentially bringing us to this goal. The phase 2 AZALEA-TIMI 71 study was stopped early because of an "overwhelming" reduction in major and clinically relevant nonmajor bleeding shown with the factor XI inhibitor abelacimab (Anthos) compared to rivaroxaban for patients with atrial fibrillation. Other factor XI inhibitors are in phase 2 and phase 3 trials.

Finally, a thorough mechanistic explanation of how AF and its risk factors contribute to thrombus formation is yet to be elucidated. The prior mechanistic model that LAA stasis from AF leads to thromboembolic phenomena is likely oversimplified as we begin to understand the importance of atrial myopathy and substrate formation as it relates to stroke. Understanding this will determine our future approach to preventing thromboembolic phenomena.

References

1. Abed HS, Wittert GA, Leong DP, Shirazi MG, Bahrami B, Middeldorp ME, Lorimer MF, Lau DH, Antic NA, Brooks AG, Abhayaratna WP, Kalman JM, Sanders P. Effect of weight reduction and cardiometabolic risk factor management on symptom burden and severity in patients with atrial fibrillation: a randomized clinical trial. JAMA. 2013;310(19):2050–60. https://doi.org/10.1001/jama.2013.280521.
2. Alonso A, Krijthe BP, Aspelund T, Stepas KA, Pencina MJ, Moser CB, Sinner MF, Sotoodehnia N, Fontes JD, Janssens ACJW, Kronmal RA, Magnani JW, Witteman JC, Chamberlain AM, Lubitz SA, Schnabel RB, Agarwal SK, McManus DD, Ellinor PT, et al. Simple risk model predicts incidence of atrial fibrillation in a racially and geographically diverse population: the CHARGE-AF consortium. J Am Heart Assoc. 2013;2(2) https://doi.org/10.1161/JAHA.112.000102.

3. Arkin JM, Kowey PR. Does atrial fibrillation pattern affect stroke risk? Data dredging to help the clinician. Eur Heart J. 2015;36(5):265–6. https://doi.org/10.1093/eurheartj/ehu420. Oxford University Press
4. Aune D, Feng T, Schlesinger S, Janszky I, Norat T, Riboli E. Diabetes mellitus, blood glucose and the risk of atrial fibrillation: a systematic review and meta-analysis of cohort studies. Nutr. Metab. Cardiovasc. Dis. 2018;32(5):501–11.
5. Boriani G, Diemberger I, Martignani C, Biffi M, Branzi A. The epidemiological burden of atrial fibrillation: a challenge for clinicians and health care systems. Eur Heart J. 2006;27(8):893–4. https://doi.org/10.1093/eurheartj/ehi651.
6. Brachmann J, Morillo CA, Sanna T, Di Lazzaro V, Diener HC, Bernstein RA, Rymer M, Ziegler PD, Liu S, Passman RS. Uncovering atrial fibrillation beyond short-term monitoring in cryptogenic stroke patients: three-year results from the cryptogenic stroke and underlying atrial fibrillation trial. Circ Arrhythm Electrophysiol. 2016;9(1) https://doi.org/10.1161/CIRCEP.115.003333.
7. Caples SM, Mansukhani MP, Friedman PA, Somers VK. The impact of continuous positive airway pressure treatment on the recurrence of atrial fibrillation post cardioversion: a randomized controlled trial. Int J Cardiol. 2019;278:133–6. https://doi.org/10.1016/j.ijcard.2018.11.100.
8. Chebbout R, Heywood EG, Drake TM, Wild JRL, Lee J, Wilson M, Lee MJ. A systematic review of the incidence of and risk factors for postoperative atrial fibrillation following general surgery. Anaesthesia. 2018;73(4):490–8. https://doi.org/10.1111/anae.14118.
9. Filardo G, Damiano RJ, Ailawadi G, Thourani VH, Pollock BD, Sass DM, Phan TK, Nguyen H, da Graca B. Epidemiology of new-onset atrial fibrillation following coronary artery bypass graft surgery. Heart. 2018;104(12):985–92. https://doi.org/10.1136/heartjnl-2017-312150.
10. Fink T, Vogler J, Heeger CH, Sano M, Sciacca V, Reissmann B, Wohlmuth P, Keelani A, Schütte C, Eitel C, Eitel I, Maurer T, Rottner L, Rillig A, Mathew S, Metzner A, Ouyang F, Kuck KH, Tilz RR. Impact of left atrial appendage closure on LAA thrombus formation and thromboembolism after LAA isolation. JACC Clin Electrophysiol. 2020;6(13):1687–97. https://doi.org/10.1016/j.jacep.2020.07.003.
11. Frost L, Hune LJ, Vestergaard P. Overweight and obesity as risk factors for atrial fibrillation or flutter: the Danish diet, cancer, and health study. Am J Med. 2005;118(5):489–95. https://doi.org/10.1016/j.amjmed.2005.01.031.
12. Ghelani KP, Chen LY, Norby FL, Soliman EZ, Koton S, Alonso A. Thirty-year trends in the incidence of atrial fibrillation: the ARIC study. J Am Heart Assoc. 2022;11(8) https://doi.org/10.1161/JAHA.121.023583.
13. Hart RG, Pearce LA, Rothbart RM, Mcanulty JH, Asinger RW, Halperin JL. Stroke with intermittent atrial fibrillation: incidence and predictors during aspirin therapy. J Am Coll Cardiol. 1999;35(1):183–7.
14. Hart RG, Pearce LA, Aguilar MI. Adjusted-dose warfarin versus aspirin for preventing stroke in patients with atrial fibrillation. Ann Intern Med. 2007;147(8):590–2. https://doi.org/10.7326/0003-4819-147-8-200710160-00018.
15. Healey JS, Lopes RD, Granger CB, Alings M, Rivard L, McIntyre WF, Atar D, Birnie DH, Boriani G, Camm AJ, Conen D, Erath JW, Gold MR, Hohnloser SH, Ip J, Kautzner J, Kutyifa V, Linde C, Mabo P, et al. Apixaban for stroke prevention in subclinical atrial fibrillation. N Engl J Med. 2023; https://doi.org/10.1056/nejmoa2310234.
16. Hohnloser SH, Pajitnev D, Pogue J, Healey JS, Pfeffer MA, Yusuf S, Connolly SJ. Incidence of stroke in paroxysmal versus sustained atrial fibrillation in patients taking oral anticoagulation or combined antiplatelet therapy. An ACTIVE W substudy. J Am Coll Cardiol. 2007;50(22):2156–61. https://doi.org/10.1016/j.jacc.2007.07.076.
17. Holmqvist F, Guan N, Zhu Z, Kowey PR, Allen LA, Fonarow GC, Hylek EM, Mahaffey KW, Freeman JV, Chang P, Holmes DN, Peterson ED, Piccini JP, Gersh BJ. Impact of obstructive sleep apnea and continuous positive airway pressure therapy on outcomes in patients with atrial fibrillation—results from the Outcomes Registry for Better Informed Treatment of Atrial

Fibrillation (ORBIT-AF). Am Heart J. 2015;169(5):647–654.e2. https://doi.org/10.1016/j.ahj.2014.12.024.

18. Hsu JC, Reynolds MR, Song Y, Doros G, Lubitz SA, Gehi AK, Turakhia MP, Maddox TM. Outpatient prescription practices in patients with atrial fibrillation (from the NCDR PINNACLE registry). Am J Cardiol. 2021;155:32–9. https://doi.org/10.1016/j.amjcard.2021.06.011.
19. Jackevicius CA, Lu L, Ghaznavi Z, Warner AL. Bleeding risk of direct oral anticoagulants in patients with heart failure and atrial fibrillation. Circ Cardiovasc Qual Outcomes. 2021;14(2):E007230. https://doi.org/10.1161/CIRCOUTCOMES.120.007230.
20. January CT, Wann LS, Calkins H, Chen LY, Cigarroa JE, Cleveland JC, Ellinor PT, Ezekowitz MD, Field ME, Furie KL, Heidenreich PA, Murray KT, Shea JB, Tracy CM, Yancy CW. 2019 AHA/ACC/HRS focused update of the 2014 AHA/ACC/HRS guideline for the Management of Patients with Atrial Fibrillation: a report of the American College of Cardiology/American Heart Association task force on clinical practice guidelines and the Heart Rhythm Society in collaboration with the Society of Thoracic Surgeons. Circulation. 2019;140(2):e125–51. https://doi.org/10.1161/CIR.0000000000000665.
21. Johnsrud DO, Melduni RM, Lahr B, Yao X, Greason KL, Noseworthy PA. Evaluation of anticoagulation use and subsequent stroke in patients with atrial fibrillation after empiric surgical left atrial appendage closure: a retrospective case-control study. Clin Cardiol. 2018;41(12):1578–82. https://doi.org/10.1002/clc.23066.
22. Jørgensen HS, Nakayama H, Reith J, Raaschou HO, Olsen TS. Acute stroke with atrial fibrillation. The Copenhagen stroke study. Stroke. 1996;27(10):1765–9. https://doi.org/10.1161/01.str.27.10.1765.
23. Kannel WB, Wolf PA, Benjamin EJ, Levy D. Prevalence, incidence, prognosis, and predisposing conditions for atrial fibrillation: population-based estimates 11Reprints are not available. Am J Cardiol. 1998;82(7):2N–9N. https://doi.org/10.1016/S0002-9149(98)00583-9.
24. Kirchhof P, Toennis T, Goette A, Camm AJ, Diener HC, Becher N, Bertaglia E, Blomstrom Lundqvist C, Borlich M, Brandes A, Cabanelas N, Calvert M, Chlouverakis G, Dan G-A, de Groot JR, Dichtl W, Kravchuk B, Lubiński A, Marijon E, et al. Anticoagulation with edoxaban in patients with atrial high-rate episodes. N Engl J Med. 2023;389(13):1167–79. https://doi.org/10.1056/nejmoa2303062.
25. Ko, D., Rahman, F., Schnabel, R. B., Yin, X., Benjamin, E. J., & Christophersen, I. E. (2016). Atrial fibrillation in women: epidemiology, pathophysiology, presentation, and prognosis. In Nature reviews cardiology 13, 6, 321–332). Nature publishing group. doi:https://doi.org/10.1038/nrcardio.2016.45.
26. Levine M, Goldstein JN. Bleeding complications of targeted oral anticoagulants: what is the risk? http://ashpublications.org/hematology/article-pdf/2014/1/504/1249594/bep00114000504.pdf (n.d.).
27. Li H, Song X, Liang Y, Bai X, Liu-Huo WS, Tang C, Chen W, Zhao L. Global, regional, and national burden of disease study of atrial fibrillation/flutter, 1990–2019: results from a global burden of disease study, 2019. BMC Public Health. 2022;22(1) https://doi.org/10.1186/s12889-022-14403-2.
28. Lubitz SA, Rosen AB, Ellinor PT, Benjamin EJ. Stroke risk in AF: do AF patterns matter? European Heart Journal. 2010;31(8):908–10. https://doi.org/10.1093/eurheartj/ehq074.
29. Mandalenakis Z, Rosengren A, Lappas G, Eriksson P, Gilljam T, Hansson P-O, Skoglund K, Fedchenko M, Dellborg M. Atrial fibrillation burden in young patients with congenital heart disease. Circulation. 2018;137(9):928–37. https://doi.org/10.1161/CIRCULATIONAHA.117.029590.
30. McAllen PM, Marshall J. Cardiac dysrhythmia and transient cerebral ischaemic attacks. Lancet (London, England). 1973;1(7814):1212–4. https://doi.org/10.1016/s0140-6736(73)90527-8.
31. McIntyre WF, Benz AP, Becher N, Healey JS, Granger CB, Rivard L, Camm AJ, Goette A, Zapf A, Alings M, Connolly SJ, Kirchhof P, Lopes RD. Direct oral anticoagulants for stroke prevention in patients with device-detected atrial fibrillation: a study-level meta-analysis

of the NOAH-AFNET 6 and ARTESiA trials. Circulation. 2023; https://doi.org/10.1161/circulationaha.123.067512.
32. Melduni RM, Schaff HV, Lee HC, Gersh BJ, Noseworthy PA, Bailey KR, Ammash NM, Cha SS, Fatema K, Wysokinski WE, Seward JB, Packer DL, Rihal CS, Asirvatham SJ. Impact of left atrial appendage closure during cardiac surgery on the occurrence of early postoperative atrial fibrillation, stroke, and mortality. Circulation. 2017;135(4):366–78. https://doi.org/10.1161/CIRCULATIONAHA.116.021952.
33. Mitchell GF, Vasan RS, Keyes MJ, Helen Parise M, Thomas Wang SJ, Larson MG, Ralph DSB, Kannel WB, Daniel Levy M, Benjamin EJ. Pulse pressure and risk of new-onset atrial fibrillation. www.jama.com (n.d.).
34. Miyasaka Y, Barnes ME, Gersh BJ, Cha SS, Bailey KR, Abhayaratna WP, Seward JB, Tsang TSM. Secular trends in incidence of atrial fibrillation in Olmsted County, Minnesota, 1980 to 2000, and implications on the projections for future prevalence. Circulation. 2006;114(2):119–25. https://doi.org/10.1161/CIRCULATIONAHA.105.595140.
35. Murphy NF, MacIntyre K, Stewart S, Hart CL, Hole D, McMurray JJV. Long-term cardiovascular consequences of obesity: 20-year follow-up of more than 15 000 middle-aged men and women (the Renfrew-Paisley study). Eur Heart J. 2006;27(1):96–106. https://doi.org/10.1093/eurheartj/ehi506.
36. Murphy NF, Simpson CR, Jhund PS, Stewart S, Kirkpatrick M, Chalmers J, MacIntyre K, McMurray JJV. A national survey of the prevalence, incidence, primary care burden and treatment of atrial fibrillation in Scotland. Heart. 2007;93(5):606–12. https://doi.org/10.1136/hrt.2006.107573.
37. Park DY, An S, Murthi M, Kattoor AJ, Kaur A, Ravi V, Huang HD, Vij A. Effect of weight loss on recurrence of atrial fibrillation after ablative therapy: a systematic review and meta-analysis. J Interventional Card Electrophysiol. 2022;64(3):763–71. https://doi.org/10.1007/s10840-022-01168-2.
38. Qi W, Zhang N, Korantzopoulos P, Letsas KP, Cheng M, Di F, Tse G, Liu T, Li G. Serum glycated hemoglobin level as a predictor of atrial fibrillation: a systematic review with meta-analysis and metaregression. PLoS One. 2017;12(3) https://doi.org/10.1371/journal.pone.0170955.
39. Rahimi K. Subclinical atrial fibrillation in need of more assertive evidence. European Heart Journal. 2017;38(17):1345–7. https://doi.org/10.1093/eurheartj/ehx122. Oxford University Press
40. Sanna T, Diener H-C, Passman RS, Di Lazzaro V, Bernstein RA, Morillo CA, Rymer MM, Thijs V, Rogers T, Beckers F, Lindborg K, Brachmann J. Cryptogenic stroke and underlying atrial fibrillation. N Engl J Med. 2014;370(26):2478–86. https://doi.org/10.1056/nejmoa1313600.
41. Santhanakrishnan R, Wang N, Larson MG, Magnani JW, McManus DD, Lubitz SA, Ellinor PT, Cheng S, Vasan RS, Lee DS, Wang TJ, Levy D, Benjamin EJ, Ho JE. Atrial fibrillation begets heart failure and vice versa: temporal associations and differences in preserved versus reduced ejection fraction. Circulation. 2016;133(5):484–92. https://doi.org/10.1161/CIRCULATIONAHA.115.018614.
42. Schnabel RB, Yin X, Gona P, Larson MG, Beiser AS, McManus DD, Newton-Cheh C, Lubitz SA, Magnani JW, Ellinor PT, Seshadri S, Wolf PA, Vasan RS, Benjamin EJ, Levy D. 50 year trends in atrial fibrillation prevalence, incidence, risk factors, and mortality in the Framingham heart study: a cohort study. Lancet. 2015;386(9989):154–62. https://doi.org/10.1016/S0140-6736(14)61774-8.
43. Staerk L, Wang B, Preis SR, Larson MG, Lubitz SA, Ellinor PT, McManus DD, Ko D, Weng LC, Lunetta KL, Frost L, Benjamin EJ, Trinquart L. Lifetime risk of atrial fibrillation according to optimal, borderline, or elevated levels of risk factors: cohort study based on longitudinal data from the Framingham heart study. BMJ (online). 2018;361 https://doi.org/10.1136/bmj.k1453.
44. Steinberg BA, Hellkamp AS, Lokhnygina Y, Patel MR, Breithardt G, Hankey GJ, Becker RC, Singer DE, Halperin JL, Hacke W, Nessel CC, Berkowitz SD, Mahaffey KW, Fox KAA, Califf

RM, Piccini JP. Higher risk of death and stroke in patients with persistent vs. paroxysmal atrial fibrillation: results from the ROCKET-AF trial. Eur Heart J. 2015;36(5):288–96. https://doi.org/10.1093/eurheartj/ehu359.

45. Szymanski FM, Filipiak KJ, Platek AE, Hrynkiewicz-Szymanska A, Kotkowski M, Kozluk E, Kiliszek M, Sierdzinski J, Opolski G. Presence and severity of obstructive sleep apnea and remote outcomes of atrial fibrillation ablations – a long-term prospective, cross-sectional cohort study. Sleep Breath. 2015;19(3):849–56. https://doi.org/10.1007/s11325-014-1102-x.
46. Traaen GM, Aakerøy L, Hunt T-E, Øverland B, Bendz C, Sande LØ, Aakhus S, Fagerland MW, Steinshamn S, Anfinsen O-G, Massey RJ, Broch K, Ueland T, Akre H, Loennechen JP, Gullestad L. Effect of continuous positive airway pressure on arrhythmia in atrial fibrillation and sleep apnea: a randomized controlled trial. Am J Respir Crit Care Med. 2021;204(5):573–82. https://doi.org/10.1164/rccm.202011-4133OC.
47. Tsao CW, Aday AW, Almarzooq ZI, Alonso A, Beaton AZ, Bittencourt MS, Boehme AK, Buxton AE, Carson AP, Commodore-Mensah Y, Elkind MSV, Evenson KR, Eze-Nliam C, Ferguson JF, Generoso G, Ho JE, Kalani R, Khan SS, Kissela BM, et al. Heart disease and stroke statistics-2022 update: a report from the American Heart Association. Circulation. 2022;145(8):E153–639). Lippincott Williams and Wilkins. https://doi.org/10.1161/CIR.0000000000001052.
48. Walkey AJ, Greiner MA, Heckbert SR, Jensen PN, Piccini JP, Sinner MF, Curtis LH, Benjamin EJ. Atrial fibrillation among Medicare beneficiaries hospitalized with sepsis: incidence and risk factors. Am Heart J. 2013;165(6):949–955.e3. https://doi.org/10.1016/j.ahj.2013.03.020.
49. Wanahita N, Messerli FH, Bangalore S, Gami AS, Somers VK, Steinberg JS. Atrial fibrillation and obesity-results of a meta-analysis. Am Heart J. 2008;155(2):310–5. https://doi.org/10.1016/j.ahj.2007.10.004.
50. Wang TJ, Parise H, Levy D, D'agostino RB, Wolf PA, Vasan RS, Benjamin EJ Obesity and the risk of new-onset atrial fibrillation. www.jama.com (n.d.).
51. Wolf PA, Abbott RD, Kannel WB. Atrial fibrillation as an independent risk factor for stroke: the Framingham study. Stroke. 1991;22(8):983–8. https://doi.org/10.1161/01.str.22.8.983.
52. Xian Y, O'Brien EC, Liang L, Xu H, Schwamm LH, Fonarow GC, Bhatt DL, Smith EE, Olson DWM, Maisch L, Hannah D, Lindholm B, Lytle BL, Pencina MJ, Hernandez AF, Peterson ED. Association of preceding antithrombotic treatment with acute ischemic stroke severity and in-hospital outcomes among patients with atrial fibrillation. JAMA. 2017;317(10):1057–67. https://doi.org/10.1001/jama.2017.1371.
53. Xiong Z, Liu T, Tse G, Gong M, Gladding PA, Smaill BH, Stiles MK, Gillis AM, Zhao J. A machine learning aided systematic review and meta-analysis of the relative risk of atrial fibrillation in patients with diabetes mellitus. Front Physiol. 2018;9(JULY) https://doi.org/10.3389/fphys.2018.00835.
54. Yao X, Gersh BJ, Holmes DR, Melduni RM, Johnsrud DO, Sangaralingham LR, Shah ND, Noseworthy PA. Association of surgical left atrial appendage occlusion with subsequent stroke and mortality among patients undergoing cardiac surgery. JAMA. 2018;319(20):2116–26. https://doi.org/10.1001/jama.2018.6024.
55. Zhao E, Chen S, Du Y, Zhang Y. Association between sleep apnea hypopnea syndrome and the risk of atrial fibrillation: a meta-analysis of cohort study. Biomed Res Int. 2018;2018:1–8. https://doi.org/10.1155/2018/5215868.

Suggested Readings

Ghelani KP, Chen LY, Norby FL, Soliman EZ, Koton S, Alonso A. Thirty-year trends in the incidence of atrial fibrillation: the ARIC study. J Am Heart Assoc. 2022;11(8) https://doi.org/10.1161/JAHA.121.023583.

January CT, Wann LS, Alpert JS, Calkins H, Cigarroa JE, Cleveland JC, Conti JB, Ellinor PT, Ezekowitz MD, Field ME, Murray KT, Sacco RL, Stevenson WG, Tchou PJ, Tracy CM, Anderson JL, Halperin JL, Albert NM, Bozkurt B, et al. 2014 AHA/ACC/HRS guideline for the management of patients with atrial fibrillation: a report of the American college of cardiology/American heart association task force on practice guidelines and the heart rhythm society. Circulation. 2014;130(23):e199–267). Lippincott Williams and Wilkins. https://doi.org/10.1161/CIR.0000000000000041.

Li H, Song X, Liang Y, Bai X, Liu-Huo WS, Tang C, Chen W, Zhao L. Global, regional, and national burden of disease study of atrial fibrillation/flutter, 1990–2019: results from a global burden of disease study, 2019. BMC Public Health. 2022;22(1) https://doi.org/10.1186/s12889-022-14403-2.

Staerk L, Wang B, Preis SR, Larson MG, Lubitz SA, Ellinor PT, McManus DD, Ko D, Weng LC, Lunetta KL, Frost L, Benjamin EJ, Trinquart L. Lifetime risk of atrial fibrillation according to optimal, borderline, or elevated levels of risk factors: cohort study based on longitudinal data from the Framingham heart study. BMJ (online). 2018;361 https://doi.org/10.1136/bmj.k1453.

Tsao CW, Aday AW, Almarzooq ZI, Alonso A, Beaton AZ, Bittencourt MS, Boehme AK, Buxton AE, Carson AP, Commodore-Mensah Y, Elkind MSV, Evenson KR, Eze-Nliam C, Ferguson JF, Generoso G, Ho JE, Kalani R, Khan SS, Kissela BM, et al. Heart disease and stroke statistics-2022 update: a report from the American Heart Association. Circulation. 2022;145(8):E153–639). Lippincott Williams and Wilkins. https://doi.org/10.1161/CIR.0000000000001052.

Chapter 2
Current Indications and Evidence for Left Atrial Appendage Closure

Nour Tashtish, Luis Augusto Palma Dallan, Judith A. Mackall, and Mauricio Arruda

Abbreviations

AF	Atrial fibrillation
DAPT	Dual antiplatelet therapy
LAA	Left atrial appendage
LAAO	Left atrial appendage occlusion
OAC	Oral anticoagulation
TEE	Transesophageal echocardiography

Highlights

- Atrial fibrillation (AF) is highly prevalent, and it significantly increases the risk of stroke and peripheral embolism-related deaths.
- Thromboembolic risk, major bleeding history, and high fall risk were the most common procedural indications for left atrial appendage occlusion (LAAO).
- LAAO is appropriate for non-valvular AF patients with high thromboembolic risk (CHA_2DS_2-VASc score ≥2 for men and ≥3 for women) and high bleeding risk (HAS-BLED score ≥3 for both genders).
- Percutaneous LAAO is indicated for non-valvular patients who are not undergoing cardiac surgery and have contraindications to long-term anticoagulation.
- Surgical ligation or amputation of the LAA can be safely performed in patients with AF undergoing any type of cardiac surgery.

N. Tashtish · L. A. P. Dallan · J. A. Mackall · M. Arruda (✉)
Division of Cardiology, Harrington Heart & Vascular Institute, University Hospitals Cleveland Medical Center, Cleveland, OH, USA
e-mail: Nour.tashtish@uhhospitals.org; luisaugusto.palmadallan@uhhospitals.org; Mauricio.arruda@uhhospitals.org

S. J. Filby et al. (eds.), *A Contemporary Manual of Left Atrial Appendage Closure*, https://doi.org/10.1007/978-3-031-68441-8_2

Introduction

Adults with atrial fibrillation (AF) have a higher risk of morbidity and mortality. Prior studies had demonstrated that, in approximately 90% of instances with non-valvular AF, the atrial appendage represented the location of atrial thrombus development, and the most common clinical manifestation of embolization is ischemic stroke caused by embolization of left atrial thrombi [11].

Among atrial fibrillation (AF) patients not receiving oral anticoagulation (OAC), the occurrence of left atrial appendage (LAA) thrombus varies between 5% and 27%. Even after commencing anticoagulant therapy, approximately 8% of individuals retain LAA thrombus [18].

The utilization of oral anticoagulant (OAC) therapy comes with an increased risk of bleeding. Therefore, recommendations for its utilization should carefully balance the potential benefits against the risks particularly with patients who have thrombocytopenia or a history of recurrent or severe bleeding or are at risk of falls.

With the recent advancements in evidence demonstrating the safety and efficacy of left atrial appendage occlusion (LAAO), major guidelines and international consensus protocols now recognize LAAO as a suitable treatment option (class of recommendation IIa) (2023 American guideline and 2020 European guideline [6]).

Indications for Percutaneous LAAO

Transcatheter LAAO is appropriate for non-valvular AF patients with high thromboembolic risk and high bleeding risk:

- CHA_2DS_2-VASc score ≥2 for men and ≥3 for women.
- HAS-BLED score ≥3 for both genders.

Patients with high thromboembolic risk have indication for thromboembolic prophylaxis; however, if one or more of the following conditions apply, patients may have a contraindication to long-term anticoagulation and may therefore have an indication for LAA occlusion (Table 2.1).

In addition, patients should not be suitable for long-term OAC, need to have an adequate life expectancy for a minimum of 1 year, and should have adequate quality of life to benefit from LAAO. There should always be patient-provider discussion for shared decision-making.

Surgical LAA Closure

Although the indications for surgical and nonsurgical closure are similar, the approach of LAA closure can be different based on the patient medical conditions.

Table 2.1 Indication for LAA closure

Coagulation defect associated with bleeding
Thrombocytopenia associated with bleeding
Recurrent bleeding, including gastrointestinal, genitourinary, or respiratory sites
History of severe bleeding, including intracranial hemorrhage
History of prior falls resulting in injury or high risk of the patient falling despite safety measures
Strong indication for combined use of dual antiplatelet and anticoagulant therapy
Intolerance of anticoagulant therapy
Poor compliance with anticoagulation therapy
Patients with lifestyle or occupational risk for bleeding

In patients with AF undergoing surgery for conditions like mitral valve or maze procedures, with a CHA_2DS_2-VASc score of at least 2, consideration is given for LAAO. Surgical LAAO can be accomplished through various techniques, including amputation and closure, stapler closure, double-layer linear closure from within the atrium, and epicardial device closure. Following surgical LAAO, long-term anticoagulation is typically prescribed, unless contraindicated. In cases where anticoagulation is not feasible, patients are usually required to take dual antiplatelet therapy for up to 6 weeks postoperatively.

Both a randomized trial and observational studies provide evidence supporting the effectiveness of LAAO for specific patients with AF undergoing cardiac surgery. In LAAOS III trial, which involved 4770 individuals with AF undergoing cardiac surgery for other indications and having a CHA2DS2-VASc score of at least 2, participants were randomly assigned to either the occlusion or no-occlusion group, with an average follow-up period of 3.8 years. The majority of participants continued oral anticoagulation post-procedure. Stroke or systemic embolism occurred in 114 participants (4.8%) in the occlusion group compared to 168 (7.0%) in the no-occlusion group (hazard ratio [HR] 0.67, 95% CI 0.53–0.85). Incidence rates of perioperative major bleeding, hospitalization for heart failure, and death were similar between the two groups [16].

In an observational study of 75,782 patients undergoing cardiac surgery, LAAO was associated with a reduced risk of ischemic stroke or systemic embolism (1.14 versus 1.59 events per 100 patient-years; HR 0.73, 95% CI 0.56–0.96) and mortality (3.01 versus 4.30 events per 100 patient-years; HR 0.71, 95% CI 0.60–0.84). LAAO was also associated with modestly higher rates of AF-related outpatient visits and hospitalizations [17].

In another retrospective cohort study of 10,524 Medicare recipients with AF undergoing cardiac surgery, surgical LAAO ($n = 3892$) compared with no occlusion ($n = 6632$) was significantly associated with a lower risk of readmission for thromboembolism at 3 years (4.2 versus 6.2%; HR 0.67; 95% CI 0.56–0.81). Among patients discharged without anticoagulation, LAAO was associated with a lower risk of thromboembolism (4.2 versus 6.0%; HR 0.26; 95% CI 0.17–0.40), but not among patients discharged with anticoagulation (4.1 versus 6.3%; HR 0.88; 95% CI

0.56–1.39). In the cohort of patients discharged with oral anticoagulation, surgical LAAO was not associated with thromboembolism but was associated with a lower risk for hemorrhagic stroke, presumably related to eventual discontinuation of oral anticoagulation among the LAAO patients. In patients without AF, there is no established role for LAAO [4].

The feasibility of stand-alone thoracoscopic LAA appendectomy was addressed in a study of 30 patients with AF and prior thromboembolism who had contraindications to oral anticoagulation [10]. Thoracoscopic LA appendectomy was not associated with increased mortality or major complications. At a mean follow-up of 16 months, no patients had experienced a recurrence of thromboembolism. Patients with no contraindication to anticoagulation are treated with anticoagulation indefinitely. Patients who are unable to tolerate long-term anticoagulation are typically managed with a regimen consisting of anticoagulation (usually a direct oral anticoagulant or DOAC) in combination with aspirin (81–325 mg daily) for a period ranging from 6 weeks to 3 months post-procedure. Subsequently, transesophageal echocardiography (TEE) is conducted to assess the extent of occlusion.

For patients with an absolute contraindication to oral anticoagulants, they are prescribed dual antiplatelet therapy (DAPT), comprising once-daily aspirin (81–325 mg) alongside clopidogrel (75 mg), during the pre-TEE phase, which typically spans from 6 weeks to 3 months. Upon confirmation of complete occlusion of the left atrial appendage (LAA) via TEE and when long-term anticoagulation is not viable, anticoagulation is ceased, and aspirin is continued indefinitely. If any leakage is observed subsequent to surgical LAAO, it is recommended to continue oral anticoagulation optimally.

This approach is supported by the results of an observational study of 72 patients undergoing surgical LAAO. The study found that the risk of stroke or systolic embolism was higher in patients with incomplete LAA closure compared with those with complete closure (24 versus 2% during the 44-month mean follow-up), despite similar rates of anticoagulation and recurrent AF. Among patients with incomplete closure, those with stroke or systemic embolism had smaller LAA neck diameters (2.8 versus 7.1 mm) than those without these adverse outcomes [2].

Percutaneous LAA Closure

Several randomized clinical trials such as PROTECT AF, PREVAIL, and PRAGUE-17 demonstrated efficacy and safety of LAAO devices compared with long-term anticoagulation.

The WATCHMAN, WATCHMAN FLX, the Amplatzer Cardiac Plug, and the Amplatzer Amulet are the leading implanted LAA endovascular devices worldwide [15].

A total of 933 patients underwent random assignment to percutaneous left atrial appendage (LAA) closure, while 583 patients were randomly assigned to receive oral anticoagulation and were subsequently monitored for an average duration of

39 months. The average age of participants was 73.3 years, with a mean CHA2DS2-VASc score of 4.1. The implanted devices included WATCHMAN, Amulet, and WATCHMAN FLX.

The analysis revealed no significant disparity in the rate of all-stroke or systemic embolism between the groups (6.1% versus 5.8%; risk ratio [RR] 0.98, 95% CI 0.65–1.48). However, LAA closure demonstrated a reduced risk of hemorrhagic stroke (0.5% versus 2.4%; RR 0.22, 95% CI 0.08–0.58), cardiovascular death (5.4% versus 8.2%; RR 0.65, 95% CI 0.44–0.95), and all-cause mortality (14.3% versus 17.8%; RR 0.78, 95% CI 0.62–0.99). Major bleeding incidence was comparable between the two groups (RR 0.89, 95% CI 0.66–1.20), although non-procedure-related major bleeding was lower with LAA closure (RR 0.53, 95% CI 0.38–0.74). Procedure-related complications were observed in 6.8% of cases.

Within the realm of percutaneous left atrial appendage (LAA) closure devices, the results of randomized trials have shown that LAA closure with the WATCHMAN device provided stroke prevention in non-valvular AF that was comparable to warfarin, with additional reductions in major bleeding, particularly hemorrhagic stroke, and mortality. The Amulet device has been established as non-inferior to the WATCHMAN device, as demonstrated in the Amulet Investigational Device Exemption (IDE) study. The choice between the WATCHMAN FLX and AMULET devices primarily hinges on anatomical considerations and the operator's level of comfort and experience. The first-generation WATCHMAN device was comprehensively evaluated in two randomized trials (PROTECT AF and PREVAIL) in patients with non-valvular AF eligible for oral anticoagulation [1, 7]. The five-year outcomes of the PREVAIL trial, combined with the five-year outcomes of the PROTECT AF trial, were reported in 2017 [12].

The PROTECT AF trial, a non-inferiority study, involved 707 patients diagnosed with atrial fibrillation (AF) and a CHADS2 score of ≥1. They were randomly allocated in a 2:1 ratio to either receive the device or undergo long-term warfarin therapy (with an international normalized ratio maintained between 2 and 3). The patients were observed for a period of 18 months [7]. The occurrence of the composite outcome, consisting of stroke, systemic embolism, or cardiovascular death, showed similar rates between the intervention and control groups, at 3 versus 4.9 events per 100 patient-years, respectively (rate ratio 0.62; 95% Bayesian credible interval 0.35–1.25). However, the primary safety endpoint, encompassing major bleeding, pericardial effusion, procedure-related stroke, or device embolization, was more frequent in the device group. An additional analysis of the PROTECT AF trial revealed that patients treated with the closure device experienced an improvement in health-related quality-of-life measures at the 12-month mark, while these measures declined among patients treated with warfarin.

The safety profile of the WATCHMAN device was examined in the PREVAIL study, where 407 patients were randomly assigned to receive either WATCHMAN or warfarin. These participants had a CHADS2 score of ≥2. At the 18-month follow-up, the first co-primary efficacy endpoint, which was a composite of stroke, systemic embolism, and cardiovascular/unexplained death, did not meet the non-inferiority criteria when comparing WATCHMAN to warfarin (0.64 versus 0.063;

rate ratio 1.07; 95% CI 0.57–1.89). However, the second co-primary efficacy endpoint, which focused on stroke or systemic embolism occurring more than 7 days post-randomization, did achieve non-inferiority (0.025 versus 0.020; risk difference 0.0053; 95% CI −0.0190–0.0273). Early safety events were observed in 2.2% of patients in the WATCHMAN arm, which was significantly lower than in the PROTECT AF study, meeting the predefined safety performance goal. In a nonrandomized study involving 400 patients, newer-generation WATCHMAN devices were found to be both effective and safe (PINNACLE FLX study) [7]. Furthermore, for patients with absolute contraindications to oral anticoagulation, left atrial appendage (LAA) closure with the WATCHMAN device was assessed in 150 patients. In the prospective multicenter, nonrandomized ASAP study, patients with a CHADS2 score of ≥1 were treated with WATCHMAN along with 6 months of a thienopyridine (clopidogrel or ticlopidine), in addition to lifelong aspirin [13]. During a mean follow-up of 14.4 months, stroke or systemic embolism occurred at a rate of 2.3% per year. This rate was lower than predicted rates for $CHADS_2$-matched cohorts of individuals taking either aspirin (7.3%) or clopidogrel (5%).

The EWOLUTION study, which examines real-world outcomes with the WATCHMAN device, reported a procedural success rate of 98.5%, with only 2.8% experiencing serious procedural complications within 7 days [3]. At the one-year follow-up, the incidence of ischemic stroke was 1.1%, signifying an 84% reduction compared to the historical estimate derived from CHA2DS2-VASc scores.

The Amplatzer device, being shorter than the WATCHMAN device, may offer advantages for individuals with shorter appendages. In a randomized trial comparing these devices, the Amulet device demonstrated non-inferiority to the WATCHMAN device in terms of primary safety and efficacy endpoints, albeit with a higher occurrence of procedure-related complications.

The Amulet Investigational Device Exemption (IDE) trial enrolled 1878 patients diagnosed with atrial fibrillation (AF) (mean CHA2DS2-VASc score of 4.6) who were randomly assigned to receive either the Amulet or WATCHMAN percutaneous left atrial appendage occlusion (LAAO) device [9]. The rate of ischemic stroke or systemic embolism at 18 months was comparable between the Amulet and WATCHMAN devices (2.8% for both). Major bleeding and all-cause death exhibited no significant differences between the two groups (10.6 versus 10% and 3.9 versus 5.1%, respectively).

In the aMAZE trial, which involved 610 patients with persistent atrial fibrillation (AF), participants were randomly assigned to undergo LAA ligation with LARIAT plus pulmonary vein antral isolation (a type of catheter ablation of AF) or pulmonary vein antral isolation alone and were followed to assess efficacy in rhythm control (i.e., freedom from antiarrhythmic medications) and safety [14]. The primary effectiveness endpoint, defined as freedom from antiarrhythmic drug therapy at 12 months, was achieved in 64.3% of the LAA ligation/pulmonary vein antral isolation group, compared to 59.9% in the pulmonary vein antral isolation alone group, although the criterion for superiority was not met. The primary safety endpoint occurred in 3.4% of the LAA ligation/pulmonary vein antral isolation group. At 12 months post-procedure, the majority of patients in the LARIAT plus catheter ablation group exhibited residual communication between the left atrium and left atrial appendage of ≤1 mm (85%).

Recommendations

According to the 2023 ACC/AHA/ACCP/HRS guidelines for the diagnosis and management of atrial fibrillation [8], as well as the 2020 consensus statement by the European Heart Rhythm Association and the European Association of Percutaneous Cardiovascular Interventions [5], left atrial appendage occlusion (LAAO) is deemed acceptable for non-valvular patients who have a contraindication to oral anticoagulation or are unwilling/unable to take oral anticoagulants, as seen in Table 2.2.

In contrast, the approval criteria set by the US Food and Drug Administration (FDA) are somewhat more permissive compared to the guidelines outlined by the European Society of Cardiology. The FDA's criteria extend eligibility beyond patients requiring oral anticoagulation and encompass other indications for non-pharmacologic therapy, such as lifestyle considerations and labile international normalized ratio.

The recommendations for cardiac surgery-LAA exclusion/excision are stronger based on the 2023 American guidelines, as seen in Table 2.3.

Table 2.2 Recommendations for percutaneous approaches to occlude the LAA based on the 2023 ACC/AHA/ACCP/HRS guidelines for the diagnosis and management of atrial fibrillation

In patients with AF, a moderate to high risk of stroke (CHA2DS2-VASc score ≥2), and a contraindication to long-term oral anticoagulation due to a nonreversible cause, percutaneous LAAO is reasonable. Class of recommendation 2a, level of evidence B-NR.
In patient with AF and a moderate to high risk of stroke and a high risk of major bleeding on oral anticoagulation, percutaneous LAAO may be a reasonable alternative to oral anticoagulation based on patient preference, with careful consideration of procedural risk and with the understanding that the evidence for oral anticoagulation is more extensive. Class of recommendation 2b, level of evidence B-R.

Table 2.3 Recommendations for cardiac surgery-LAA exclusion/excision are stronger based on the 2023 ACC/AHA/ACCP/HRS guidelines for the diagnosis and management of atrial fibrillation

In patients with AF undergoing cardiac surgery with a CHA_2DS_2-VASc score ≥2 or equivalent stroke risk, surgical LAA exclusion, in addition to continued anticoagulation, is indicated to reduce the risk of stroke and systemic embolism. Class of recommendation 1, level of evidence A.
In patients with AF undergoing cardiac surgery and LAA exclusion, a surgical technique resulting in absence of flow across the suture line and a stump of <1 cm as determined by intraoperative transesophageal echocardiography should be used. Class of recommendation 1, level of evidence A.
In patients with AF undergoing cardiac surgery with CHA_2DS_2-VASc score ≥2 or equivalent stroke risk, the benefit of surgical LAA exclusion in the absence of continued anticoagulation to reduce the risk of stroke and systemic embolism is uncertain. Class of recommendation 2b, level of evidence A.

Future Perspectives

There are many ongoing trials addressing the question of whether the indications for LAAO should be expanded, as seen in the timeline of the major clinical trials in Fig. 2.1 (for OAC eligible patients—OPTION trial, CHAMPION-AF trial, and CATALYST trial; for OAC-contraindicated patients—ASAP-TOO trial, STROKE-CLOSE trial, and CLOSURE-AF trial). Some of the most expected trials are the CHAMPION-AF trial and the CATALYST trial, both with expected inclusion of >2500 patients and performing a direct comparison by randomizing non-valvular AF patients to DOAC or LAAO, respectively, with the WATCHMAN FLX or the AMULET devices. Those trials may have a major impact in the LAAO indication depending on its results. While the final results for those trials are still pending, additional data analysis is still warranted (such as meta-analysis) to better understand which patients would have the best indication for LAAO, but the most recent guidelines indeed have provided better class of recommendations and are reassuring for the safety and effectiveness of LAAO.

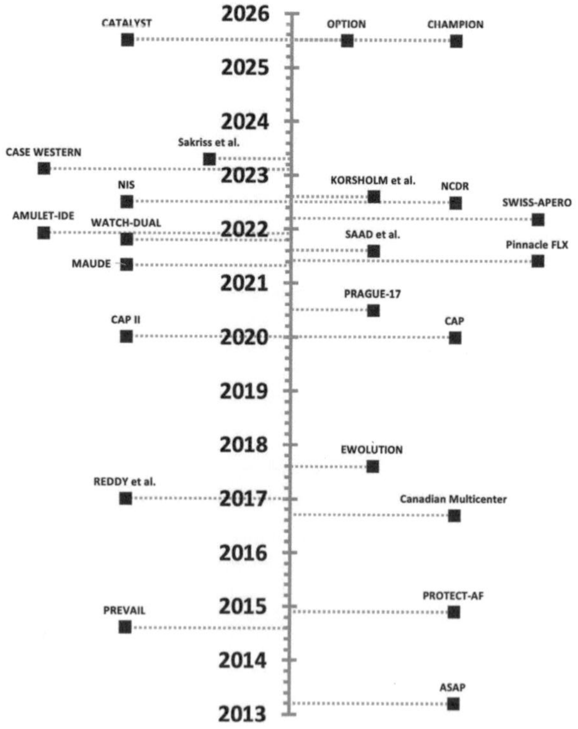

Fig. 2.1 Timeline of the major clinical trials

Conclusions

Patients undergoing cardiac surgery: In patients with AF with indication for anticoagulation who are undergoing cardiac surgery for another indication and do not have a contraindication to long-term anticoagulation, concurrent surgical LAAO is classified as class of recommendation 1 by the American guidelines. If there is a contraindication to long-term anticoagulation, concurrent surgical LAAO is designated as class of recommendation 2b by the American guidelines.

Patients not undergoing cardiac surgery: For individuals diagnosed with nonvalvular AF requiring anticoagulation but having a contraindication to long-term anticoagulation, the left atrial appendage occlusion (LAAO) procedure is categorized as class of evidence 2a by the American guidelines.

References

1. Alli O, Doshi S, Kar S, et al. Quality of life assessment in the randomized PROTECT AF (Percutaneous closure of the left atrial appendage versus warfarin therapy for prevention of stroke in patients with atrial fibrillation) trial of patients at risk for stroke with nonvalvular atrial fibrillation. J Am Coll Cardiol. 2013;61:1790–8. https://doi.org/10.1016/J.JACC.2013.01.061.
2. Aryana A, Singh SK, Singh SM, et al. Association between incomplete surgical ligation of left atrial appendage and stroke and systemic embolization. Heart Rhythm. 2015;12:1431–7. https://doi.org/10.1016/J.HRTHM.2015.03.028.
3. Boersma LV, Ince H, Kische S, et al. Evaluating real-world clinical outcomes in atrial fibrillation patients receiving the WATCHMAN left atrial appendage closure technology. Circ Arrhythm Electrophysiol. 2019;12:e006841. https://doi.org/10.1161/CIRCEP.118.006841.
4. Friedman DJ, Piccini JP, Wang T, et al. Association between left atrial appendage occlusion and readmission for thromboembolism among patients with atrial fibrillation undergoing concomitant cardiac surgery. JAMA. 2018;319:365. https://doi.org/10.1001/JAMA.2017.20125.
5. Glikson M, Wolff R, Hindricks G, et al. EHRA/EAPCI expert consensus statement on catheter-based left atrial appendage occlusion – an update. EuroIntervention. 2020;15:1133–80. https://doi.org/10.4244/EIJY19M08_01.
6. Hindricks G, Potpara T, Kirchhof P, et al. 2020 ESC guidelines for the diagnosis and management of atrial fibrillation developed in collaboration with the European Association for Cardio-Thoracic Surgery (EACTS): the Task Force for the diagnosis and management of atrial fibrillation of the European Society of Cardiology (ESC) Developed with the special contribution of the European Heart Rhythm Association (EHRA) of the ESC. Eur Heart J. 2021;42:373–498. https://doi.org/10.1093/EURHEARTJ/EHAA612.
7. Holmes DR, Kar S, Price MJ, et al. Prospective randomized evaluation of the watchman left atrial appendage closure device in patients with atrial fibrillation versus long-term warfarin therapy: the PREVAIL trial. J Am Coll Cardiol. 2014;64:1–12. https://doi.org/10.1016/J.JACC.2014.04.029.
8. Joglar JA, Chung MK, Armbruster AL, Benjamin EJ, Chyou JY, Cronin EM, Deswal A, Eckhardt L, Goldberger ZD, Gopinathannair R, Gorenek B, Hess PL, Hlatky M, Hogan G, Ibeh C, Indik JH, Kido K, Kusumoto F, Link MS, Linta KT, Marcus GM, McCarthy PM,

Patel N, Patton KK, Perez MV, Piccini JP, Russo AM, Sanders P, Streur MM, Thomas KL, Times S, Tisdale JE, Valente AM, Van Wagoner DR. 2023 ACC/AHA/ACCP/HRS guideline for the diagnosis and management of atrial fibrillation: a report of the American College of Cardiology/American Heart Association Joint Committee on Clinical Practice Guidelines. Circulation. 2024;149:e1–e156. https://doi.org/10.1161/CIR.0000000000001193.
9. Lakkireddy D, Thaler D, Ellis CR, et al. Amplatzer Amulet left atrial appendage occluder versus watchman device for stroke prophylaxis (Amulet IDE): a randomized, controlled trial. Circulation. 2021;144:1543–52. https://doi.org/10.1161/CIRCULATIONAHA.121.057063.
10. Ohtsuka T, Ninomiya M, Nonaka T, et al. Thoracoscopic stand-alone left atrial appendectomy for thromboembolism prevention in nonvalvular atrial fibrillation. J Am Coll Cardiol. 2013;62:103. https://doi.org/10.1016/j.jacc.2013.01.017.
11. Osmancik P, Herman D, Neuzil P, et al. Left atrial appendage closure versus direct oral anticoagulants in high-risk patients with atrial fibrillation. J Am Coll Cardiol. 2020;75:3122–35. https://doi.org/10.1016/J.JACC.2020.04.067.
12. Reddy VY, Doshi SK, Kar S, et al. 5-year outcomes after left atrial appendage closure from the PREVAIL and PROTECT AF trials on behalf of the PREVAIL and PROTECT AF investigators. J Am Coll Cardiol. 2017;70(24):2964–75.
13. Reddy VY, Möbius-Winkler S, Miller MA, et al. Left atrial appendage closure with the watchman device in patients with a contraindication for oral anticoagulation the ASAP study (ASA Plavix feasibility study with watchman left atrial appendage closure technology). J Am Coll Cardiol. 2013;61(25):2551. https://doi.org/10.1016/j.jacc.2013.03.035.
14. Sharples LD, Mills C, Da CY, et al. Five-year results of Amaze: a randomized controlled trial of adjunct surgery for atrial fibrillation. Eur J Cardiothorac Surg. 2022;62:181. https://doi.org/10.1093/EJCTS/EZAC181.
15. Turagam MK, Osmancik P, Neuzil P, et al. Left atrial appendage closure versus oral anticoagulants in atrial fibrillation: a meta-analysis of randomized trials. J Am Coll Cardiol. 2020;76:2795–7. https://doi.org/10.1016/J.JACC.2020.08.089.
16. Whitlock RP, Belley-Cote EP, Paparella D, et al. Left atrial appendage occlusion during cardiac surgery to prevent stroke. N Engl J Med. 2021;384:2081–91. https://doi.org/10.1056/NEJMOA2101897/SUPPL_FILE/NEJMOA2101897_DATA-SHARING.PDF.
17. Yao X, Gersh BJ, Holmes DR, et al. Association of surgical left atrial appendage occlusion with subsequent stroke and mortality among patients undergoing cardiac surgery. JAMA. 2018;319:2116–26. https://doi.org/10.1001/JAMA.2018.6024.
18. Zhan Y, Joza J, Al Rawahi M, et al. Assessment and management of the left atrial appendage thrombus in patients with nonvalvular atrial fibrillation. Can. J. Cardiol. 2018;34:252–61. https://doi.org/10.1016/J.CJCA.2017.12.008.

Chapter 3
Anatomy of the Left Atrial Appendage

Sundeep Kumar and Sergio Thal

The left atrial appendage (LAA) is a small, three-dimensional structure with a fingerlike projection located in the left atrium of the heart. It is a remnant of embryonic development and embryologically derived from the primitive atrium. The formation of the left atrial appendage is part of the intricate process of heart development during embryogenesis. The outer surface of LAA is covered by the visceral layer of the pericardium. The LAA exhibits greater distensibility and compliance when compared to the main body of the left atrium. LAA contains smooth and trabeculated portions. The trabecular portion of the left atrial appendage (LAA) represents the residual structure of the embryonic left atrium formed in the third week of gestation, while the smooth-walled left atrial cavity emerges at a later stage, originating from the extension of the pulmonary veins.

The left atrial appendage has a well-defined orifice, a neck region that further extends into the body of the appendage. The ostium of LAA is most commonly elliptical in as much as two-thirds of cases [1]. The primary axis of LAA is not straight and instead exhibits variation with a curved or spiral configuration. In most people, the LAA projects in an anterosuperior direction to lie over the left ventricle, and in the minority, it is pointed behind the pulmonary trunk in the transverse sinus [2]. The tip of LAA may be directed inferomedially and oriented towards the free wall of the left ventricle. The great cardiac vein lies near LAA in the atrioventricular

S. Kumar
University Hospitals Harrington Heart & Vascular Institute, Case Western Reserve University, Cleveland, OH, USA
e-mail: Sundeep.Kumar@UHhospitals.org

S. Thal (✉)
University Hospitals Harrington Heart & Vascular Institute, Division of Cardiovascular Medicine, Cardiac Electrophysiology, Case Western Reserve University, Cleveland, OH, USA

Ahuja Medical Center, Cleveland, OH, USA
e-mail: Sergio.thal@uhhospitals.org

S. J. Filby et al. (eds.), *A Contemporary Manual of Left Atrial Appendage Closure*, https://doi.org/10.1007/978-3-031-68441-8_3

groove, which also houses the left circumflex artery. The LAA is separated from the left superior pulmonary vein by the ridge of Marshall.

The wall of the left atrial appendage is muscular and lined by a single layer of endothelium. This muscularity allows the appendage to contract and pump blood. The LAA also serves a reservoir function and can be enlarged in patients with heart failure and atrial fibrillation. The internal surface of the walls is lined with pectinate muscles, which are muscular ridges that contribute to the contraction and mixing of blood. Prominent pectinate muscle can sometimes be confused for thrombus and may require advanced imaging for distinction from thrombus. Pectinate muscles typically exhibit repetition, are hyper-refractile, and are regularly organized, differentiating them from thrombus.

The left atrial appendage (LAA) presents with diverse shapes, and its morphology can differ from one individual to another. The most frequent configuration of the LAA consists of two lobes, with three lobes being less common, and a single lobe being the least frequent. Shape and morphology analysis becomes particularly crucial during the planning phase of interventional procedures like left atrial appendage occlusion (LAAO). Although there may be some variability in its shape, the left atrial appendage (LAA) is typically categorized into a few common forms as below.

1. *Chicken wing*: This is the most common variety and relatively straightforward shape in which the LAA has a curved, winglike appearance (Fig. 3.1). This type is associated with the lowest risk of stroke.
2. *Cactus*: In this shape, the LAA has multiple lobes or protrusions, resembling the arms of a cactus (Fig. 3.2).
3. *Windsock*: The LAA is elongated and tubular, resembling a windsock (Fig. 3.3).
4. *Cauliflower*: This shape is characterized by multiple irregular outgrowths, somewhat like the surface of a cauliflower (Fig. 3.4). This shape is most associated with thrombus formation.
5. *Amorphous or irregular*: In some cases, the LAA may not have a distinct, easily categorizable shape, and its structure may be more irregular.

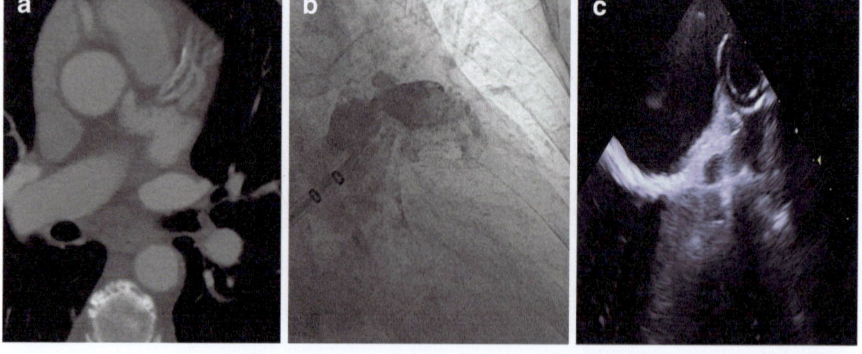

Fig. 3.1 Left atrial appendage chicken wing morphology with computed tomography (**a**), cine angiography (**b**), and intracardiac echocardiogram (**c**) images

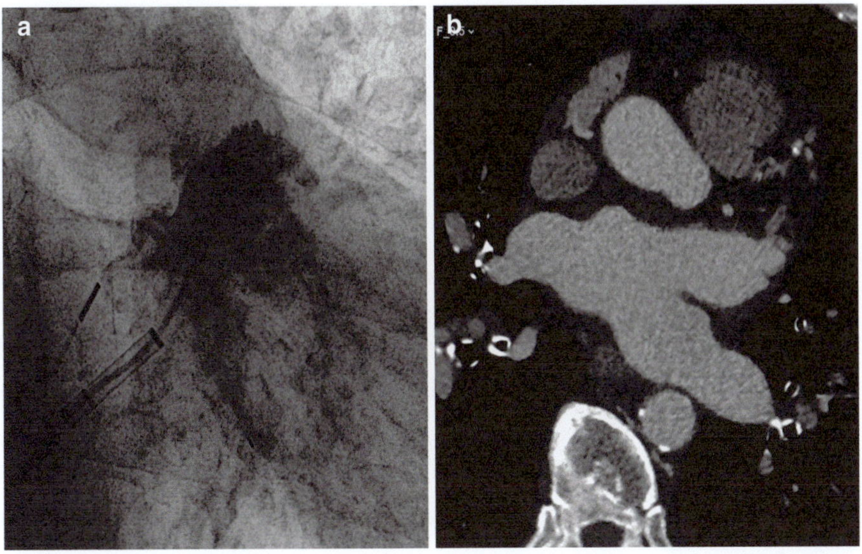

Fig. 3.2 Left atrial appendage Cactus morphology Cine angiography (**a**) and computed tomography images (**b**)

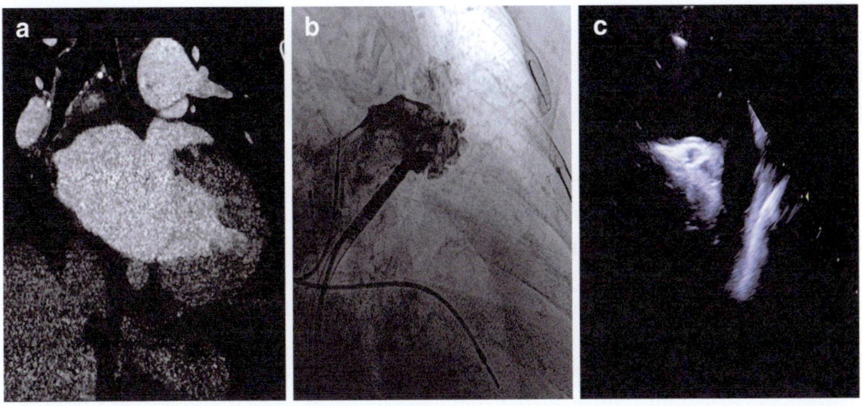

Fig. 3.3 Left atrial appendage Winsock morphology with computed tomography (**a**), cine angiography (**b**), and intracardiac echocardiogram (**c**) images

The varied morphology of the left atrial appendage emphasizes that the same approach for choosing a closure device for LAA may not be appropriate. Variations in the morphology of the left atrial appendage (LAA) have the potential to modify the risk of thromboembolism by influencing blood flow velocities across different LAA subtypes. For example, individuals exhibiting chicken-wing LAA morphology are statistically less likely to experience embolic events, even when accounting for comorbidities and CHADS2 score [3].

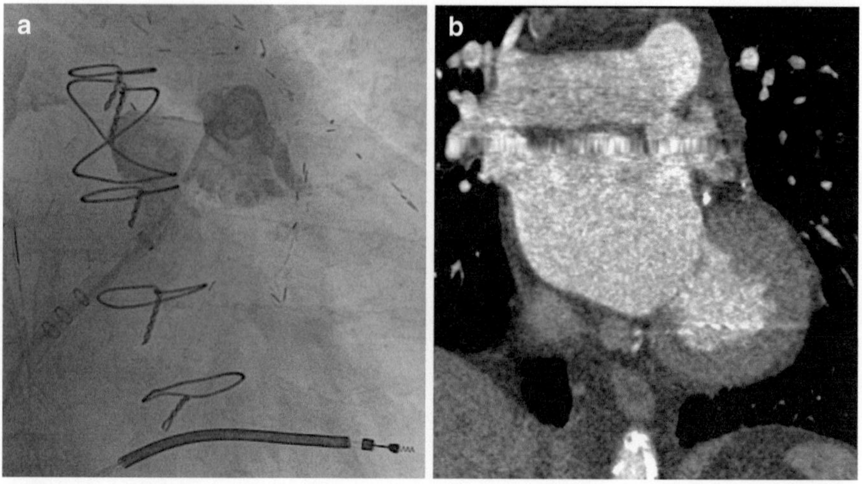

Fig. 3.4 Left atrial appendage Cauliflower morphology Cine angiography (**a**) and computed tomography (**b**) images

Procedural Perspective

The orifice of LAA can vary in shape, most commonly oval, and less commonly triangular and semicircular [4]. The knowledge of orifice anatomy is critical as implanting an improperly shaped left atrial appendage occluder (LAAO) device as choosing an inappropriate size can lead to a suboptimal seal. The goal of LAAO is the complete exclusion of the left atrial appendage. Due to variable anatomy, device selection needs careful attention for safe and successful procedural outcomes. Considerable differences in anatomy exist based on CT and MRI data [5, 6]. Various anatomical considerations, including the configuration, ostial diameter, and extent and arrangement of septal trabeculations, could influence the results shortly after the LAA closure procedure as well as the long-term follow-up outcomes. Many centers utilize transesophageal echocardiogram (TEE) or cardiac computed tomography for anatomical evaluation and pre-procedural planning. During the procedure, intracardiac echo and TEE are used by operators for procedural guidance. The ostium of LAA is measured at the level of the left circumflex artery to the point 1–2 cm below the left superior pulmonary vein limb. The depth of LAA is chosen from the center of the ostium to the tip of the appendage. In general, the LAA closure device chosen for closure is wider than the largest orifice diameter of LAA, enough to facilitate device compression by 8–20%. Frequently, the patient's volume status can influence the size of the left atrial appendage (LAA), and measurements are typically reassessed during the procedure to prevent mismatch between device diameter and LAA size, which could result in an incomplete seal. When the maximum depth of LAA is shorter than the length of the device that will allow full closure, then technically, LAAO using the Watchman™ device is not suitable.

In some cases, complications may arise in periprocedural settings due to interaction with anatomical structures. The left circumflex coronary artery lies in the proximity of the LAA orifice, which can be at risk from peri-device trauma [7]. The phrenic nerve lies on the exterior surface of LAA and is at risk for damage with epicardial closure of LAA. The anterolateral wall of LAA is thinnest, and caution is needed during cardiac procedure to avoid damage and resultant pericardial effusion.

References

1. Su P, McCarthy KP, Ho SY. Occluding the left atrial appendage: anatomical considerations. Heart. 2008;94(9):1166–70. https://doi.org/10.1136/hrt.2006.111989. Epub 2007 May 8
2. Beigel R, Wunderlich NC, Ho SY, Arsanjani R, Siegel RJ. The left atrial appendage: anatomy, function, and noninvasive evaluation. JACC Cardiovasc Imaging. 2014;7(12):1251–65. https://doi.org/10.1016/j.jcmg.2014.08.009.
3. Di Biase L, Santangeli P, Anselmino M, Mohanty P, Salvetti I, Gili S, Horton R, Sanchez JE, Bai R, Mohanty S, Pump A, Cereceda Brantes M, Gallinghouse GJ, Burkhardt JD, Cesarani F, Scaglione M, Natale A, Gaita F. Does the left atrial appendage morphology correlate with the risk of stroke in patients with atrial fibrillation? Results from a multicenter study. J Am Coll Cardiol. 2012;60(6):531–8. https://doi.org/10.1016/j.jacc.2012.04.032.
4. Li CY, Gao BL, Liu XW, Fan QY, Zhang XJ, Liu GC, Yang HQ, Feng PY, Wang Y, Song P. Quantitative evaluation of the substantially variable morphology and function of the left atrial appendage and its relation with adjacent structures. PLoS One. 2015;10(7):e0126818. https://doi.org/10.1371/journal.pone.0126818. PMID: 26230395; PMCID: PMC4521946
5. Heist EK, Refaat M, Danik SB, Holmvang G, Ruskin JN, Mansour M. Analysis of the left atrial appendage by magnetic resonance angiography in patients with atrial fibrillation. Heart Rhythm. 2006;3(11):1313–8. https://doi.org/10.1016/j.hrthm.2006.07.022. Epub 2006 Aug 3
6. Wang Y, Di Biase L, Horton RP, Nguyen T, Morhanty P, Natale A. Left atrial appendage studied by computed tomography to help planning for appendage closure device placement. J Cardiovasc Electrophysiol. 2010;21(9):973–82. https://doi.org/10.1111/j.1540-8167.2010.01814.x.
7. Shoji T, Sato Y, Togashi D, et al. ST-segment elevation during percutaneous left atrial appendage closure. J Am Coll Cardiol Case Rep. 2024;29(4):102216.

Chapter 4
Pre-procedural Planning for Left Atrial Appendage Closure: Transesophageal Echocardiography

Takahiro Tsushima and Brian D. Hoit

Highlights

- TEE has been the gold-standard imaging modality for the conventional LAAO procedure; however, cardiac CT (Chaps. 1, 2, 3, 4 and 5) is increasingly recognized as an excellent imaging modality for pre-procedural planning.
- During the pre-procedural TEE, it is imperative to take note of the presenting rhythm, the alterations of left ventricular preload, and the timing of TEE imaging acquisition (at left ventricular end-systole vs. end-diastole).
- It is necessary to understand the anatomy of the LAA and the relationship between each region of the LAA (ostium, neck, body, and apex) and neighboring structures such as coronary arteries and mitral valvular annulus.
- It should be noted that each LAAO device requires specific measurements to determine appropriately the size of patient's LAA.

Introduction

The anatomy of the left atrial appendage (LAA) is highly variable, making the careful assessment of the LAA critical to obtain accurate sizing, select the appropriate left atrial appendage occlusion (LAAO) device, and plan the procedural approach.

T. Tsushima
Harrington Heart & Vascular Institute, University Hospitals Cleveland Medical Center, Cleveland, OH, USA
e-mail: takahiro.tsushima2@uhhospitals.org

B. D. Hoit (✉)
University Hospitals Harrington Heart & Vascular Institute, Cleveland, OH, USA

Department of Physiology and Biophysics, Case Western Reserve University, Cleveland, OH, USA
e-mail: Brian.hoit@uhhospitals.org

S. J. Filby et al. (eds.), *A Contemporary Manual of Left Atrial Appendage Closure*, https://doi.org/10.1007/978-3-031-68441-8_4

Under-sizing of the LAAO device has a risk of device migration or embolization, whereas oversizing can cause cardiac perforation, mechanical injury to adjacent vessels and structures, and the development of pericardial effusion that may progress to acute cardiac tamponade. Transesophageal echocardiography (TEE) has been the gold-standard imaging modality for the conventional LAAO procedure [1]. In this chapter, we will review pre-procedural assessment with TEE for conventional LAAO device implantation.

Patient's Conditions Affecting TEE Assessment

The size and morphology of the LAA are essential components of the pre-procedural assessment. The shape and size of the LAA orifice differ significantly between atrial fibrillation (AF) and normal sinus rhythm (NSR) [2, 3]. Ernst et al. compared the morphology of LAA using postmortem LAA casts; LAA volumes, minimum and maximum orifice dimensions, were larger in casts from patients in AF than those from patients in NSR (7060 mm^3 vs. 4645 mm^3, 17 mm vs. 14 mm, and 23 mm vs. 20 mm, respectively; all $p < 0.01$) [2]. Spencer et al. also evaluated the size of the LAA with TEE during general anesthesia before and after a 500–1000 ml infusion of intravenous normal saline [3]. The average increase in the LAA orifice and depth was 1.9 mm ($p < 0.001$) and 2.5 mm ($p < 0.001$), respectively, after the intravenous fluid bolus [3]. Such a 10% size increase can correspond to the upsizing of the LAAO device, so it is recommended to measure the LAA size during maximal filling of the LAA (typically with mean left atrial pressure > 12 mmHg) at the end of left ventricular systole [4, 5].

During the TEE procedure, it is imperative to note the presenting rhythm, the alterations of LV loading (as occurs with both moderate sedation and general anesthesia), the fluid status (patients are usually dehydrated during TEE procedure), and the timing of TEE imaging acquisition (at left ventricular end-systole vs. end-diastole).

Anatomy of LAA and Neighboring Structures (Fig. 4.1)

It is also crucial to understand the anatomy of the LAA. The LAA is anatomically divided into four regions: the ostium, neck, body, and apex [4, 6]. Although the ostium is generally oval in shape, a very eccentric LAA ostium has a risk of peri-device leakage [4]. The wall of LAA ostium and neck can be very thin, which can increase the risk of LAA perforation during the LAAO device implantation [4]. The ostium is adjacent to the mitral valvular annulus inferiorly and is separated from the

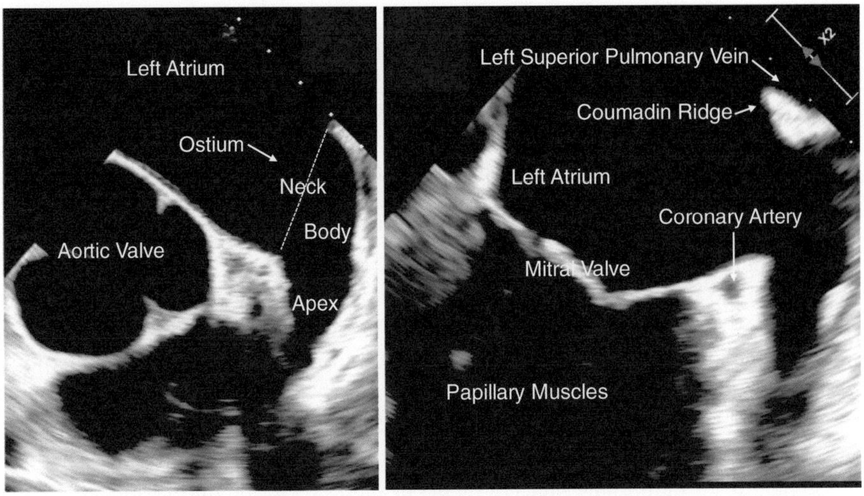

Fig. 4.1 Anatomy of LAA and neighboring structures

left superior pulmonary vein by the ligament of Marshall, otherwise known as the Coumadin ridge [4, 6]. Given that most of the LAAO-indicated patients are elderly and may have significant mitral valvular diseases and/or mitral annular calcification, mitral valve function before and after the LAAO device implantation should be evaluated, especially when using larger LAAO devices [5].

The ostium opens to the LAA neck, the tubular junction between the ostium and the body [4, 6]. Passing beneath the LAA neck are the left anterior descending and left circumflex arteries, great cardiac vein, and lymphatics [4]. The sinus node artery originates from either the left anterior descending or left circumflex coronary artery in up to 30% of adult patients [4, 7, 8]. To avoid myocardial ischemia and acute sinus node dysfunction during the LAAO device implantation, the distances between the LAA neck and these neighboring vessels warrant careful evaluation.

The body and apex of LAA can have several lobes (two to four lobes, most commonly two) or outpouching spaces from the main tubular body of the LAA [4, 6]. It is crucial to identify the main anchoring lobe correctly. Usually, the main tubular body is defined as the LAA lobe that has the longest straightening distance from the LAA ostium without significant directional change [8]. The main lobe needs enough length to accommodate the selected LAAO device [4, 6]. An increase in the number of the LAA lobes is positively and independently related to the development of the LAA thrombus [6]. If a mass or thrombus inside the LAA body and apex cannot be fully differentiated from the pectinate muscle of the LAA, an ultrasound-enhancing agent or a three-dimensional TEE with multiplane reconstruction may be helpful.

Comprehensive TEE Evaluation for the LAA Anatomy (Fig. 4.2)

While a baseline TEE is recommended before commencing on the occlusion procedure, some experienced centers perform the baseline TEE at the time of the procedure, a practice discouraged for new centers and inexperienced operators in the SCAI/HRS Expert Consensus Statement [1].

A comprehensive TEE procedure for the LAAO device implantation should include (1) the morphology of the LAA (ostium, neck, body, and apex) in standard rotational imaging planes; (2) the number and location of accessory LAA lobes; (3) the adjacent structures (e.g., the left circumflex coronary artery, mitral annulus); (4) the interatrial septum (atrial septal aneurysm [ASA], secundum ASD, and/or patent foramen ovale [PFO]); (5) the documentation of baseline pericardial effusion; and (6) the presence of spontaneous echocardiographic contrast, sludge, or thrombus [4–6].

Standardized multiplane measurements of the LAA at the mid-esophageal level should be performed at 0°, 45°, 90°, and 135° views to determine the maximal diameter of the anticipated LAAO device landing zone and the anchoring LAA depth on 2D TEE imaging [4, 6]. Biplane imaging can be used from any angles, and

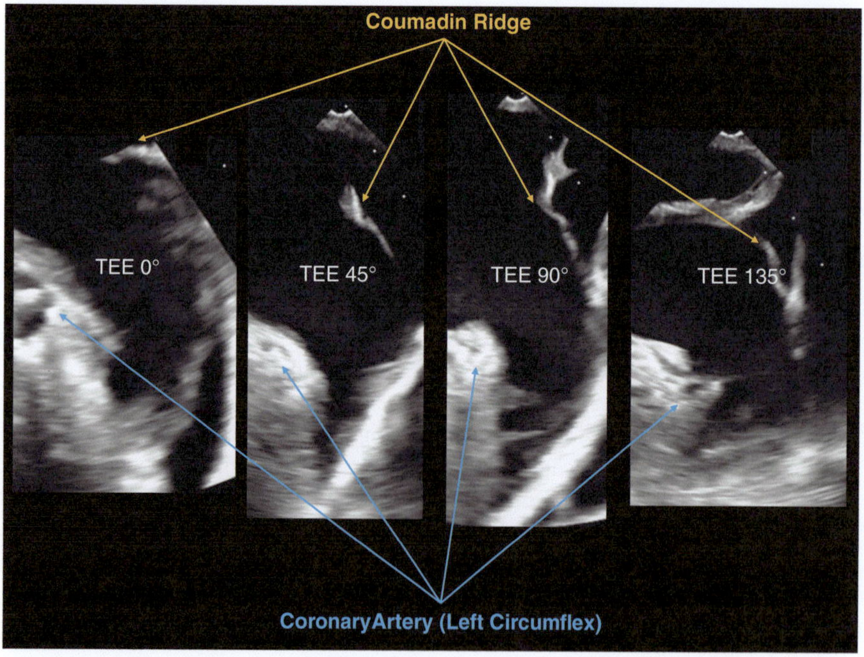

Fig. 4.2 Comprehensive TEE evaluation for the LAA anatomy. A comprehensive TEE procedure for the LAAO device implantation should include (1) the morphology of the LAA in standard rotational imaging planes; (2) number and location of accessory LAA lobes; (3) adjacent structures; (4) inter-atrial septum; (5) documentation of baseline pericardial effusion; and (6) presence of spontaneous echocardiographic contrast, sludge, or thrombus

slight anteflexion may help acquisition of the appropriate views. Because the LAA ostium is oval in shape in most cases, the largest diameter of the LAA ostium is often found on 120°–135° planes [4, 6]. Because of the tomographic limitation of 2D imaging, 3D TEE with multiplane reconstruction may provide more accurate measurement especially in patients with complex LAA morphology [4, 6].

Pre-Procedural TEE Measurement Specific for the Indicated LAAO Device (Figs. 4.3 and 4.4)

For non-disc lobe LAAO devices such as Watchman (Boston Scientific, Maple Grove, MN), the LAAO landing zone is measured from the left circumflex artery to a point 2 mm below the tip of the left superior pulmonary vein limbus [4, 6, 9] (Fig. 4.3). The LAA depth is measured from the plane of the LAA orifice to the LAA apex [4, 6, 9] (Fig. 4.3). After obtaining multiplane measurements as mentioned above, the largest LAA landing zone diameter is selected for the LAAO device size [4, 6, 9]. Typically, the device is oversized in comparison to the largest measured LAA diameter by 8–20% [4, 6, 9]. The LAA anatomic exclusion criteria and possible exclusion criteria for the older Watchman device were well established [9, 10]. New Watchman devices (Watchman FLX Pro and Watchman FLX) not only are shorter in length but also have a conformable shape, so measurements of the usable length of the LAA may not have to be orthogonal to the LAA orifice [11]. The below findings should be carefully assessed with pre-procedural TEE.

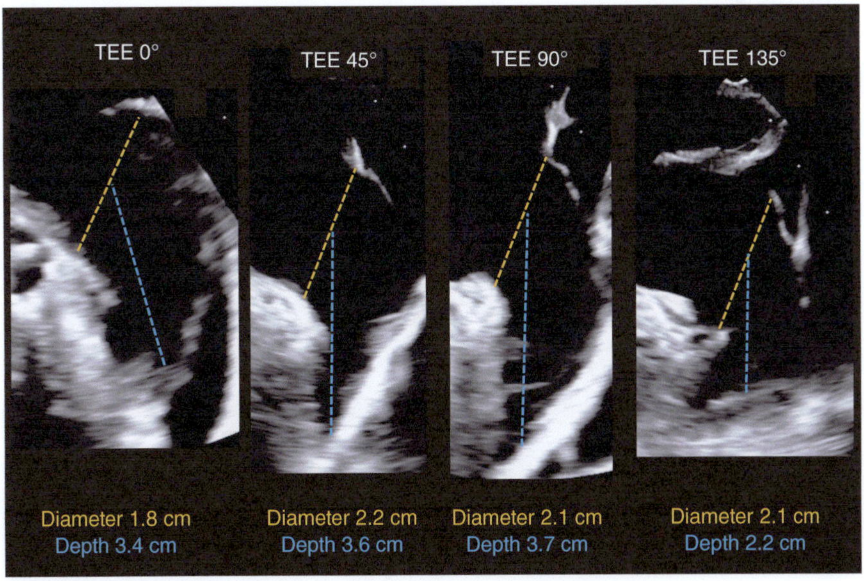

Fig. 4.3 Pre-procedural TEE measurement specific for the Watchman device

LAA Anatomic Exclusion Criteria for the Watchman Device

- LAA orifice diameter that is either too small (<14.0 mm) or too large (>36.0 mm).
- LAA depth that is too shallow (LAA depth less than the largest LAA orifice diameter).
- History of ASD or PFO repair or a closure device is present.

Other Echocardiographic Exclusion Criteria for the Watchman Device

- Presence of intracardiac thrombus or cardiac tumor.
- Reduced left ventricular ejection fraction <30%.
- High-risk PFO with an ASA excursion distance >15 mm or length > 15 mm.
- Large interatrial shunt (early, within 3 beats and substantial passage of bubbles, i.e., > 20).
- Complex atheroma with mobile plaque of the descending and/or aortic arch.
- Significant mitral stenosis (mitral valve area < 1.5 cm^2).
- Pericardial effusion with thickness > 2–5 mm (relative contraindication).

Like the Watchman device, disc lobe LAAO devices, such as the Amulet device (Abbott, Minneapolis, MN), have a LAA size measured at 0°, 45°, 90°, and 135° views at the mid-esophageal level [4, 6, 9, 10]. However, in the case of the Amulet device, it is recommended to focus on the “short axis” (technically the minor diameter axis for oval

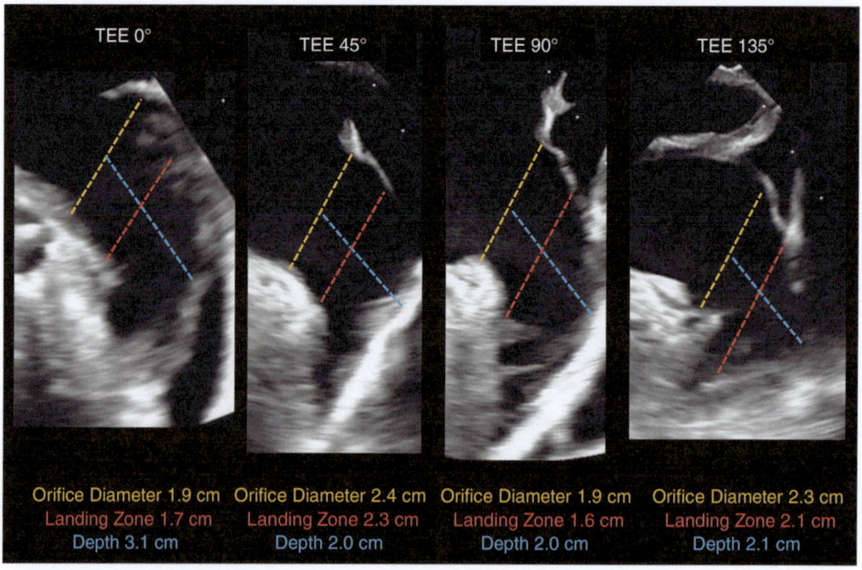

Fig. 4.4 Pre-procedural TEE measurement specific for the Amulet device

LAA orifice, usually between 30° and 60°) and the "long axis" (technically the major diameter axis for oval LAA orifice, usually between 120° and 150°) [4, 6, 9, 10] (Fig. 4.4). The LAA ostial diameter is defined as the line from the pulmonary vein ridge to the circumflex artery (Fig. 4.4). The landing zone diameter is then measured 10–12 mm distal to the ostium at an angle perpendicular to the neck axis [4, 6, 9, 10] (Fig. 4.4). Both the ostial and landing zone LAA diameter measurements are usually wider on the "long-axis" view compared with the "short-axis" view. The Amulet device selection is based primarily on the landing zone diameter measurement [4, 6, 9].

LAA Anatomic Exclusion Criteria for the Amulet Device

- The LAA landing zone diameter cannot be too large (>31 mm) or too small (<11 mm).
- Minimal depth is 10 mm for 16–22 mm Amulet devices.
- Minimal depth is 12 mm for 25–34 mm Amulet devices.

Other Echocardiographic Exclusion Criteria for the Amulet Device

- Presence of intracardiac thrombus or cardiac tumor.
- Large interatrial shunt, defined as >20 bubbles that appear within 3 beats on agitated saline injection.
- Atrial septal aneurysm with excursion >15 mm or length >15 mm beyond the plane of the atrial septum.
- Complex atheroma with mobile plaque in the aortic arch or the descending aorta.
- Significant mitral stenosis (mitral valve area < 1.5 cm^2).
- Pericardial effusion with thickness >2mm.
- The placement of the device would interfere with any intracardiac or intravascular structure.

Potential Patient Groups Requiring Careful TEE Assessment Prior to LAAO Implantation

- History of complex congenital heart disease and previous complex pediatric cardiac surgery.
- History of adult cardiac surgery especially with surgical LAA ligation or resection.
- History of prosthetic mitral valve procedure or surgery. These patients may have a dilated LAA, and the distance between the ostium of the LAA and the neigh-

boring structures (e.g., mitral annular plane and left upper pulmonary vein) can be shorter. There are insufficient data regarding procedural safety with either Watchman or Amulet LAAO device for this specific population [12].

- Malposition of the esophagus due to scaphoid or excavatum-type thoracic deformity or previous surgery for upper gastrointestinal disease. When the esophagus is positioned in an unusual location, the LAA can be completely obscured by intervening structures [13].
- Congenital absence of the LAA [14, 15].

Conclusions

In conclusion, TEE has been the gold-standard imaging modality for the conventional LAAO procedure; however, cardiac CT (Chaps. 1, 2, 3, 4 and 5) is increasingly recognized as an excellent imaging modality for pre-procedural planning. During the pre-procedural TEE, it is imperative to take note of the presenting rhythm, the alterations of left ventricular preload, and the timing of TEE imaging acquisition (at left ventricular end-systole vs. end-diastole). It is necessary to understand the anatomy of the LAA and the relationship between each cavity of the LAA (ostium, neck, body, and apex) and neighboring structures such as coronary arteries and mitral valvular annulus. Finally, it should be noted that each LAAO device requires specific measurements to determine the size of patient's LAA appropriately.

References

1. Saw J, Holmes DR, Cavalcante JL, Freeman JV, Goldsweig AM, Kavinsky CJ, Moussa ID, Munger TM, Price MJ, Reisman M, Sherwood MW, Turi ZG, Wang DD, Whisenant BK. SCAI/HRS expert consensus statement on transcatheter left atrial appendage closure. Heart Rhythm. 2023 May;20(5):e1–e16. https://doi.org/10.1016/j.hrthm.2023.01.007.
2. Ernst G, Stöllberger C, Abzieher F, Veit-Dirscherl W, Bonner E, Bibus B, Schneider B, Slany J. Morphology of the left atrial appendage. Anat Rec. 1995 Aug;242(4):553–61. https://doi.org/10.1002/ar.1092420411.
3. Spencer RJ, DeJong P, Fahmy P, Lempereur M, Tsang MYC, Gin KG, Lee PK, Nair P, Tsang TSM, Jue J, Saw J. Changes in left atrial appendage dimensions following volume loading during percutaneous left atrial appendage closure. JACC Cardiovasc Interv. 2015;8(15):1935–41. https://doi.org/10.1016/j.jcin.2015.07.035.
4. Wunderlich NC, Beigel R, Swaans MJ, Ho SY, Siegel RJ. Percutaneous interventions for left atrial appendage exclusion: options, assessment, and imaging using 2D and 3D echocardiography. JACC Cardiovasc Imaging. 2015;8(4):472–88. https://doi.org/10.1016/j.jcmg.2015.02.002.
5. Wang DD, Forbes TJ, Lee JC, Eng MH. Echocardiographic imaging for left atrial appendage occlusion: transesophageal echocardiography and Intracardiac echocardiographic imaging. Interv Cardiol Clin. 2018;7(2):219–28. https://doi.org/10.1016/j.iccl.2018.01.001.

6. Hahn RT, Saric M, Faletra FF, Garg R, Gillam LD, Horton K, Khalique OK, Little SH, Mackensen GB, Oh J, Quader N, Safi L, Scalia GM, Lang RM. Recommended standards for the performance of transesophageal echocardiographic screening for structural heart intervention: from the American Society of Echocardiography. J Am Soc Echocardiogr. 2022 Jan;35(1):1–76. https://doi.org/10.1016/j.echo.2021.07.006.
7. Berdajs D, Patonay L, Turina MI. The clinical anatomy of the sinus node artery. Ann Thorac Surg. 2003;76(3):732–5.; discussion 735–6. https://doi.org/10.1016/s0003-4975(03)00660-x.
8. Su P, McCarthy KP, Ho SY. Occluding the left atrial appendage: anatomical considerations. Heart. 2008;94(9):1166–70. https://doi.org/10.1136/hrt.2006.111989.
9. Vainrib AF, Harb SC, Jaber W, Benenstein RJ, Aizer A, Chinitz LA, Saric M. Left atrial appendage occlusion/exclusion: procedural image guidance with transesophageal echocardiography. J Am Soc Echocardiogr. 2018;31(4):454–74. https://doi.org/10.1016/j.echo.2017.09.014.
10. Lakkireddy D, Thaler D, Ellis CR, Swarup V, Sondergaard L, Carroll J, Gold MR, Hermiller J, Diener HC, Schmidt B, MacDonald L, Mansour M, Maini B, O'Brien L, Windecker S. Amplatzer amulet left atrial appendage occluder versus watchman device for stroke prophylaxis (amulet IDE): a randomized. Controlled Trial Circulation. 2021;144(19):1543–52. https://doi.org/10.1161/CIRCULATIONAHA.121.057063.
11. Kar S, Doshi SK, Sadhu A, Horton R, Osorio J, Ellis C, Stone J Jr, Shah M, Dukkipati SR, Adler S, Nair DG, Kim J, Wazni O, Price MJ, Asch FM, Holmes DR Jr, Shipley RD, Gordon NT, Allocco DJ. Reddy VY; PINNACLE FLX investigators. Primary outcome evaluation of a next-generation left atrial appendage closure device: results from the PINNACLE FLX trial. Circulation. 2021;143(18):1754–62. https://doi.org/10.1161/CIRCULATIONAHA.120.050117.
12. Martellini A, Meucci F, Mattesini A, Ristalli F, Stolcova M, Di Mario C. Percutaneous watchman FLX implantation in a patient with previous mitral valve surgery and large-sized left atrial appendage. Eur Heart J Case Rep. 2020;4(5):1–2. https://doi.org/10.1093/ehjcr/ytaa192.
13. Kilcullen NM, Woo JK, Abbara S, Barrett CD, Baggish A. The missing left atrial appendage. J Cardiovasc Comput Tomogr. 2012;6(1):60–1. https://doi.org/10.1016/j.jcct.2011.07.002.
14. Enomoto Y, Hashimoto G, Sahara N, Hashimoto H, Niikura H, Nakamura K, Iijima R, Hara H, Suzuki M, Noro M, Moroi M, Sugi K, Nakamura M. Congenital absence of left atrial appendage diagnosed by multimodality imaging. Int Heart J. 2018;59(2):439–42. https://doi.org/10.1536/ihj.17-094.
15. Saleh M, Balakrishnan R, Castillo Kontak L, Benenstein R, Chinitz LA, Donnino R, Saric M. Congenital absence of the left atrial appendage visualized by 3D echocardiography in two adult patients. Echocardiography. 2015;32(7):1206–10. https://doi.org/10.1111/echo.12882.

Chapter 5
Pre-procedural Planning for Left Atrial Appendage Closure with Cardiac Computed Tomography Angiography

Luis Augusto Palma Dallan, Amit Gupta, Robert Gilkeson, and Steven J. Filby

Abbreviations

3D	Three-dimensional
AF	Atrial fibrillation.
CTA	Computed tomography angiography.
ICE	Intracardiac echocardiography.
LAA	Left atrial appendage.
LAAC	Left atrial appendage closure.
TEE	Transesophageal echocardiography.
VMI_{low}	Low-energy virtual monoenergetic images.

Highlights

- CTA may be performed for planning left atrial appendage closure (LAAC) as a noninvasive alternative to transesophageal echocardiography (TEE).
- Commercially available software packages provide sizing measurements, and information about surrounding cardiac structures may improve device selection strategy over TEE.

L. A. P. Dallan · S. J. Filby
Division of Cardiology, Harrington Heart & Vascular Institute, University Hospitals Cleveland Medical Center, Cleveland, OH, USA
e-mail: luisaugusto.palmadallan@uhhospitals.org; steven.filby@uhhospitals.org

A. Gupta (✉) · R. Gilkeson
Division of Cardiothoracic Imaging, Department of Radiology, University Hospitals Cleveland Medical Center, Cleveland, OH, USA

Department of Radiology, Case Western Reserve University School of Medicine, Cleveland, OH, USA
e-mail: amit.gupta@uhhospitals.org; Robert.gilkeson@uhhospitals.org

S. J. Filby et al. (eds.), *A Contemporary Manual of Left Atrial Appendage Closure*, https://doi.org/10.1007/978-3-031-68441-8_5

- CTA-planned LAAC may improve procedure efficiency and can be incorporated into a same-day imaging strategy.

Introduction

The size and shape of the left atrial appendage (LAA) widely vary among individuals. Imaging guidance for the LAAC (left atrial appendage closure) procedure is of utmost importance to procedural success, as it helps guide the choice of device, size of device, and device delivery system. Failure in device sizing or inadequate device positioning may result in peri-device leakage or even in device embolization. LAAC approval was predicated upon trials designed with transesophageal echocardiography (TEE) preplanning. TEE has thus since served as the gold standard for the LAAC procedure, and this has persevered, in part, because of the extensive availability of TEE and the widespread experience with this imaging modality. However, TEE has some notable disadvantages compared with cardiac computed tomography angiography (CTA). CTA may offer a superior, noninvasive alternative with better anatomical segmentation for the LAA and its surrounding structures. CTA may also improve device sizing accuracy over TEE when used in experienced centers.

Computed Tomography Angiography (CTA)

A multidetector CT scanner with at least 64 detector rows is required for a high-quality scan. After appropriate fasting, patients receive an IV normal saline bolus (250 or 500 mL) via pressure bag on pre-imaging (no more than 15 min immediately prior to imaging) to increase LA preloading and thus to avoid underestimation of the LAA size. The scan can be performed with either prospective or retrospective electrocardiogram (ECG) gating due to dynamic changes in the LAA size over the cardiac cycle. Our center performs CT imaging as per single contrast bolus and dual-phase imaging protocol. Bolus tracking in the left atrium is used to trigger the imaging acquisition. Images are acquired from the carina to the diaphragm at expiratory breath hold. Retrospective ECG gating in the arterial phase (because of variable heart rate in AF patients) and delayed scan using prospective triggering or helical high-pitch acquisition (to decrease total radiation exposure) is utilized, as previously described. Late systolic phase coned images (40% in the arterial phase and 35% in the delayed phase) are reconstructed for the interpretation. Typically, delayed phase scan starts 15 s after the arterial phase to facilitate optimal left atrial appendage thrombus assessment (Fig. 5.1). Whenever dual-energy CT technology is available, we also utilize the low-energy virtual monoenergetic images (VMI_{low}) on the delayed phase to boost the contrast, therefore enabling improved visualization of the LAA, and make a more confident distinction between the true thrombus and circulatory stasis (Fig. 5.2). Further specifications of a CTA preplanning protocol workflow are detailed in Table 5.1.

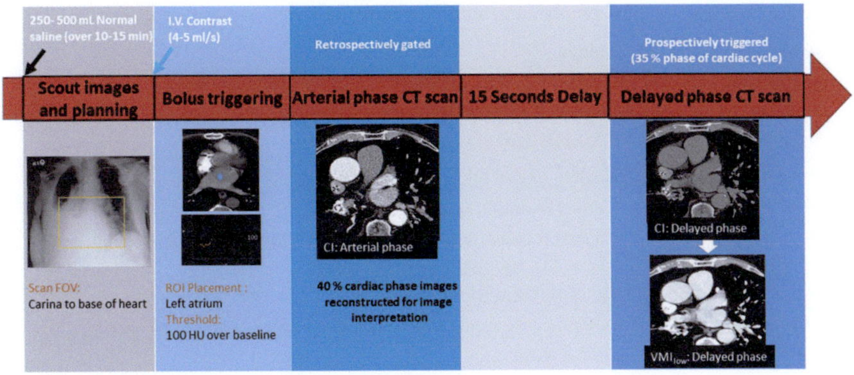

Fig. 5.1 Single contrast injection and dual-phase imaging protocol for left atrial appendage evaluation. *CI* conventional CT images; VMI_{low} low-energy virtual monoenergetic images

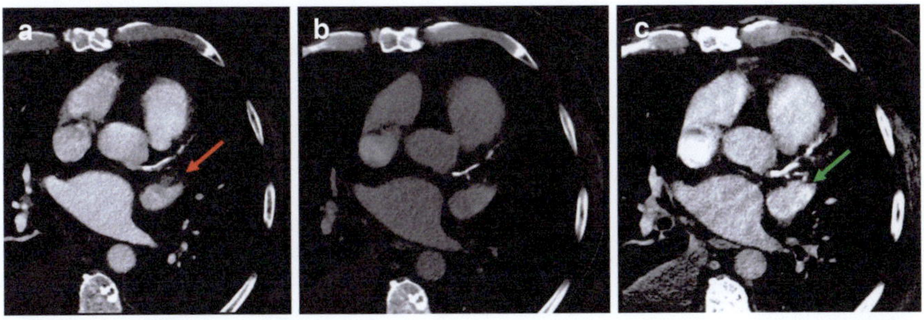

Fig. 5.2 A 79-year-old male with history of atrial fibrillation presents for preimplantation planning cardiac CT before LAA occluder device placement. On the initial arterial phase, axial CT image (A), there is a filling defect in the anterior aspect of the left atrial appendage (red arrow), which may be due to thrombus or circulatory stasis. The delayed phase CT image (B) demonstrates resolution of the filling defect, although the assessment is difficult due to very poor contrast opacification. The low-energy virtual monoenergetic image (VMI_{low}) reconstruction from the delayed phase (C) provides the necessary contrast boost and makes more confident diagnosis of circulatory stasis (green arrow) and exclusion of thrombus

CTA provides accurate three-dimensional (3D) images of the LAA and allows for detailed visualization of cardiac structures. CTA measurements for LAA landing zone should be performed utilizing 3D multiplanar reformatting images at the level of the circumflex artery in the mid-to-late systolic phase of the cardiac cycle to ensure maximal contrast opacification of the LAA.

The LAA is seldom circular, and sizing disparities in an elliptically shaped LAA may lead to inaccurate sizing of the device if a maximal diameter is used for device sizing. In these cases, average diameter, area-derived diameter, or perimeter may provide more accurate device measurements (Fig. 5.3). Multiplanar imaging with CTA allows the operator to manipulate the oblique angles appropriately to select the maximal dimensions. This aids in the assessment of the LAA given its inherent highly variable anatomy and varying orientations and lobes. CTA also provides a reliable LAA diameter to guide optimal device selection, and it should be noted that

Table 5.1 Example of CTA preplanning workflow protocol

Cardiac-gated scans	Values
Tube potential	100 kV for BMI <30 120 kV if BMI >30
Tube current	170, 145 mA
Scan direction	Cranial to caudal
Scan volume	Carina to diaphragm
Size	Images reconstructed to 0.75 and 0.7 mm with 40% overlap, 512 × 512 mm matrix, FOV 25 cm
Detector collimation	128 × 0.6 mm Siemens
Cardiac phase reconstruction	Relative triggering 35% of RR interval or absolute triggering 250 ms after R wave
Contrast bolus tracking	Cardiac definition (Siemens) Bolus tracked with ROI in left atrium and threshold of 100HU
Scan 1	Gated retrospectively at 35% recon phase full FOV
Scan 2	Gated prospectively at 40% recon phase coned FOV at 50 s postinjection
Delayed imaging phase	Images acquired 15 s after arterial phase
IV contrast injection (5 cc/s)	5 cc/sec, extended bolus 70 mL IsoVue 370, with 50 cc NS chaser
Heart rate	No restriction
Beta-blocker and nitrates	Not required

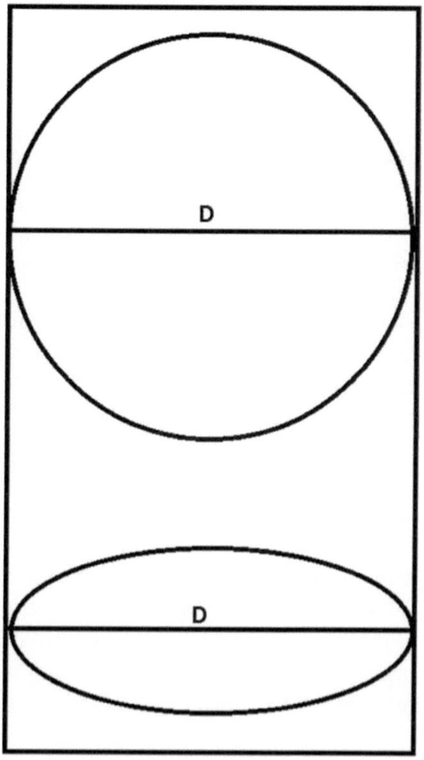

Fig. 5.3 Example of the importance of the area-derived diameter for the WATCHMAN™ sizing. Of note, diameter disparities due to the elliptical shape of the LAA may lead to inaccurate sizing. In this figure, the circle (top) and the ellipse (bottom) shapes both have the same diameter (D). Therefore, if sizing was performed based solely on diameter, then both shapes would have an inaccurate same sizing, even though the elliptical area is much smaller than the circle area

Table 5.2 Characteristics of CTA

Noninvasive
Capaçity for 3-dimensional rendering
Excellent spatial resolution
Fast image acquisition
Precise delineation of LAA anatomy and interatrial septum
Manipulation of oblique angles for assessment of the maximum LAA ostium diameter.
Depiction of anatomy of surrounding structures
Accuracy in LAA thrombus exclusion (negative predictive value 87–99%)

LAA measurements on cardiac CT tend to be 2–3 mm larger than TEE. Multiplanar imaging with CTA allows the operator to manipulate the oblique angles properly to select the maximal dimensions.

CTA characteristics are depicted in Table 5.2.

Pre-procedural Imaging

The pre-procedural imaging plan for LAAO can be divided in three major steps:

Step 1: Assessing the LAA anatomy and contraindications for device placement
Step 2: Device sizing/selection
Step 3: Transseptal puncture planning

Step 1: Assessing the LAA anatomy and contraindications for device placement

Pre-procedural cardiac CTA imaging should be ideally acquired within 2 weeks of the device implant. It can also be performed on the same day of the procedure for centers seeking a same-day imaging + implant strategy.

The first step is to evaluate the morphology of the left atrial appendage. There are four main types of LAA morphology described in the literature, based on the number of lobes, bend angle, and presence of dominant lobe—windsock, chicken-wing, cactus, and broccoli or cauliflower—as seen in Fig. 5.4. The windsock type has a single dominant lobe, which is the easiest to measure and the most conducive to LAAO implantation. The "chicken-wing type" is the most common type and confers the lowest risk of stroke. This type has a dominant lobe and a sharp kink (<100°) which leads to short usable length (limiting device selection) proximal to the bend and increased procedure complexity. The cactus type has a dominant lobe and multiple secondary lobes without a bend and is usually amenable to straightforward measurement and device implantation. The broccoli or cauliflower type is the least common, with complex multi-lobulated and no dominant lobe, presenting a challenge for identifying the landing zone and a potentially high risk for device embolization.

In our center, delayed contrast images are reviewed first as the presence of LAA thrombus is an absolute contraindication to closure, as previously demonstrated in

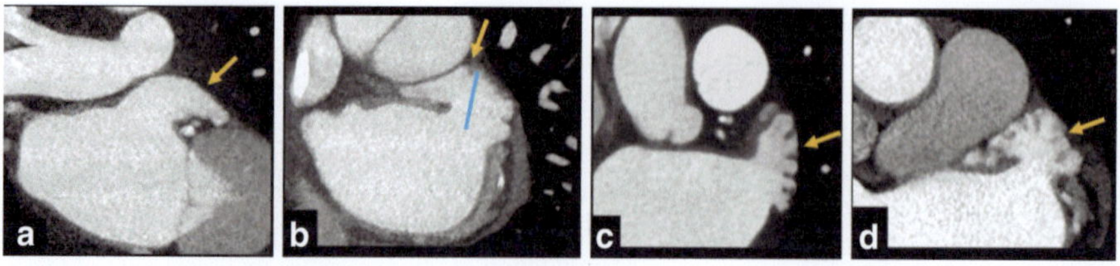

Fig. 5.4 Morphology of the left atrial appendage. **Panel A**: the windsock type (dominant lobe with an angle of more than 100° from the ostium). **Panel B**: the chicken-wing type (sharp bend with an angle of more than 100° from the ostium; blue line shows the usable length). **Panel C**: the cactus type (several small lobes arising from a dominant lobe). **Panel D**: the broccoli type (complex morphology with no single dominant lobe)

Fig. 5.2. The acquisition of delayed series is recommended to allow adequate contrast mixing, avoiding overinterpretation of the thrombus in the LAA. CTA has high rates of sensitivity (~96%) and specificity (~92%) for LAA thrombus detection and an impressive negative predictive value of 87–99%. Reconstructive segmentation for device sizing should be performed at scan increments ideally between 0.5 and 1.5 mm slice thicknesses with late-pass delayed scan to exclude LAA thrombus.

Step 2: Device sizing/selection

A CT scanner with a minimum of 64-slice resolution yields adequate imaging for LAAC planning. Various software packages such as Aquarius™ iNtuition Workstation (TeraRecon Inc.) and the 3mensio™ software (Pie Medical Imaging, Maastricht, Netherlands) can be used for pre-procedural planning. Recently purpose-built LAAC software packages such as TruPlan™ software (Circle Cardiovascular Imaging Inc., Calgary) and FEops HEARTguide™ software (FEops NV, Ghent, Belgium) have been developed which allow for greater procedural specificity.

In general, current workstation software provides a multiplanar reconstruction once the oblique plane is defined from the level of the circumflex artery to a point 1–2 cm from the tip of the limbus. A step-by-step approach is outlined in Table 5.3. Some software packages may provide automatic LAA measurements and device size selection upon identification of the landing zone. They may be also able to simulate the final position of the device in the LAA with the predicted compression and final shape. Understanding LAA anatomy may aid in appropriate device selection, particularly in challenging anatomies.

Step 3: Transseptal planning

CTA also allows detailed transseptal puncture planning, as depicted in Fig. 5.5. For this, the interatrial septum is first aligned in two of three planes with one plane axis across the septum and the other through the appendage. In this way, the interatrial septum may be surveyed allowing for the most ideal puncture site to be chosen for coaxial device delivery. The correct orientation of the catheter should be coplanar with the axis of the principal LAA lobe, and generally an inferior and posterior

Table 5.3 Brief step-by-step approach for LAAC planning using CTA

1. Select the appropriate arterial gated phase, typically 35% R-R phase)
2. Find the appendage. Scrolling cranial to caudal in the axial view, the appendage may be identified just below the proximal left pulmonary artery. Compare images with delayed contrast phase to rule out LAA thrombus
3. Align the same axis across the LAA ostium in two of three planes (e.g., sagittal and coronal planes), to find the ostium en face in the third view (true axial plane)
4. Outline the LAA ostium in the true axial plane and obtain measurements. Though some workstation software will automatically draw the LAA ostium, in our practice manual landing zone assessment is routinely done
5. Measure the depth of the LAA by tracing a perpendicular line from the landing plane to the distalmost aspect of the most usable lobe
6. Select device and size. Usually more than one device size fits within the recommended compression range. Our approach is to choose a device size based on an area-derived diameter with a target compression of 15–25%
7. Find the angle of deployment. This may be performed by manipulation of 3D reconstruction images to find the angle that best demonstrates ostial coaxiality and appendage depth. Some software packages have a dedicated workflow to facilitate this function
8. Plan the transseptal puncture
9. Assess for other features such as baseline pericardial effusion

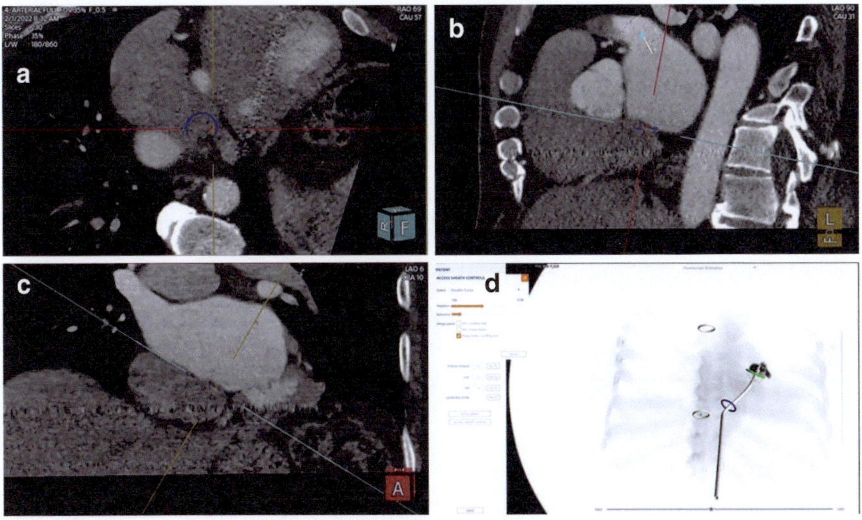

Fig. 5.5 Example of simulation of the transseptal puncture preplanning using the TruPlan™ software workstation for LAAC with the WATCHMAN™ device. **Panel A**: axial view. **Panel B**: sagittal view. **Panel C**: coronal view. **Panel D**: angiography simulation

transseptal puncture is best for LAAC. However, the interatrial septum may not have ideal thickness at this location. In addition, some LAA anatomies are suitable for mid-septal or even anterior puncture. By selective image processing, it is possible to simulate multiple sites of transseptal punctures, to understand the optimal site where that catheter should cross the interatrial septum, and even to select the ideal delivery catheter for a given LAA anatomy.

Comparison of Dedicated Software Workstations for LAAC

Software packages that are purpose-built for LAAC may have advantages especially for implanters that are less experienced with CTA. These programs allow for semi-automatic LAA anatomy depiction, device sizing, transseptal puncture planning, simulation of the final device position and compression, and thrombus exclusion. In a recent publication, a comparison between two commercially available software workstations for LAAC with WATCHMAN™ device was performed using TeraRecon™ and TruPlan™ software packages. Procedural success, number of devices, and adverse events were evaluated. However, the study did not show a difference regarding safety and outcomes.

TruPlan™ Workstation Software

TruPlan™ workstation software (Fig. 5.6) is dedicated to the WATCHMAN™ FLX device, providing a full workflow plan to ensure the most precise implantation of the device. Upon landing zone identification, it automatically provides device size

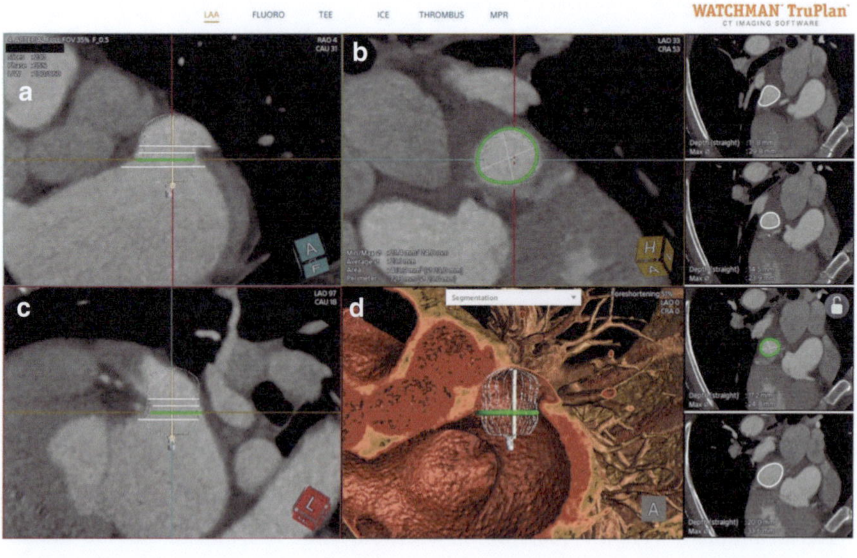

Fig. 5.6 Cardiac CTA pre-procedural planning using multiplanar images with the TruPlan™ software for the WATCHMAN™ device. **Panel A**: coronal view. **Panel B**: axial view. **Panel C**: sagittal view. **Panel D**: 3D simulation of the WATCHMAN™ device position in the LAA

selection choice with predicted compression based on LAA maximal diameter, average diameter, area-derived diameter, and perimeter. LAA device depth is automatically depicted at 15 mm but may also be manually estimated, and a 3D-rendering is shown to help assess LAA morphology. The interatrial septum may be assessed for morphology and thickness as well as best angle of entry to access the LAA.

The TruPlan™ software has many features that may contribute to accurate pre-procedural planning. Sizing and compression estimates are derived automatically, and device selection can be chosen based on several measurements, including area-derived diameter, maximum diameter, average diameter, and perimeter. Usually there are two device sizes that fit within the recommended 10–30% compression range, and in this situation, the decision is at the operator's discretion. We select device size based on a target compression of 15–25% using area-derived diameter, though average diameter and perimeter may also be used. Once selected, TruPlan™ digitally superimposes the device onto the CTA image of the LAA. This overlay may aid in the decision-making process, as the device may be virtually repositioned in the appendage to predict how the LAA tissue may interact with the device.

TruPlan™ software also simulates device shape at the predicted compression, illustrating how the device may appear during implant. There are six different workflows that may add value in challenging cases: LAA, Fluoro, TEE, ICE, Thrombus, and MPR. These workflows assist with important steps of the LAAC such as the ideal transseptal puncture strategy, the ideal angulation of the imaging intensifier, and the optimal final position and compression of the LAA device.

The LAA workflow is used for appendage measurement and for landing zone identification. The Fluoro workflow allows for device selection and for simulation of device position and compression. The device also may be manually repositioned in this workflow for final decision-making. The Fluoro workflow provides a perspective of the fluoroscopic simulation and prediction of the best image intensifier angle for device deployment. Both the TEE and ICE workflows may be best suited for training. The TEE workflow allows the operator to visualize a perspective of the TEE simulation with LAA images in different angles. Similarly, the ICE workflow provides a perspective of the intracardiac echocardiogram (ICE) simulation with LAA images in different views. The MPR (multiplanar reconstruction) workflow allows different approaches to better visualize the LAA, including three-dimensional images, such as draw, trim, flange, segment, etc. Finally, the Thrombus workflow allows delayed phase imaging to be shown side by side with the left atrial phase imaging to facilitate thrombus evaluation. In this workflow, attenuation assessment, available under the Tools menu, can be used to assess concerning areas.

FEops HEARTguide™ Simulation

FEops HEARTguide™ is a CT-based preoperative planning tool providing patient-specific simulations to optimize the planning for structural heart disease interventions. It can support both LAAO and TAVI interventions. The simulation provides accurate prediction of the interaction between the specific anatomy and the device, as depicted in Fig. 5.7.

For LAAC interventions, both the Amulet™ and WATCHMAN™ devices can be simulated. The simulation output provides the measurements of the dimension of the device after the deployment and a graphical representation of the "apposition plot": the deformed 3D device is displayed with a color map, identifying the distance between its surface and the surrounding anatomy. This feature can potentially identify device malapposition. FEops HEARTguide™ allows implant simulation of different size devices (according to the artificial intelligence-supported anatomical analysis) and at different depths.

The CT process starts with the anatomical analysis consisting of the assessment of the LAA morphology through landmark identification (measurements). Then the anatomy is reconstructed in 3D, and the landmarks are displayed. It is possible to rotate, zoom, and pan the three-dimensional (3D) reconstruction to better investigate the anatomy. Fluoroscopic angles are displayed to find the most suitable angulation for the fluoroscopy implant orientation. In this way, the optimal implant angle and landing zone can be determined with minimal parallax. Transseptal puncture visualization is also provided. Following the anatomical analysis and reconstruction, patient-specific cardiac CT-based computer simulations of different device sizes and implant positions are generated with FEops™ HEARTguide, and the operator can plan the optimal procedure matching the targeted pre-procedural computational model.

FEops HEARTguide™ simulation requires the CT images to be uploaded on the online platform, so that the FEops team can work on them and provide measurements and different simulation options for both optimal and suboptimal implant scenarios. For this, good-quality CT images are required, since the simulation cannot be performed if the images are not good enough to guarantee an accurate anatomical reconstruction and a reliable prediction of the anatomy/device interaction.

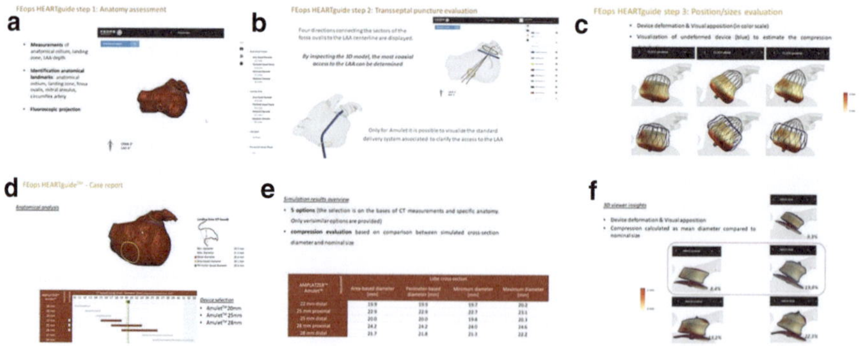

Fig. 5.7 Example of a step-by-step approach: cardiac CTA computational simulation of the LAAC using the FEops™ HEARTguide software for the Amulet™ device. **Panel A**: anatomy assessment. **Panel B**: transseptal puncture evaluation. **Panel C**: position/size evaluation. **Panel D**: anatomical analysis. **Panel E**: simulation results overview. **Panel F**: 3D viewer insights

The main differentiating characteristic of FEops HEARTguide™ is the possibility to provide a realistic device/anatomy interaction, not just a compressed overlay of the device as with TruPlan™. This makes it possible to predict device seal and anchor and may be particularly useful in challenging anatomies. FEops HEARTguide™ also offers a standardized and scalable solution: the anatomical analysis is artificial intelligence supported, and the simulations are the results of validated computational models that guarantee that the provided insights are not operator dependent. All the steps of the process are subject to a quality control step, performed by an expert analyst with extensive experience in the field, who followed an additional quality control training.

Clinical Evidence for CTA

There have been several pivotal studies highlighting the advantages of CTA for LAAC. However, most of the data for CTA comes from single-center experience. Saw, Wang, and colleagues have performed the pivotal studies first demonstrating the utility of CTA for LAAC preplanning, including its impact on early operator learning curve. From those studies, CTA has been increasingly adopted and has become a noninvasive alternative to TEE for LAAC preplanning.

Wang and colleagues studied the application of 3D CTA imaging guidance to WATCHMAN™ implantation and its impact on early operator learning curve in 53 consecutive patients in a single center and concluded that 3D CTA planning provides a comprehensive and customized LAA assessment specific to each patient. In this analysis, CTA appeared not only to be accurate but also to help reduce the learning curve for LAAC.

In another single-center study, measurements of CTA, TEE, and fluoroscopy of the LAAC in 50 consecutive patients were compared. The authors concluded that all three imaging modalities correlated with the Amplatzer™ landing zone and WATCHMAN™ ostium measurements, with CTA providing the largest measurements, followed by TEE and fluoroscopy. Saw and colleagues also published in 2016 a review article addressing the role of CTA for LAAC. They determined the practical utility of CTA, while it offers unique imaging planes and preplanning anatomic LAA assessment and can identify pre-existing LAA thrombus.

A recent study evaluated the strategy of CTA and intracardiac echocardiogram (ICE) for LAAC in a single-center, prospective analysis of 71 patients who underwent LAAC over an 18-month period. Procedural success, correlation of CTA preprocedural device sizing with final device size utilization, adverse events, length of procedure, and length of stay were evaluated. The authors concluded that a strategy of CTA and ICE is a safe and feasible protocol for LAAC regarding adequate device sizing and can be used for a strategy of same-day discharge. In addition, if ICE is the selected imaging guidance strategy, it should incorporate CTA preplanning, since CTA yields more information than TEE. Therefore, the limitations from ICE imaging can be supported by the advanced imaging from CTA.

Although there are no guidelines regarding specific CTA sizing strategy, excellent results have been previously described using area-based diameter for device sizing. A recent single-center, prospective study included 115 patients who underwent cardiac CTA and WATCHMAN™ device implantation and demonstrated that cardiac CTA LAA ostium area-based sizing algorithm was highly accurate (95.6%) at predicting WATCHMAN™ device size and demonstrated excellent clinical outcomes with a lower device utilization per case than what was reported in literature.

Another single-center, prospective study including 71 patients who underwent cardiac CTA and WATCHMAN™ device implantation collected and analyzed baseline characteristics, procedural data, and clinical outcomes. The device size predicted by cardiac CTA was calculated based on the area-derived diameter and corresponded with the final device used in all cases, and the procedure success rate for this series was 100%. We concluded that cardiac CTA-guided pre-procedural planning resulted in accurate device sizing in this patient sample and may be used in conjunction with ICE and conscious sedation for a same-day discharge strategy in select patients.

Another recent paper addressed the pre-procedural determination of device size in LAAC using three-dimensional cardiac computed tomography. In this retrospective study, they reviewed 62 patients with Amplatzer™ Cardiac Plug and Amulet™ LAAC devices. The minimal, maximal, average, area-derived, and perimeter-derived diameters of the LAA landing zone were measured using CT-based images. Predicted device sizes using sizing charts were compared with actual successfully implanted device sizes. The authors concluded that when using cardiac CT-based measurements for LAAC planning, the perimeter-derived diameter was the most accurate parameter to predict the device size. Of note, the eccentricity of the LAA ostium was a critical factor responsible for the discrepancy among the CT-based measurements, and the perimeter-derived diameter was advantageous in patients with a highly eccentric LAA ostium.

Comparison Between CTA and TEE

TEE may underestimate the landing zone diameter, while CT provides a more reliable LAA diameter to guide optimal selection of the device due to its superior spatial resolution. A strategy of pre-procedural planning using cardiac CTA has advantages over TEE, such as increasing LAAC procedural efficiency, facilitating accurate device sizing, avoiding general anesthesia, being safer in the COVID pandemic era, and finally translating into reduced hospital stay and cost. The advantages are listed in Table 5.4.

A study reported that CTA predicted accurate LAAC device size 75.7% of the time using a 64-slice scanner. Furthermore, in that series, CTA outperformed both TEE (51.4%) and angiography (48.6%) for appropriate device sizing. The authors

Table 5.4 Advantages of CTA over TEE

Increased LAAC procedural efficiency
No sedation
More accurate device sizing
Better assessment of surrounding structures
Improved safety particularly in the COVID era
Translate into reduced hospital stay
Cost reduction when associated with same-day discharge strategy

Table 5.5 Situations in which pre-procedural planning with CTA should be avoided

Patient refusal
Impaired renal function (GFR < 30)
Severe contrast allergy
Pregnancy (especially in the first trimester)
LAA diameter greater than 40 mm
Multi-lobed LAA
Some cases of prior cardiac surgery with subsequent new anatomical abnormalities (e.g., left internal mammary artery adherent to the LAA)
Chest wall abnormalities such as pectus excavatum deformity and history of thoracic radiation exposure
For the Lariat device: it is contraindicated in patients with a history of pericarditis or cardiac surgery, recent myocardial infarction in the last 3 months, chest wall abnormalities such as pectus excavatum, and a history of thoracic radiation exposure

concluded that cardiac CTA offered several other advantages over TEE in LAAC planning as it provided accurate ostial and depth measurements of the left atrial appendage due to the ability to reformat images. Other recent studies have reported that CTA helps improve device sizing and contributes to a more efficient and safer LAAC procedure than the use of TEE to predict the device size.

A recent subanalysis of the SWISS-APERO trial evaluated the impact of pre-procedural CTA on top of peri-procedural TEE to plan LAAC. In this multicenter prospective study, the investigators included 219 LAAC preceded by CTA; 42.1% were assigned to CTA unblinded group and 57.9% to the blinded group. The authors concluded that unblinding of the interventionists to pre-procedural CTA images was independently associated with a ~3× higher rate of short-term procedural success and ~2× higher rate in the long-term follow-up.

When to Avoid CTA for Pre-procedural Planning

There are some clinical scenarios in which CTA should not be selected for LAAC pre-procedural planning strategy, as seen in Table 5.5 and Fig. 5.8.

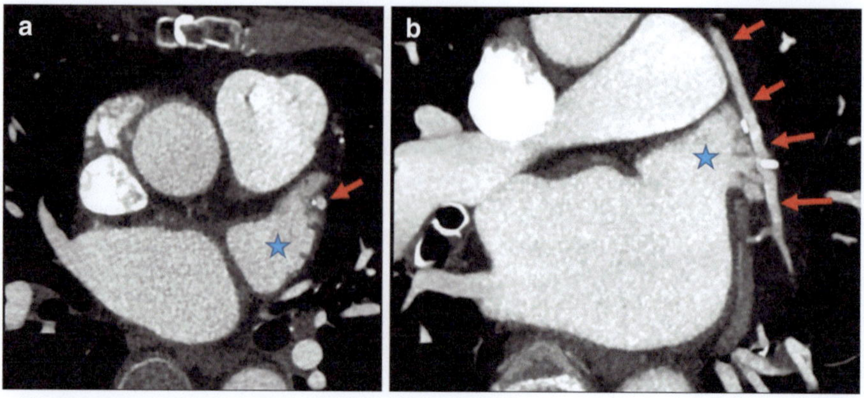

Fig. 5.8 Potential contraindication to hybrid endocardial-epicardial device placement. **Panel A**: axial CT. **Panel B**: coronal multiplanar reconstruction showing the LIMA-to-LAD bypass graft (red arrows) in close approximation with the LAA (blue star)

Future Directions for CT Imaging

The field of transcatheter LAAC has evolved tremendously in the last two decades, with marked improvements in safety, efficacy, and device iterations. Ongoing trials and evolving practices indicate significant future advancements to come. 3D printing and computer simulation based on artificial intelligence (AI) hold much promise in this field, especially with the challenging anatomies operators face.

Advances in AI decision-making solutions could result in improved procedural efficiency and a trend toward better procedural outcomes. The recently published PREDICT-LAA trial was a prospective, multicenter, randomized trial in which 200 patients were 1:1 randomized to standard planning vs. cardiac CT simulation-based planning of LAA closure with the Amulet™ device. The AI-enabled CT-based anatomical analyses and computer simulations were provided by FEops™ HEARTguide. The composite primary endpoint, defined as contrast leakage distal to the Amulet lobe and/or presence of DRT, was observed in 41.8% in the standard group vs. 28.9% in the CT + simulation group. In addition, use of computer simulations resulted in improved procedural efficiency with use of fewer Amulet™ devices and fewer device repositioning in the CT + simulation group.

The fusion of 3D multidetector computed tomography (3D-MDCT) onto real-time fluoroscopy screen to guide the LAAC procedure also holds promise. "Fluoro-CT fusion" will be addressed in a later chapter.

Conclusions

CTA pre-procedural planning is a safe and feasible strategy for LAAC which allows for accurate device sizing and allows for a streamlined procedure with improved scheduling logistics. New software workstations have multiple features to help the CT interpreter to select not only the best device type but also the best implantation strategy based on each patient's unique anatomical shape of the LAA. The workstation may also help the operator to navigate through the procedure with the most adequate transseptal puncture prediction, to select the best deployment angle into the LAA and to predict eventual pitfalls based on the precise anatomy of the LAA. Further operator's experience is warranted to determine whether the software workstation-simulated positions and depths could be achieved in practice and to understand the role of artificial intelligence in future versions of the software and its impact in clinical practice.

References and Suggested Readings

1. Buysschaert I, Viaene D. Clinical impact of preprocedural CT-based 3D computational simulation of left atrial appendage occlusion with amulet. J Interv Cardiol. 2021;2021:9972228. https://doi.org/10.1155/2021/9972228. PMID: 34385893; PMCID: PMC8328713
2. Cho I, Kim WD, Lee OH et al. Pre-procedural determination of device size in left atrial appendage occlusion using three-dimensional cardiac computed tomography, 12 August 2021, PREPRINT (Version 1) available at Research Square [https://doi.org/10.21203/rs.3.rs-795122/v1].
3. Dallan LAP, Bezerra HG, Cochet A, Kobayashi A, Attizzani GF, Rashid I, Rajagopalan S, Simon DI, Shishehbor MH, Arruda M, Filby SJ. Safety, efficacy, and cost-effectiveness of same-day discharge for left atrial appendage occlusion. J Invasive Cardiol. 2022;34(2):E124–31.
4. Dallan LAP, Arruda M, Yoon SH, Rana MA, Mogalapalli A, Carneiro HA, Reed J, Rashid I, Rajagopalan S, Filby SJ. Novel computed tomography angiography-based sizing methodology for WATCHMAN FLX device in left atrial appendage closure. J Cardiovasc Electrophysiol. 2022;33(8):1781–7.
5. De Backer O, Iriart X, Kefer J, et al. Impact of computational modeling on transcatheter left atrial appendage closure efficiency and outcomes. J Am Coll Cardiol Intv. 2023;16(6):655–66.
6. Filby SJ, Dallan LAP, Cochet A, et al. Left atrial appendage occlusion using cardiac CT angiography and Intracardiac echocardiography: a prospective, Single-Center Study. J Invasive Cardiol. 2021;33(11):E851–6.
7. Freitas-Ferraz AB, Bernier M, Vaillancourt R, et al. Safety of transesophageal echocardiography to guide structural cardiac interventions. J Am Coll Cardiol. 2020;75:3164–73.
8. Hur J, Young JK, Lee HJ, et al. Left atrial appendage thrombi in stroke patients: detection with two-phase cardiac CT angiography versus transesophageal echocardiography. Radiology. 2009;251:683–90. https://doi.org/10.1148/radiol.2513090794.
9. Lopez-Minguez JR, Gonzalez-Fernandez R, Fernandez-Vegas C, Millan-Nunez V, Fuentes-Canamero ME, Nogales-Asensio JM, Doncel-Vecino J, Yuste Dominguez M, Garcia Serrano L, Sanchez Quintana D. Comparison of imaging techniques to assess appendage anatomy and measurements for left atrial appendage closure device selection. J Invasive Cardiol. 2014;26:462–7.
10. Nadeem F, Igwe C, Stoycos S, et al. A new WATCHMAN sizing algorithm utilizing cardiac CTA. Cardiovasc Revasc Med. 2021;33:13–9. https://doi.org/10.1016/j.carrev.2021.01.009.
11. Ribeiro J, Teixeira R, Puga L, et al. Comparison of intracardiac and transesophageal echocardiography for guidance of percutaneous left atrial appendage occlusion: a meta-analysis. Echocardiography. 2019;00:1–8.
12. Saw J, Lopes JP, Reisman M, et al. Cardiac computed tomography angiography for left atrial appendage closure. Can J Cardiol. 2016;32:1033.e1–9.
13. Saw J, Fahmy P, Spencer R, et al. Comparing measurements of CT angiography, TEE, and fluoroscopy of the left atrial appendage for percutaneous closure. J Cardiovasc Electrophysiol. 2016;27:414–22.

14. Saw J, Holmes DR, Cavalcante JL, et al. SCAI/HRS expert consensus statement on transcatheter left atrial appendage closure. J Soc Cardiovasc Angiogr Interv. 2023;2:100577. https://doi.org/10.1016/j.jscai.2022.100577.
15. Wang DD, Eng M, Kupsky D, et al. Application of 3-dimensional computed tomographic image guidance to Watchman implantation and impact on early operator learning curve: single-center experience. JACC Cardiovasc Interv. 2016;9:2329–40.

Chapter 6
Pre-procedural Planning for Left Atrial Appendage Closure: Cardiac Magnetic Resonance

Cody R. Johnson, Mohammed A. Alghammass, Luis Augusto Palma Dallan, Steven J. Filby, and Amit Gupta

Abbreviations

AF	Atrial fibrillation
CMR	Cardiac magnetic resonance imaging
LAA	Left atrial appendage
LAAO	Left atrial appendage occlusion
MRA	Magnetic resonance angiography
TEE	Transesophageal echocardiography
3D	Three-dimensional

Highlights
- Cardiac MRI (CMR) may be performed for planning left atrial appendage closure (LAAC) as a noninvasive alternative to transesophageal echocardiography (TEE) or CTA.
- When compared to CT, CMR offers advantages such as avoidance of contrast medium administration and radiation exposure.

C. R. Johnson · A. Gupta (✉)
Division of Cardiothoracic Imaging, Department of Radiology, University Hospitals Cleveland Medical Center, Cleveland, OH, USA

Department of Radiology, Case Western Reserve University School of Medicine, Cleveland, OH, USA
e-mail: amit.gupta@uhhospitals.org

M. A. Alghammass · L. A. P. Dallan · S. J. Filby
Division of Cardiology, Harrington Heart & Vascular Institute, University Hospitals Cleveland Medical Center, Cleveland, OH, USA
e-mail: luisaugusto.palmadallan@uhhospitals.org; steven.filby@uhhospitals.org

S. J. Filby et al. (eds.), *A Contemporary Manual of Left Atrial Appendage Closure*, https://doi.org/10.1007/978-3-031-68441-8_6

- CMR provides extensive structural, morphological, and functional assessment of the cardiac chambers, valves, coronary arteries, myocardium, and surrounding anatomical structures.

Introduction

In circumstances where therapeutic anticoagulation poses challenges in atrial fibrillation management, left atrial appendage occlusion (LAAO) presents a viable alternative. Prudent pre-procedural planning holds substantial importance for the successful execution of LAAO, given the considerable anatomical variability observed within the left atrial appendage across patient cohorts. While transesophageal echocardiography (TEE) has traditionally served as the primary modality for pre-procedural assessment, recent emphasis has been placed on modalities like computed tomography (CT) and cardiac magnetic resonance imaging (CMR) for this purpose [1, 2]. Notably, a retrospective analysis of the National Cardiovascular Data LAAO Registry spanning the period 2016–2021, which included patients who underwent attempted LAAO with Watchman or Watchman FLX, showed that only 18% ($n = 20{,}851$) of 114,348 procedures incorporated CT or MRI in pre-procedural planning. This analysis showed that pre-procedural CT/MRI was associated with increased likelihood of device success, implant success, and procedural success [3]. In some patients, cardiac computed tomography angiography (CTA) may not be feasible due to allergic reactions to iodinated contrast or in the setting of severe chronic renal dysfunction or acute kidney injury. CMR is an imaging modality that can effectively offer a noninvasive alternative to CTA or TEE for pre-procedural planning prior to LAAO, and it is appealing from the standpoint of incurring no ionizing radiation exposure. The LAA can be clearly identified, segmented, and measured on CMR and helps guide the choice of device, size of device, and device delivery system. See Table 6.1 for the characteristics of CMR. Failure of adequate device sizing or inadequate device positioning may result in unwanted complications such as peri-device leakage or device embolization.

Table 6.1 Characteristics of CMR

Noninvasive
Capacity for three-dimensional rendering
Excellent soft tissue contrast
Precise delineation of LAA anatomy and interatrial septum
Manipulation of oblique angles for assessment of the maximum LAA ostium diameter
Depiction of anatomy of surrounding structures
Accuracy in LAA thrombus exclusion (negative predictive value 100% on long TI sequence)

Cardiac Magnetic Resonance Imaging (CMR)

CMR encompasses a variety of pulse sequence techniques that facilitate comprehensive assessment of cardiac morphology and anatomy, function, quantification, and tissue characterization. Morphology can be assessed using either "dark blood" or "bright blood" techniques. Function is analyzed by using cine imaging with steady-state free precession (SSFP) or gradient echo (GRE) sequences. Flow quantification can be determined by phase contrast imaging. Tissue characterization can be evaluated by myocardial T1, T2, and T2* mapping sequences as well as delayed contrast enhancement sequences. In addition, more specialized sequences can be obtained which help to serve as clinical problem-solving tools. One such sequence is the so-called long time-to-inversion (TI) sequence to evaluate for thrombus. Additional sequences that can be performed include perfusion sequences and magnetic resonance angiography (MRA) sequences.

Clinical Applications of CMR

The clinical utility of CMR is vast and includes myocardial viability, ischemic and nonischemic cardiomyopathy, valvular and pericardial disease, and assessment of congenital heart disease. It has also been increasingly used for anatomic assessment and pre-procedural planning to include LAAO. The ability to obtain 3D thin slice image acquisitions in the heart allows for improved spatial resolution as compared to traditional MR images which have excellent tissue contrast but relatively limited spatial resolution as compared to CTA and TEE. Furthermore, the ability to acquire long TI sequences has robust clinical applications in detecting thrombus with a negative predictive value of 100% in one study. This sequence has been shown to be superior to conventional cine sequences and is not affected by the strength of the magnet used (1.5T or 3T) or the presence of atrial fibrillation. Contrast-enhanced sequences, cine sequences, and perfusion sequences tend to be more limited in the setting of arrythmias, motion/breathing, and flow-related artifacts. According to the 2019 joint consensus document by the American College of Cardiology on Appropriate Use Criteria for Multimodality Imaging in the Assessment of Cardiac Structure and Function in Nonvalvular Heart Disease, CMR received a numerical rating of 5 out of a possible 9 which indicates that it "may be appropriate" for pre-procedural evaluation for LAAO. This rating is in comparison with TEE and CTA which received scores ranging from 7 to 9 which is considered to be "appropriate."

Cardiac Magnetic Resonance Imaging of LAA Pre-procedural Imaging

At our institution, a Siemens Aera 1.5 Tesla (T) scanner is used. In addition to necessary localizer sequences for image planning, our protocol includes black blood axial and sagittal half-Fourier acquisition single-shot turbo spin echo (HASTE) sequences, 2-chamber and 4-chamber bright black stack true fast imaging with steady-state free precession (TRUFISP), a 4-chamber time-resolved angiography with interleaved stochastic trajectories (TWIST; with real-time monitoring of contrast entering the LA to begin image acquisition), followed by a gated MRA in 2-chamber orientation, 4-chamber and 2-chamber TI 600 PSIR sequences for thrombus detection, and finally a 3D whole-heart sequence in 2-chamber orientation which was used for multiplanar reconstructions and LAA measurements. Figure 6.1 summarizes our institution's MR protocol. A full technical description of each MR sequence is beyond the scope of this chapter; however, Table 6.2 provides pertinent details on the sequences that we find to be the most useful.

Once images are obtained, the initial evaluation at our institution begins with an evaluation for LAA thrombus, as the presence of a thrombus is an absolute contraindication to the procedure. The long inversion time sequence (TI 600) should be used for this assessment. After ruling out LAA thrombus, a methodical approach should begin with an evaluation of the overall morphology of the LAA. There are four main types of LAA morphology described in the literature, based on the number of lobes, bend angle, and presence of dominant lobe: windsock, chicken-wing, cactus, and broccoli or cauliflower. The windsock type has a single dominant lobe, which is the easiest to measure and the most conducive to LAAO implantation. The "chicken-wing type" is the most common type and confers the lowest risk of stroke. This type has a dominant lobe and a sharp kink (<100°) which leads to short usable length (limiting device selection) proximal to the bend and increased procedure complexity. The cactus type has a dominant lobe and multiple secondary lobes without a bend and is usually amenable to straightforward measurement and device implantation. The broccoli or cauliflower type is the least common, with complex multi-lobulated and no dominant lobe, presenting a challenge for identifying the landing zone and a potentially high risk for device embolization.

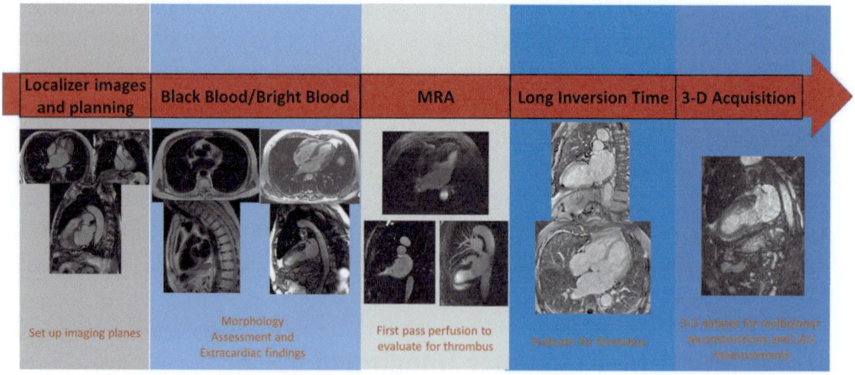

Fig. 6.1 Our institution's protocol for LAAO pre-procedural CMR. First, localizer sequences are obtained for planning dedicated cardiac imaging planes. Subsequent to this, we obtain both axial and sagittal black and bright blood sequences for overall anatomic assessment and morphology. After the injection of gadolinium contrast material, first-pass perfusion sequences are obtained to evaluate for thrombus. Long inversion time (TI = 600 ms) sequences are also used to clear the LAA of thrombus. Finally, a 3D acquisition is obtained that allows for multiplanar reconstructions in different planes to provide measurements of the LAA

Table 6.2 Our institution's LAAO pre-procedural planning CMR imaging protocol

Sequence	Clinical utility	Technical details
Axial and sagittal HASTE	Overall cardiac morphology and evaluation of extra-cardiac structures	Black blood; all slice data is obtained after a single 90°-excitation pulse
2-chamber and 4-chamber TRUFISP	Closer evaluation of cardiac morphology	Bright blood; free breathing, resolution 2.1 mm × 2.1 mm, slice thickness 4 mm
4-chamber TWIST	Real-time monitoring of contrast entering the LA to begin image acquisition	Low flip angle (20 degrees) allows for high temporal resolution and allows for fast image acquisition during the contrast bolus
ECG-gated 2-chamber and 4-chamber MRA	Evaluation of contrast opacification within the LAA and detection of slow flow	Takes advantage of different k-space sampling techniques for rapid imaging that allows for high temporal and spatial resolution
TI 600	Evaluation of LAA thrombus	Inversion time 600 ms, flip angle 40 degrees
3-D TRUFISP	Enhanced spatial resolution for LAA device sizing measurements; allows for multiplanar reformats	Utilizing a diaphragmatic navigator to time image acquisition with breathing; resolution is 0.7 mm × 0.7 mm; slice thickness 1.5 mm; flip angle 90 degrees

Table 6.3 Our institution's approach to LAAO CMR

1. On the long inversion time sequence (TI 600), find the left atrial appendage. Scrolling cranial to caudal in the axial view, the appendage may be identified just below the proximal left pulmonary artery. Look for a homogeneously "nulled" hypointense signal within the appendage to rule out thrombus
2. Select the appropriate 3D gated sequence which is usually acquired in a sagittal plane
3. Using a multiplanar reformatting tool, begin in the straight axial plane (Fig. 6.2). Then, align the axis in the axial plane along the course of the left circumflex coronary artery within the atrioventricular groove (Fig. 6.3). Look at the sagittal oblique (formerly true sagittal) image, and align the imaging plane with the Coumadin ridge (Fig. 6.4). Cross-check on the double oblique coronal (formerly true coronal) image that the plane is perpendicular to the LAA ostium (Fig. 6.5). The double-oblique axial (formerly the true axial) image should now show the LAA ostium en face
4. Outline the LAA ostium in the double-oblique plane and obtain measurements (Fig. 6.6). Though some workstation software will automatically draw the LAA ostium, in our practice, manual landing zone assessment is routinely done
5. Measure the depth of the LAA by tracing a perpendicular line from the landing plane to the distalmost aspect of the most usable lobe
6. Select device and size. Usually more than one device size fits within the recommended compression range. Our approach is to choose a device size based on an area-derived diameter with a target compression of 15–25%
7. Find the angle of deployment. This may be performed by manipulation of 3D reconstruction images to find the angle that best demonstrates ostial coaxiality and appendage depth. Some software packages have a dedicated workflow to facilitate this function
8. Plan the transseptal puncture

After evaluating the morphology of the LAA, appropriate measurements can then be obtained to allow for device sizing. Table 6.3 provides a step-by-step algorithm for obtaining the appropriate measurements and is then summarized as a diagram in Fig. 6.7.

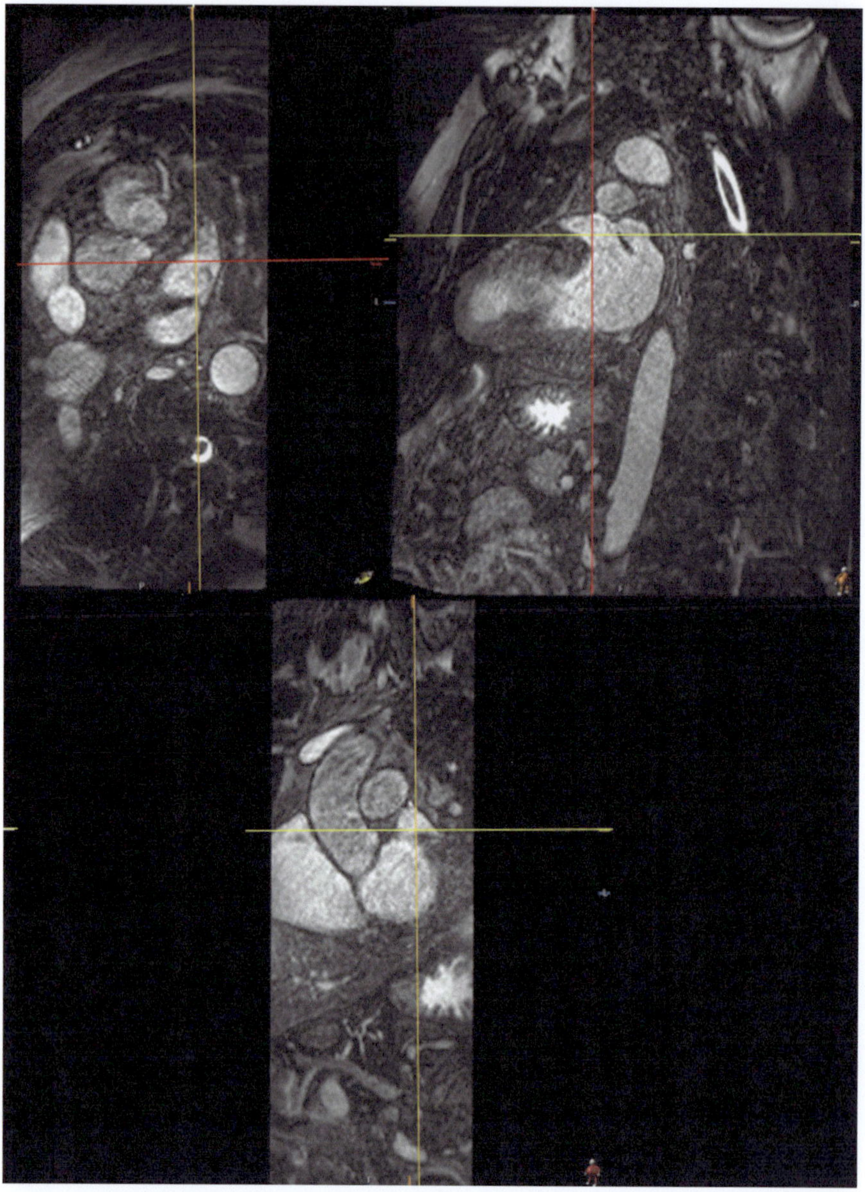

Fig. 6.2 Using a multiplanar reformatting tool, begin in the straight axial plane

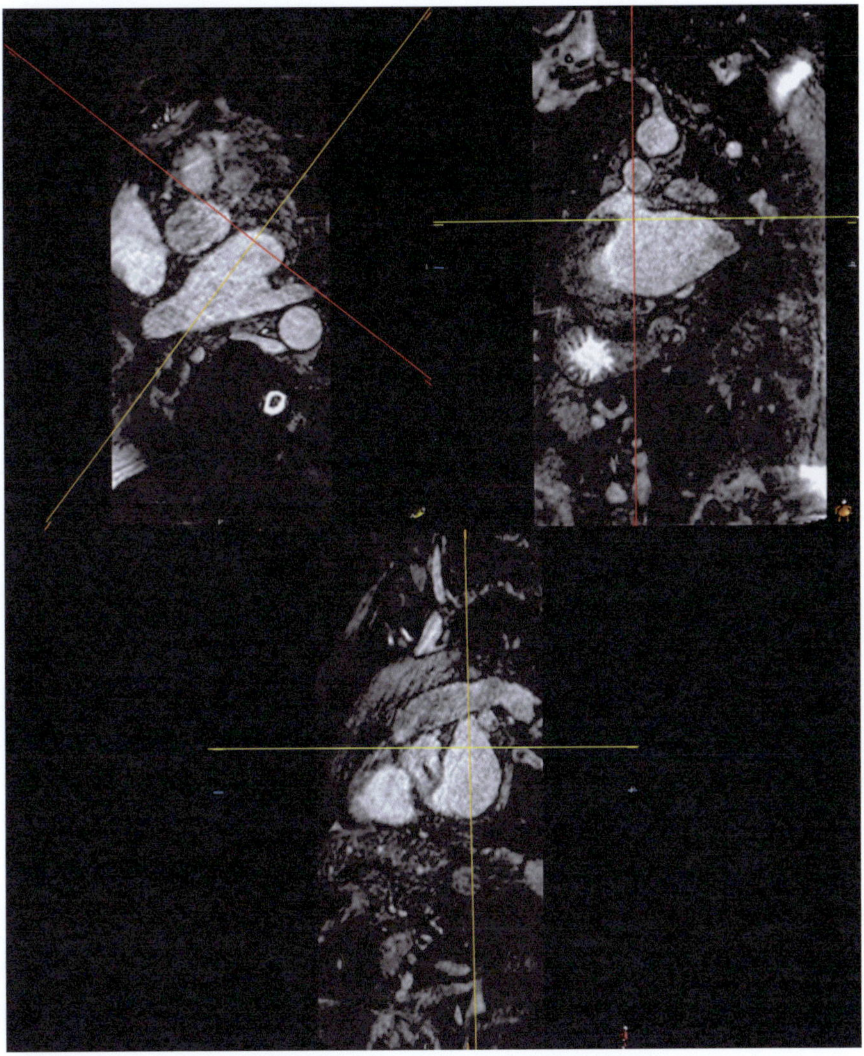

Fig. 6.3 Align the crosshair axis in the axial plane along the course of the left circumflex coronary artery/the atrioventricular groove

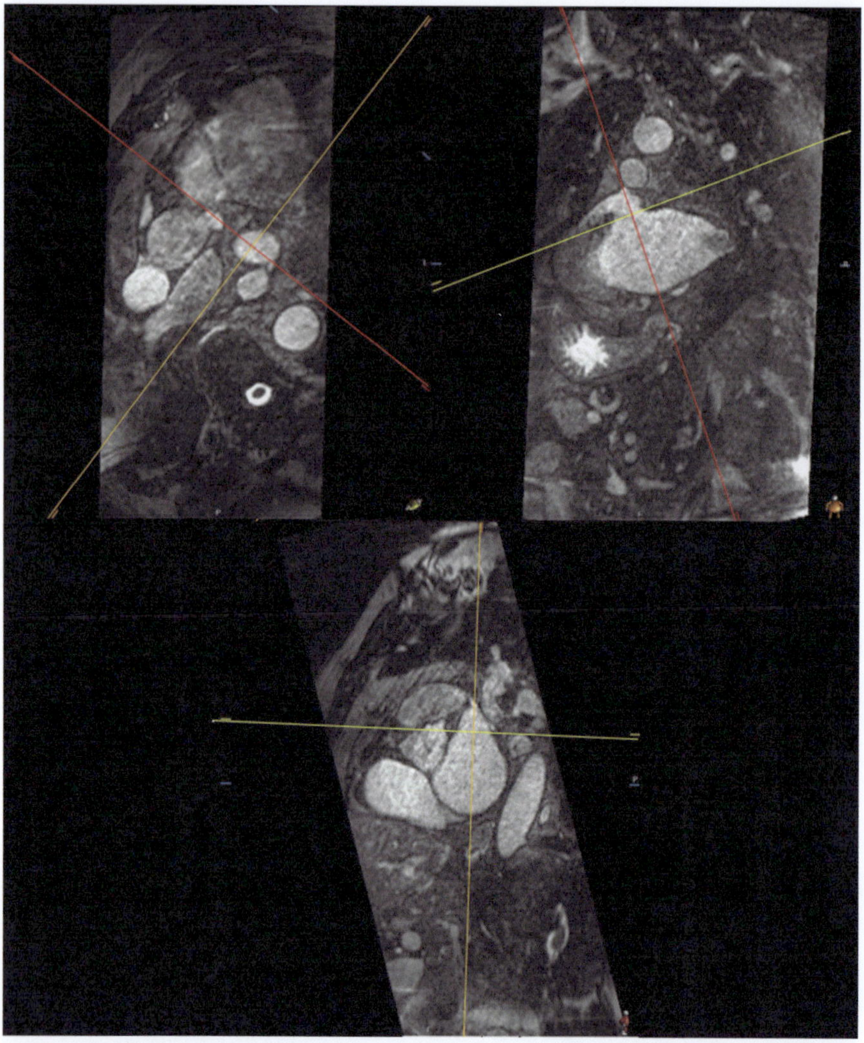

Fig. 6.4 Look at the sagittal oblique (formerly true sagittal) image, and align the crosshair imaging plane with the Coumadin ridge

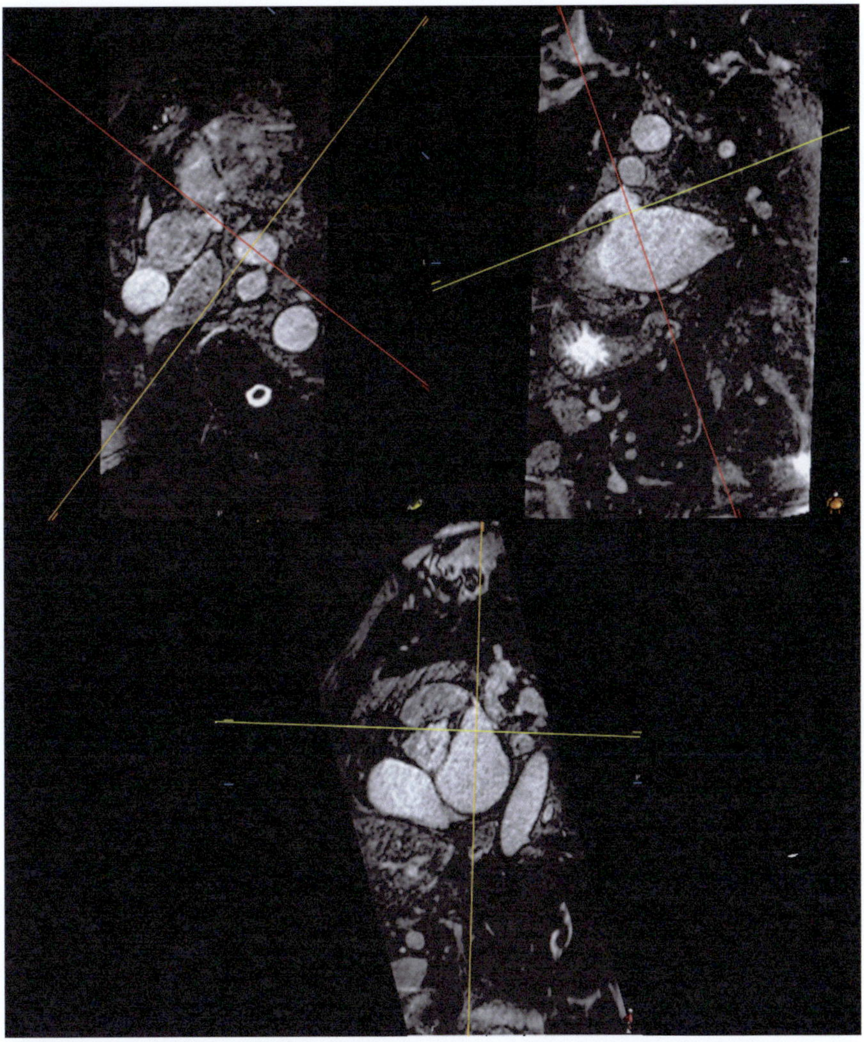

Fig. 6.5 Cross-check on the double-oblique coronal (formerly true coronal) image that the plane is perpendicular to the LAA ostium

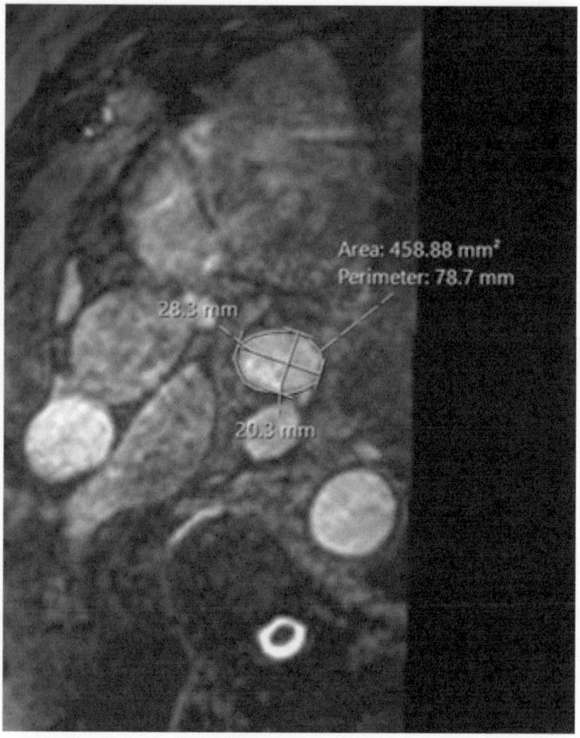

Fig. 6.6 Outline the LAA ostium in the double-oblique plane and obtain measurements. In this example, the area, perimeter, and long-/short-axis diameters of the LAA are measured

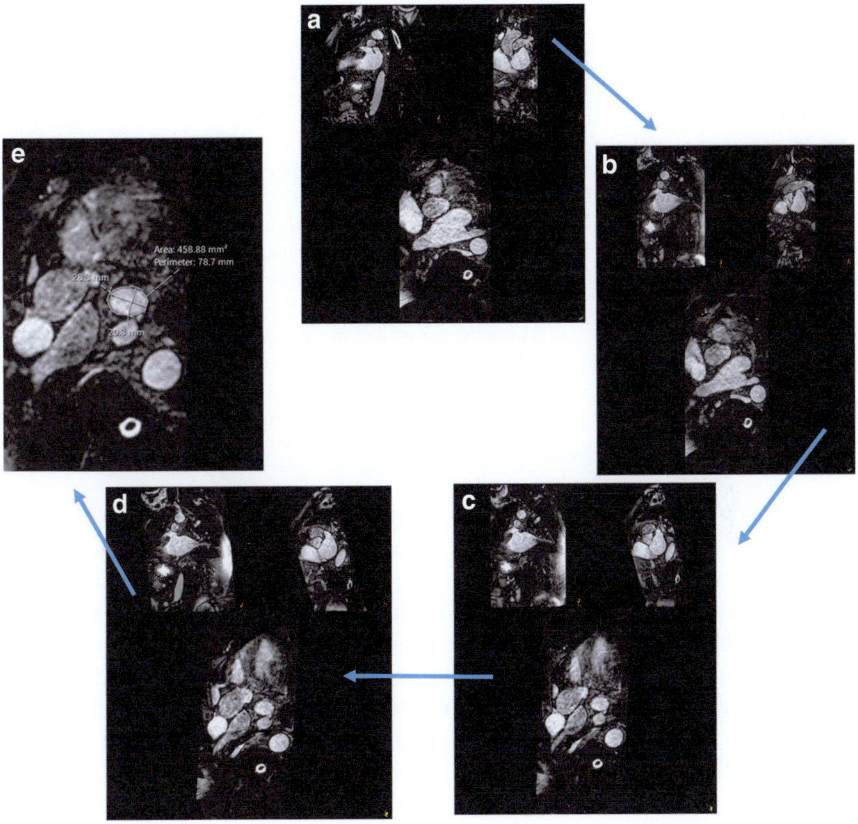

Fig. 6.7 Initial evaluation begins with a 3D dataset that can be acquired with or without intravenous contrast (**a**). The left atrioventricular groove should first be identified. Sometimes, this can be easily identified by locating the left circumflex coronary artery, though this may not always be seen on non-contrast MRI sequences if the vessel is small in caliber. The axial imaging plane should be aligned along the axis of the left atrioventricular groove. Next, the oblique sagittal (formerly the true sagittal) images should clearly show the left atrial appendage (**b**). The oblique sagittal image should then align the crosshairs between the left atrioventricular groove (most easily identified by the left circumflex coronary artery) and the Coumadin ridge. At this point, the double-oblique axial image should show the left atrial appendage orifice (**c**). Minor corrections may be needed by aligning the double-oblique coronal image with the plane of the left atrial appendage orifice (**d**). Once the imaging planes have been established, measurements of the LAA can commence (**e**)

Clinical Evidence for CMR in LAAO Pre-procedural Planning

Existing literature suggests that procedural imaging prior to LAAO is associated with increased likelihood of successful implantation. While the existing body of literature on the use of CMR in LAAO pre-procedural planning remains sparse, the available data shows promising potential. According to 1 small pilot study of

Table 6.4 Imaging modalities for the assessment of the left atrial appendage

	CT	TEE	CMR
Successful prediction of device size	75.7–97.2%	51.4–64%	80%
Pros	Fast Excellent spatial resolution	Portable and can be performed during the LAAO procedure Allows for assessment of real-time physiology	Excellent tissue contrast and characterization Ability to image in any desired plane Excellent temporal resolution
Cons	Ionizing radiation Need for iodinated contrast	Limited assessment in patients with poor acoustic windows Need for sedation	Long acquisition times Susceptible to numerous artifacts and potentially contraindicated in patients with certain devices

13 patients which investigated the use of non-contrast CMR for LAAO planning, the shape of the LAA and the landing zone can accurately be determined for the assessment of the dimensions required for device selection. In this small study, the CMR assessment of the LAA was compared directly to fluoroscopically derived measurements. This study also showed that CMR can reasonably predict the optimal angulation for the C-arm during the procedure which has the potential to streamline LAAO and decrease radiation exposure to patients. Nonetheless, it highlighted constraints in device sizing due to the current limitations in the available sizing charts.

Another prospective single-center study demonstrated that pre-procedural planning with CMR had a success rate of 80% for predicting device size prior to LAAO. In this study, a 3-month follow-up CTA showed successful LAAO in 100% of the patients, clearly showing that pre-procedural planning with CMR is feasible. Table 6.4 provides a comparison of the different imaging modalities for LAA assessment with their respective strengths and limitations.

Another interesting study tested an MRI-based training model for LAAO, aiming to address patient-specific anatomical variability in transseptal puncture (TSP) site selection. Utilizing patient-specific MRI data, silicone models of LAAs were 3D-printed, allowing demonstration of TSP impact on LAA access. The model showcased the technical feasibility of occluder deployment and facilitated the practice of catheter handling even in nonoptimal puncture scenarios. This non-contrast MRI-derived model offers a means to evaluate TSP influence on patient-specific LAA shapes, aiding pre-procedural planning for LAA closure procedures, with potential implications for device sizing and initial TSP estimation. Finally, successful, noninvasive detection of left atrial appendage thrombus with CMR has also been clearly established with studies dating back more than 20 years.

MRI Limitations

Magnetic resonance imaging (MRI) is generally regarded as a ubiquitous and safe imaging modality. Despite its widespread availability in most parts of the United States, there are limitations and contraindications that may restrict its applicability in cardiac patients. The relatively limited availability of MR scanners in rural areas may preclude their routine use in pre-procedural planning in lieu of other available options like CTA or TEE. With regard to safety concerns, it should be remembered that the magnetic forces generated around an MRI scanner are many thousands of times greater than the earth's own magnetic field and that any ferromagnetic objects within range of the scanner can become high-speed ballistics without warning. Because of this, the magnetic forces involved can pose safety threats to patients and to technologists that work around them. Medical institutions equipped with MRI capabilities routinely employ patient safety protocols, including comprehensive checklists, completed before commencing any MRI examination in order to screen individuals for any potential contraindications, including implanted devices or surgical hardware. Individuals with implanted permanent cardiac devices such as pacemakers, implantable cardioverter defibrillators (ICDs), and cardiac resynchronization therapy defibrillators (CRTDs) necessitate the presence of a qualified technician or physician to program these devices into an "MRI safe" mode due to the induction of currents that can occur during exams and within the MRI scanner room itself. Many current devices are considered safe to scan under certain conditions that are set forth by the manufacturer, and these devices are termed MR conditional. Devices that are not listed as MR conditional can be scanned in extenuating clinical circumstances but require informed patient consent. Non-MRI compatible devices remain an absolute contraindication. In addition, the presence of multiple leads within the cardiac chambers as well as the device itself along the chest wall can result in extensive artifact formation on the final images which may limit evaluation in some cases. Furthermore, challenges such as obesity and claustrophobia can present additional barriers to undergoing MRI scans in this patient population. Finally, the time involved with image acquisition for MRI exams is greater than that for CTA and requires the cooperation of patients to coordinate breath holds and remain relatively still during the exam.

Future Directions for MR Imaging

As MRI scanners increase in number over time and reach relatively underserved areas, it is likely that they will be increasingly used for pre-procedural planning, particularly in subsets of patients for whom TEE or CTA is difficult or contraindicated. Imaging protocols and improved image acquisition techniques can continue to be optimized and result in decreasing exam times. Finally, as artificial intelligence algorithms proliferate, their use in CMR may be further expanded through which operator and reporting physician efficiency can be increased.

Conclusions

CMR pre-procedural planning is an effective strategy for LAAC which allows for accurate device sizing and avoidance of unwanted complications. 3D MR acquisition techniques are able to provide spatial resolution approaching that of CTA, and long inversion time sequences are very effective at excluding thrombi within the LAA. The unique anatomic shape and ostium of the LAA can be accurately assessed which allows for the selection of not only the best device type but also the best implantation strategy based on each patient's anatomy. Much like CTA, workstation software may help the operator to navigate through the procedure for adequate transseptal puncture prediction and the best deployment angle into the LAA, as well as potential pitfalls and complications depending on each patient. As CMR becomes more widely available, streamlined protocols become the standard, and the potential role of artificial intelligence in future versions of planning software is investigated further, the effectiveness of this tool in preprocedural planning can be optimized for effective, safe, and efficient patient care.

References and Suggested Readings

1. Doherty J, Kort S, Mehran R, et al. ACC/AATS/AHA/ASE/ASNC/HRS/SCAI/SCCT/SCMR/STS 2019 appropriate use criteria for multimodality imaging in the assessment of cardiac structure and function in Nonvalvular heart disease: a report of the American College of Cardiology Appropriate use Criteria Task Force, American Association for Thoracic Surgery, American Heart Association, American Society of Echocardiography, American Society of Nuclear Cardiology, Heart Rhythm Society, Society for Cardiovascular Angiography and Interventions, Society of Cardiovascular Computed Tomography, Society for Cardiovascular Magnetic Resonance, and the Society of Thoracic Surgeons. J Am Coll Cardiol. 2019;73(4):488–516. https://doi.org/10.1016/j.jacc.2018.10.038.
2. Clarke J, Higgins A, Wang Y, et al. Impact of preprocedure imaging for left atrial appendage occlusion: insights from the NCDR LAAO registry. J Am Coll Cardiol Intv. 2023;16(11):1317–28. https://doi.org/10.1016/j.jcin.2023.05.008.
3. Kitkungvan D, Nabi F, Ghosn MG, Dave AS, Quinones M, Zoghbi WA, Valderrabano M, Shah DJ. Detection of LA and LAA thrombus by CMR in patients referred for pulmonary vein isolation. J Am Coll Cardiol. 2016;9(7):809–18. https://doi.org/10.1016/j.jcmg.2015.11.029.
4. Bertsche D, Metze P, Luo E, Dahme T, Gonska B, Rottbauer W, Vernikouskaya I, Rasche V, Schneider LM. Cardiac magnetic resonance imaging for preprocedural planning of percutaneous left atrial appendage closure. Front Cardiovasc Med. 2023;10:1132626. https://doi.org/10.3389/fcvm.2023.1132626.
5. Bertsche D, Reinelt A, Metze P, Rasche V, Dahme T, Schneider L-M, et al. MRI-based 3D silicone model for left atrial appendage occluder device size determination. Int J CARS. 2022;17(Suppl 1):73–4. https://doi.org/10.1007/s11548-022-02635-x.

6. Ohyama H, et al. Comparison of magnetic resonance imaging and transesophageal echocardiography in detection of thrombus in the left atrial appendage. Stroke. 2003;10(34):2436–9. https://doi.org/10.1161/01.STR.0000090350.73614.0F.
7. Lopez-Minguez JR, Gonzalez-Fernandez R, Fernandez-Vegas C, et al. Comparison of imaging techniques to assess appendage anatomy and measurements for left atrial appendage closure device selection. J Invasive Cardiol. 2014;26:462–7.
8. Filby SJ, Dallan LAP, Cochet A, et al. Left atrial appendage occlusion using cardiac CT angiography and Intracardiac echocardiography: a prospective, single-center study. J Invasive Cardiol. 2021;33(11):E851–6. PMID: 34619655
9. Dallan LAP, Reed J, Yoon SH, Janus S, Rajagopalan S, Rashid I, Al-Kindi S, Filby SJ. Novel cardiac magnetic resonance imaging-based sizing for left atrial appendage closure. J Cardiovasc Electrophysiol. 2022;33(12):2649–50. https://doi.org/10.1111/jce.15720.
10. Eng MH, Wang DD, Greenbaum AB, et al. Prospective, randomized comparison of 3-dimensional computed tomography guidance versus TEE data for left atrial appendage occlusion (PRO3DLAAO). Catheter Cardiovasc Interv. 2018;92(2):401–7. https://doi.org/10.1002/ccd.27514.
11. Chow DH, Bieliauskas G, Sawaya FJ, et al. A comparative study of different imaging modalities for successful percutaneous left atrial appendage closure. Open Heart. 2017;4:e000627. https://doi.org/10.1136/openhrt-2017-000627.

Part II
Procedural Approach

Chapter 7
Same-Day Discharge Following Left Atrial Appendage Closure

Jason Galo, Hamza A. Lodhi, Sojin Wass, Rafey Feroze, Luis Augusto Palma Dallan, and Steven J. Filby

Abbreviations

AF	Atrial fibrillation
ICE	Intracardiac echocardiography
LAA	Left atrial appendage
LAAC	Left atrial appendage closure
TEE	Transesophageal echocardiography
SDD	Same-day discharge

Highlights
- The safety and feasibility of same-day discharge post-left atrial appendage closure.
- Implementable algorithms have demonstrated success across multiple medical centers.
- Same-day discharge presents an opportunity for substantial cost savings.

Introduction

As the experience with left atrial appendage closure (LAAC) has grown, the overall safety profile of the procedure has significantly improved. The initial reported 7-day procedural-related complication rate was 8.7% in the PROTECT-AF trial,

J. Galo · H. A. Lodhi · S. Wass · R. Feroze · L. A. P. Dallan · S. J. Filby (✉)
Division of Cardiology, Harrington Heart & Vascular Institute, University Hospitals Cleveland Medical Center, Cleveland, OH, USA
e-mail: Jason.galo@uhhospitals.org; sojin.wass@uhhospitals.org; Rafey.feroze@uhhospitals.org; Luis.dallan@uhhospitals.org; steven.filby@uhhospitals.org

S. J. Filby et al. (eds.), *A Contemporary Manual of Left Atrial Appendage Closure*, https://doi.org/10.1007/978-3-031-68441-8_7

decreasing to 4.2% in the subsequent PREVAIL trial [1, 2]. The real-world EWOLUTION study further demonstrated this trend, reporting a 7-day procedure-related complication rate of 2.7%, less than half of the landmark PROTECT-AF trial [3]. The latest SURPASS study, focused exclusively on data from the new generation Watchman FLX device and involving a large patient sample, revealed a remarkably low procedure-related event rate of 0.22% at 7 days [4]. This evolution of LAAC procedures, showcased through trials and registry, underscores the remarkable advancements in safety. These findings illuminate the transformative journey and the unprecedented safety achievements with LAAC, offering promising prospects for patient care and treatment efficacy.

The feasibility and safety of same-day discharge (SDD) have been firmly established in percutaneous coronary interventions (PCI), even with a higher overall risk of complications compared to left atrial appendage closure (LAAC) [5]. LAAC procedures exhibit more predictability due to less heterogeneity compared to PCI, further supporting the feasibility of SDD. Moreover, evidence indicates improved patient satisfaction and cost savings associated with SDD after PCI. Similarly, SDD following atrial fibrillation ablation, a procedure involving the transseptal puncture technique like LAAC, has also been well established. The evidence supporting SDD across various procedures, such as PCI and atrial fibrillation ablation akin to LAAC, underscores its feasibility, safety, and potential for enhanced patient satisfaction and cost-effectiveness.

Upon reviewing data from various procedures, taking into account patient satisfaction and cost considerations, it becomes logical to consider same-day discharge (SDD) strategies after left atrial appendage closure (LAAC). Notably, a study by Ponce et al., utilizing the Vizient Clinical Database, demonstrated a noteworthy trend, with the percentage of SDD increasing from less than 4% in cases before 2020 to 25.9% in 2021 [6].

Ensuring the Safety and Feasibility of Same-Day Discharge (SDD) Following Left Atrial Appendage Closure (LAAC)

Numerous studies conducted thus far have assessed the safety and feasibility of same-day discharge (SDD) after left atrial appendage closure (LAAC) (Table 7.1). In an early exploration of SDD after LAAC, William et al. shared their findings in 2018 from the United Kingdom [7]. Conducting a small retrospective study over a decade with 117 patients, they demonstrated successful SDD in 67% of cases. The primary devices used were ACP (St. Jude Medical, Minneapolis, MN) and Amulet (Abbott Laboratories, USA), with a complication rate during the procedure of less than 5%. In 2020, Gilhofer et al. reported a satisfying SDD experience involving 24 patients who underwent procedures using Watchman (Boston Scientific, MN) and Amulet (Abbott Laboratories, USA) [8]. Similarly, Marmagkiolis et al. detailed the safe SDD experiences of 112 US patients post-LAAC employing Watchman (Boston

Table 7.1 Comprehensive overview of seven studies on percutaneous left atrial appendage closure (LAAC)

First Author (Location) (Year)	Enrollment Period for SDD	Anesthesia Approach and Type of Imaging	Number of SDD Patients and Average Age	Control Group and Average Age	LAAO Device in SDD Patients	Major Outcomes
Williams et al. (United Kingdom) (2018)	2007–2016	Most cases: GA with TEE	$N = 117$, 75.6 (55–90) ±	None	ACP, $n = 59$; amulet, $n = 48$; Wavecrest, $n = 7$; Watchman, $n = 3$	Low complication rates (less than 5%) necessitating inpatient admission.
		Rarely: GA with ICE				
Gilhofer et al. (Vancouver general hospital, Canada) (2020)	2018–2019	GA and TEE, 87.5%; MS and ICE 12.5%	$N = 24$, 76.6 ± 7.5	None	Amulet, $n = 12$; Watchman $n = 12$	No clinical complications observed at 1 month or during long-term follow-up.
Marmagkliolis et al. (MD Anderson cancer, USA) (2021)	2016–2019	MS and TEE, 100%	$N = 112$, 73.5 ± 4.5	None	Watchman, $n = 112$	No complications during the procedure or POD1
Tan et al. (Brigham and Women's hospital, USA) (2021)	2016–2019	GA and TEE, 100%	$N = 72$, 75.7 ± 7.8	Non-SDD, 75.9 ± 8.6	Watchman, $n = 72$	Composite outcome[a]: SDD vs. non-SDD
						No significant differences at 7 and 45 days post-procedure.

(continued)

Table 7.1 (continued)

First Author (Location) (Year)	Enrollment Period for SDD	Anesthesia Approach and Type of Imaging	Number of SDD Patients and Average Age	Control Group and Average Age	LAAO Device in SDD Patients	Major Outcomes
Dallan et al. (Cleveland medical center, USA) (2022)	6/2020–12/2020	MS and ICE, 100%	$N = 23$, 74.4 ± 8.6	Non-SDD, TEE and GA, $n = 119$, 76.5 ± 8.4	Watchman 2.5, $n = 8$, Watchman FLX, $n = 15$	Procedural complications or in-hospital adverse events: SDD vs non-SDD: No significant differences at 7 days and 45 days post procedure
Piayda et al. (amulet observational postmarket study) (2021)	2015–2016	TEE, 98% ICE, 2% (anesthesia unknown)	$N = 60$, 77 ± 7	Next-day discharge (NDD), $n = 526$, 75 ± 8	Amulet, $n = 60$	Among those eligible for SDD, numerically lower rates of serious adverse events.
Gibson et al. (SURPASS of the NCDR LAAO registry)	2020–2021	N/A	$N = 3167$, 75.6	Non-SDD, $n = 13{,}266$, 76.2	Watchman FLX, $n = 3167$	SDD vs. non-SDD major adverse events: 2.78% vs. 5.22% ($P < 0.01$)
						Pericardial effusion requiring intervention: 0.04% vs. 0.64% ($P < 0.01$)
						Major bleeding: 2.00 vs, 3.9%, ($P < 0.01$).

[a]Composite of stroke, systemic embolism, major bleeding requiring transfusion, vascular complications requiring endovascular intervention, or death through 7 days (periprocedural) and 45 days post-procedure

Scientific, MN) [9]. Procedures in these studies were predominantly performed under transesophageal echocardiography (TEE). Most patients in the studies by William et al. and Gilhofer et al. received general anesthesia, while 100% of those discharged on the SDD protocol in Marmagkiolis et al.'s study received moderate sedation. It is important to note that all three studies were single-arm and lacked any comparator group.

Subsequently, as the interest in same-day discharge (SDD) after left atrial appendage closure (LAAC) grew, especially during the COVID-19 pandemic, additional studies with more comprehensive comparative data emerged. Tan et al. presented data from 190 patients who underwent TEE-guided LAAC with the Watchman device (118 conventional, 72 SDD) [10]. The study revealed no substantial differences in baseline and procedural characteristics between the two groups, and the 45-day event rate was comparable. Similarly, Dallan et al. published observational data from 142 patients undergoing ICE-guided LAAC with the Watchman device (119 conventional, 23 SDD), demonstrating no significant distinctions in baseline characteristics, procedural complications, or clinical events at 45 days between the conventional and SDD groups [11]. Notably, eligible candidates for SDD exhibited significantly shorter procedure durations. The same group later reinforced the safety of SDD at 1 year, establishing the broader and reliable application of this strategy [12]. Piayda et al. conducted an observational postmarket study on Amulet (Abbott Laboratories, USA), encompassing 60 patients who underwent SDD. Among those eligible for SDD, there were numerically lower rates of serious adverse events [13]. Additionally, Gibson et al. examined 3168 patients who received the Watchman FLX, finding that individuals eligible for SDD were significantly less prone to major adverse events, particularly major bleeding [14].

Kawamura et al. conducted a propensity score-matched analysis using the US Nationwide Readmission Database, including 961 matched pairs in each group, and showed no difference in 30 days readmission between the conventional and SDD [15]. Lastly, Khan et al. conducted a meta-analysis on seven observational studies, indicating no variance in safety outcomes and post-discharge complications between patients with SDD and those with a conventional hospital overnight stay after LAAC [16]. The expanding array of studies, including comprehensive analyses and meta-analyses, consistently support the safety and viability of SDD following LAAC, making a significant paradigm shift in post-procedural care with comparable outcomes to conventional hospital stays.

Traditionally, left atrial appendage closure (LAAC) procedures have been conducted under general anesthesia with transesophageal echocardiography (TEE), necessitating extended recovery periods. In recent times, there has been a growing trend toward utilizing intracardiac echocardiography (ICE) for LAAC, performed under conscious sedation, leading to faster recovery times. Nevertheless, the feasibility of same-day discharge (SDD) has been established irrespective of the imaging modality employed.

Implementation of Same-Day Discharge

Several factors significantly influence the feasibility and success of same-day discharge (SDD) protocols following LAAC (Table 7.2). Those who experience an acute cardiovascular condition, such as myocardial infarction (AMI), stroke, or acute decompensated heart failure (HF), may necessitate extended observation due to heightened post-procedural risks. The ability to execute a full 6-h observation before an appropriate discharge time plays a pivotal role, as it ensures sufficient monitoring to gauge post-procedural stability or recovery. Moreover, the absence of familial or caregiver-based social support post-discharge with SDD becomes a crucial consideration, impacting the patient's safety and well-being during the critical early phase after treatment. Additionally, the comfort level of the patient or their family with SDD significantly influences the decision-making process, as their confidence and acceptance of this discharge strategy are paramount for successful implementation. These factors collectively underscore the complexity involved in adopting SDD protocols for individuals post-LAAC, necessitating through assessment and tailored approaches to ensure patient safety and optimal outcomes.

Different studies examining the feasibility of SDD have revealed various factors impacting the viability of SDD. For example, Dallan et al. emphasized certain challenges, such as difficulties in obtaining post-implant TTE (transthoracic echocardiography) in the late afternoon [11]. This issue is often attributed to the limited availability of echo sonographers beyond standard business hours. To mitigate the risk of heightened device recaptures that could potentially lead to perforation, certain institutions have devised protocols. These protocols involve overnight observation for patients who exceed a specified number of recaptures. Consequently, these

Table 7.2 Barriers to same-day discharge

Difficulties in obtaining post-implant TTE in the late afternoon
Access site complications
Pericardial effusion requiring further intervention
Acute cardiovascular condition (e.g., AMI, stroke, acute decompensated HF)
The incapacity to undergo a complete 6-h observation before a suitable discharge time
Absence of familial or caregiver-based social support following discharge with SDD
Patient or family are not comfortable with SDD

AMI acute myocardial infarction, *HF* heart failure, *TTE* transthoracic echocardiogram, *SDD* same day discharge individuals become ineligible for same-day discharge. Similarly, Tan et al. identified ineligible cases due to minor access site complications or procedural complexities like pericardial effusion requiring further intervention [10]. Wass et al.'s comprehensive analysis underscored that shorter needle-to-device deployment correlated significantly with eligibility for SDD [12]. In essence, these studies collectively emphasize the multifaceted nature of barriers and indicators influencing the feasibility of SDD in LAAC procedures.

To enable safe SDD for patients following left atrial appendage closure (LAAC), the implementation of standardized institutional protocols is paramount. Several institutions have shared their experiences with these protocols, showcasing their practical application and safety. In a notable study, Dallan et al. successfully implemented their protocol in 225 patients, presenting one of the most streamlined algorithms to date. All these protocols generally adhere to similar principles, including:

1. Uncomplicated vascular access with successful closure.
2. Uncomplicated device deployment with a predefined limit on recapture attempts.
3. Device stability and the absence of pericardial effusion.
4. Adequate patient recovery from sedation and the ability to ambulate.
5. Availability of overnight caregivers and transport.

A proposed algorithm to guide the decision-making process for SDD is outlined below (Fig. 7.1).

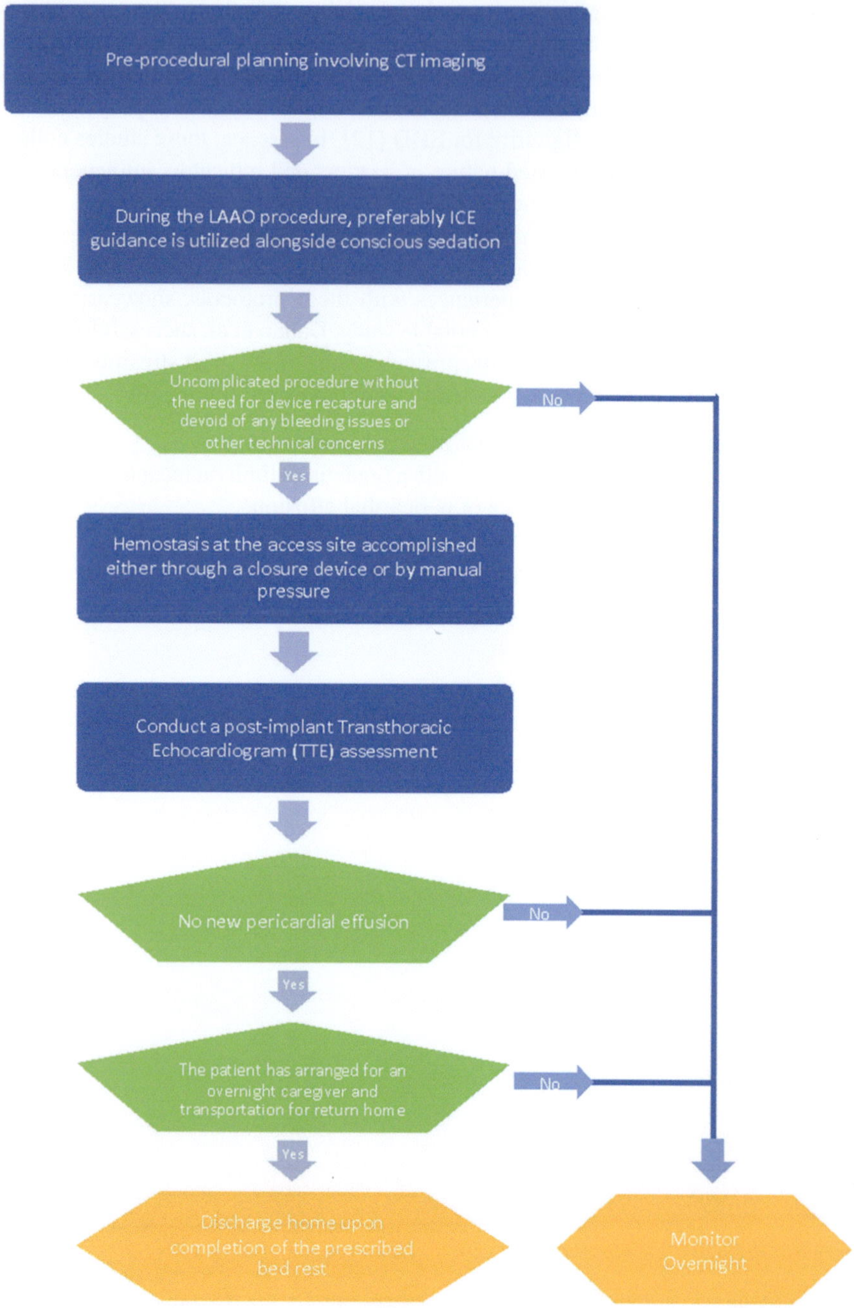

Fig. 7.1 Same-day discharge protocol algorithm

Examining the Advantages and Disadvantages of Same-Day Discharge (SDD)

Implementing same-day discharge (SDD) protocols following left atrial appendage closure (LAAC) procedures offers several potential advantages. Patients discharged on the same day as the procedure experience reduced hospital stays, leading to potential cost savings and efficient utilization of healthcare resources. Moreover, returning home on the day of the procedure can enhance patient comfort, potentially contributing to improved psychological well-being and faster recovery. SDD also reduces the risk of hospital-acquired infections and allows patients to resume their daily activities sooner than if they remained hospitalized. Additionally, this approach aligns with patient-centered care, providing personalized options and flexibility in managing post-procedure recovery. These advantages underscore the potential benefits of same-day discharge strategies after LAAC, emphasizing patient-centric care, cost-effectiveness, and efficient resource utilization within healthcare systems.

SDD protocols post-LAAC procedures offers numerous benefits but also presents potential drawbacks. Patients discharged on the same day as the procedure might face increased risks of complications or adverse events without the continuous observation provided by a longer hospital stay. Additionally, some individuals might require extended monitoring and recovery time, particularly those with pre-existing health conditions or complications during the procedure. Lack of a strong support system or access to post-discharge care could also pose challenges, impacting recovery and follow-up. Furthermore, patient discomfort or unease with quick discharge, resource limitations in healthcare facilities, and insurance coverage constraints might hinder the successful implementation of SDD protocols. These potential disadvantages highlight the importance of thorough patient assessment, robust post-discharge plans, and adequate resources to ensure the safety and effectiveness of same-day discharge strategies after LAAC.

Examining the Cost-Effectiveness of Same-Day Discharge (SDD)

One additional advantage of the same-day discharge (SDD) strategy is the potential for cost savings. The traditional approach of an overnight stay involves the occupancy of a telemetry bed, additional laboratory tests, and chest X-rays the next day, all adding to the overall procedure cost. Variations in costs may also arise depending on whether transesophageal echocardiography (TEE) or intracardiac echocardiography (ICE) guidance is utilized during the procedure, as the former requires the involvement of anesthesia team and the latter requires a single-use imaging catheter.

Dallan et al. ($n = 142$), in their single-center study, demonstrated a 15% reduction in costs with SDD compared to the conventional strategy, where ICE guidance was employed in both groups. Tan et al. ($n = 211$), drawing from data at their single

Table 7.3 Pros and cons of same-day discharge compared to conventional discharge

Pros	Cons
Increased earlier stage mobilization	Post procedural risks
Increased patient satisfaction	Lack of observation
Decreased resource utilization and cost	Inadequate recovery
Decreased hospital-based complications	Need for caregiver support
Lower risk of hospital-acquired infections	Patient comfort
Quicker return to daily activities	Resource allocation

center, reported $2500 in cost savings with SDD using TEE guidance for left atrial appendage closure (LAAC). Zahid et al. (n = 54,880), utilizing the national readmission database (2015–2019), reported cost savings of $4116 with SDD; similar findings were shown by Kawamura et al., using propensity score-matched analysis using the same cohort (n = 1922), where SDD showed $2157 in cost savings with SDD [11, 15]. Please consult Table 7.3 for a comprehensive list outlining the pros and cons of same-day discharge compared to conventional discharge.

Conclusion

Same-day discharge (SDD) following left atrial appendage closure (LAAC) is not only feasible and safe but also proves to be a cost-effective approach. Various centers have demonstrated easily implementable protocols to achieve safe SDD after LAAC. Similar to various other cardiac procedures, SDD can be employed as the preferred method of post-procedure disposition for most patients undergoing LAAC.

References

1. Reddy VY, et al. Percutaneous left atrial appendage closure vs warfarin for atrial fibrillation: a randomized clinical trial. JAMA. 2014;312(19):1988–98.
2. Holmes DR Jr, et al. Prospective randomized evaluation of the Watchman left atrial appendage closure device in patients with atrial fibrillation versus long-term warfarin therapy: the PREVAIL trial. J Am Coll Cardiol. 2014;64(1):1–12.
3. Boersma LV, et al. Implant success and safety of left atrial appendage closure with the WATCHMAN device: peri-procedural outcomes from the EWOLUTION registry. Eur Heart J. 2016;37(31):2465–74.
4. Watchman. *SURPASS early results*. 2022 [cited 2023; Available from: https://www.watchman.com/en-us-hcp/clinical-evidence/surpass.html.
5. Krishnaswamy A, et al. Same-day discharge after elective percutaneous transcatheter cardiovascular interventions. JACC Cardiovasc Interv. 2023;16(13):1561–78.
6. Ponce AC, et al. Contemporary trends in same-day versus deferred discharge after left atrial appendage occlusion. JACC Adv. 2023;2(2):100261.
7. Williams T, et al. Day-case percutaneous left atrial appendage occlusion-safety and efficacy. Catheter Cardiovasc Interv. 2018;92(7):1439–43.

8. Gilhofer TS, et al. Safety and feasibility of same-day discharge after left atrial appendage closure. Can J Cardiol. 2020;36(6):945–7.
9. Marmagkiolis K, et al. Effectiveness and safety of same day discharge after left atrial appendage closure under moderate conscious sedation. Catheter Cardiovasc Interv. 2021;97(5):912–6.
10. Tan BE, et al. Safety and feasibility of same-day discharge after left atrial appendage closure with the WATCHMAN device. Circ Cardiovasc Interv. 2021;14(1):e009669.
11. Dallan LAP, et al. Safety, efficacy, and cost-effectiveness of same-day discharge for left atrial appendage occlusion. J Invasive Cardiol. 2022;34(2):E124–31.
12. Wass SY, et al. Predictors of successful same-day discharge and 1-year outcomes after left atrial appendage closure. Catheter Cardiovasc Interv. 2022;100(7):1307–13.
13. Piayda K, et al. Clinical outcomes of patients undergoing percutaneous left atrial appendage occlusion in general anaesthesia or conscious sedation: data from the prospective global Amplatzer Amulet Occluder observational study. BMJ Open. 2021;11(3):e040455.
14. Gibson DN, et al. PO-656-04 safety and effectiveness of same day discharge after left atrial appendage occlusion with Watchman FLX. Heart Rhythm. 2022;19(5):S268.
15. Kawamura I, et al. Thirty-day readmission rate of same-day discharge protocol after left atrial appendage occlusion: a propensity score-matched analysis from the National Readmission Database. Heart Rhythm. 2022;19(11):1819–25.
16. Khan JA, et al. Same-day discharge for left atrial appendage occlusion procedure: a systematic review and meta-analysis. J Cardiovasc Electrophysiol. 2023;34(5):1196–205.

Chapter 8
Transseptal Puncture: Best Practice and Techniques

Ram Amuthan, Samer A. H. De Oliveira, and Mauricio Arruda

Highlights

- Transseptal puncture technique has been adapted for a variety of procedures including atrial fibrillation catheter ablation (Class Ia) and left atrial appendage occlusion (LAAO Class IIa) ACC/AHA/HRS atrial fibrillation guidelines. Also for mitral valve interventions.
- Understanding the anatomy of the interatrial septum (IAS).
- Real-time echocardiography imaging (TEE, ICE), transseptal needles, wires, and sheaths are key factors in the safety and effectiveness of the procedure.
- Prompt identification and management of complications during TSP.

Introduction

Transseptal left atrial puncture (TSP) was originally described in the late 1950s. It was developed at the National Institutes of Health by Dr. Ross as a new technique for the measurement of left atrial pressure [1]. Since then, the technique has been adapted for a variety of procedures, including atrial fibrillation ablation, mitral valve interventions, and left atrial appendage (LAA) closure. In this chapter we aim to review the techniques and the tools available to achieve a safe and effective TSP in the context of the deployment of left atrial appendage occlusion (LAAO) devices. We will also describe our approach to TSP, including the management of challenging transseptal access and periprocedural complications.

R. Amuthan · S. A. H. De Oliveira (✉) · M. Arruda
Division of Cardiology, Harrington Heart & Vascular Institute, University Hospitals Cleveland Medical Center, Cleveland, OH, USA
e-mail: Ram.amuthan@uhhospitals.org; Samer.deoliveira@uhhospitals.org; mauricio.arruda@uhhospitals.org

S. J. Filby et al. (eds.), *A Contemporary Manual of Left Atrial Appendage Closure*, https://doi.org/10.1007/978-3-031-68441-8_8

Interatrial Septum Anatomy

The interatrial septum (IAS) is a fibromuscular structure separating the right and the left atrium. Understanding the anatomy of the IAS is crucial to avoid complications during TSP. The IAS is an extensive structure bound superiorly and inferiorly by the caval orifices, anteroinferiorly by the coronary sinus orifice, anterosuperiorly by the aortic noncoronary sinus, and anteriorly by the tricuspid valve leaflet. The fossa ovalis (FO) is an oval depression on the infero-posterior part of the IAS. It is the embryonic septum primum and covers only 20% of the IAS [2]. It is often referred to as the true IAS by anatomists and is the primary target for a safe TSP. Puncture of the FO allows for direct communication between the two atria without impinging on the adjacent epicardial structures. Figure 8.1 illustrates the anatomical boundaries of the FO and its relationship with the surrounding structures. Several anatomic variants of the FO have been described. The operator should thus spend time understanding the anatomy of the FO prior to attempting TSP.

Anatomic Considerations with LAAO Devices

The goal is to achieve a TSP that coaxially orients the access sheath to the LAA. The LAA is usually anteriorly and superiorly oriented. Thus, a posterior TSP on the FO provides the most favorable sheath orientation to the LAA. The height of the TSP depends on the LAAO device deployed. An inferior TSP has been suggested for the WATCHMAN™ device and the Amplatzer cardiac plug, while a superior location has been suggested for the Lariat procedure. However, significant variation exists in the anatomy and orientation of the LAA, which should be considered prior to TSP.

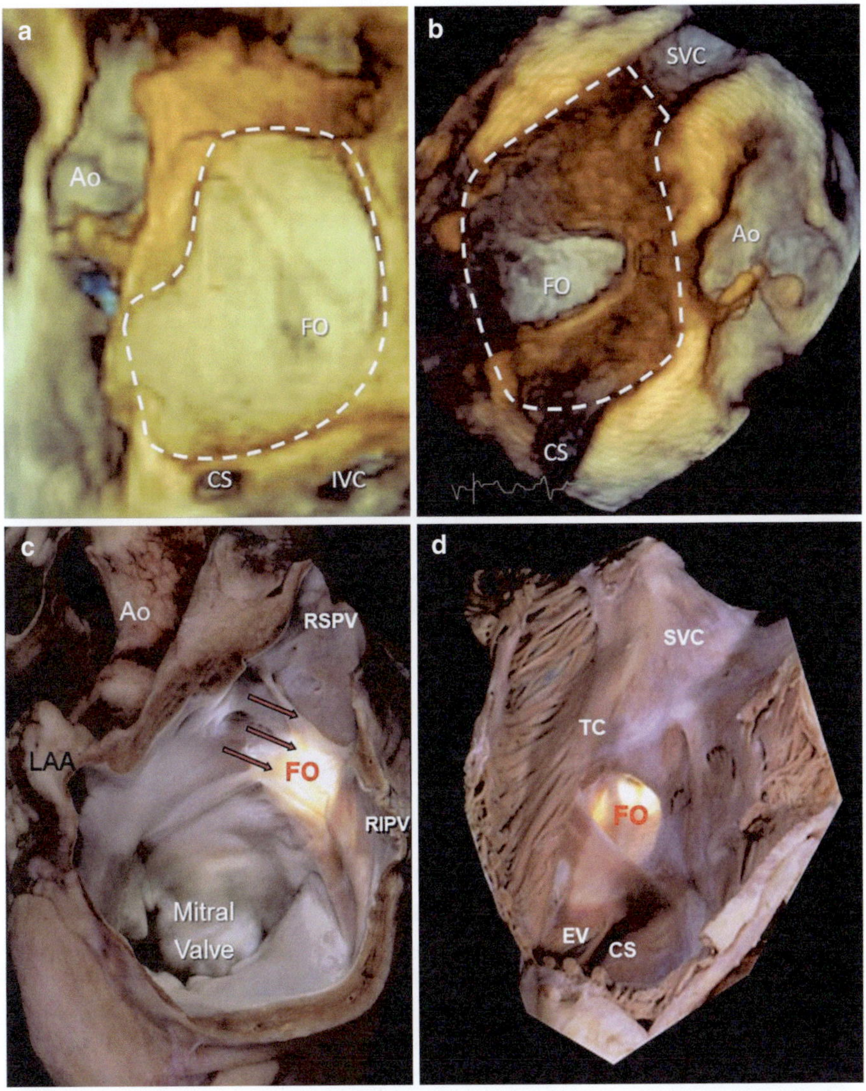

Fig. 8.1 Three-dimensional transesophageal echo showing the extensive surface (dotted line) corresponding to the medial wall of both atria seen from the left (**a**) and right (**b**) atrial perspective. (**c**, **d**) Anatomic specimens displayed in similar orientation to show the fossa ovalis transilluminated. *Ao* aorta, *CS* coronary sinus, *EV* Eustachian valve, *LAA* left atrial appendage, *RIPV* right inferior pulmonary vein, *RSPV* right superior pulmonary vein, *SVC* superior vena cava, *TC* terminal crest. Reproduced with permission from Francesco F. Faletra et al.: Revisiting Anatomy of the Interatrial Septum and its Adjoining Atrioventricular Junction

Imaging Guidance

Real-time imaging is required for a safe TSP. Fluoroscopy and echocardiography are the available imaging modalities to aid in obtaining transseptal access. Though a TSP can be performed with just fluoroscopy, echocardiography has the advantage of direct visualization of critical structures and is thus considered safer.

Several fluoroscopic techniques have been described. The placement of catheters in the coronary sinus and bundle of His helps define the anatomic landmarks of the IAS, and a pigtail catheter in the aortic root is useful to mark the position of the aorta. Left anterior oblique fluoroscopy when the transseptal assembly is dragged down from the superior vena cava to the right atrium is helpful to identify the characteristic "jumps." Two distinct jumps have been described. The first is when the assembly passes from the superior vena cava to the right atrium, and the second is when the assembly passes over the limbus of the IAS to the FO.

Both transesophageal echocardiography (TEE) and intracardiac echocardiography (ICE) can be utilized for imaging guidance. TEE, however, requires general anesthesia and a second operator. Phased array and radial transducer ICE are available. Phased array technology is widely utilized and has the advantage of better imaging of far-field structures and maneuverability which allows visualization of structures from multiple views.

Transseptal Puncture Toolkit

Depending on the LAAO device to be deployed, a 9–14 Fr transseptal access is required. A successful TSP requires a transseptal needle and a sheath to gain left atrial access. The Brockenbrough needle and the BRK series needles are used to mechanically puncture the FO. Even though there is vast clinical experience with these needles, they require mechanical pressure that, in rare cases, can lead to catastrophic complications. To avoid the use of excessive force and to navigate challenging atrial septal anatomy, radiofrequency (RF)- and laser-powered needles have been developed. The RF needle (NRG® Transseptal Needle, Boston Scientific, USA) has been shown to be effective in clinical situations where the conventional needle has failed including fibrotic and aneurysmal IAS and both synthetic and pericardial atrial septal patches. The laser-powered needle is currently not in clinical use. Currently available transseptal sheaths either have a fixed curve or are steerable. Though steerable sheaths have better outcomes in atrial fibrillation ablation, fixed curve sheaths are sufficient to gain initial transseptal access for LAAO procedures.

Guidewire-Based Transseptal Tools

The general principle underlying these tools is that once transseptal access is obtained, the guidewires assume an atraumatic shape that can be cushioned against the left atrial wall. The wires can then be safely used as rails for the insertion of

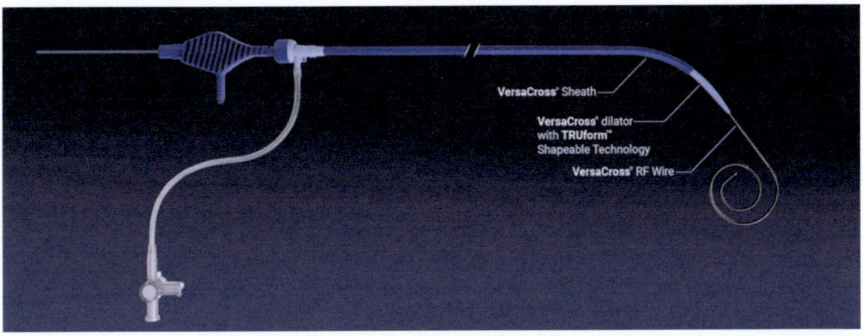

Fig. 8.2 VersaCross™ transseptal access solution which includes a RF wire and an access sheath eliminating exchanges and facilitating quick access to delivery of the WATCHMAN™ device

large-bore transseptal access sheaths. The guidewires have been incorporated with both mechanical puncture needles (SafeSept transseptal device, Pressure Products, USA) and RF needles (VersaCross™ RF Transseptal Solution, Boston Scientific, USA). The SafeSept system incorporates a 0.014-inch nitinol coated guidewire which assumes a J shape after the tip perforates the IAS and a fixed curve sheath. The VersaCross system incorporates a 0.035-inch J-tip or pigtail RF wire and a fixed curve or a steerable sheath. The wires then maintain reliable left atrial access for the delivery of transseptal sheaths, thereby reducing the risk of perforation.

Integrated Tools

The VersaCross Connect™ access solution connects the VersaCross® technology with the WATCHMAN™ sheaths for zero-exchange left-heart access and deployment of the LAAO device (Fig. 8.2). After RF transseptal puncture, the 0.035-inch guidewire is then used to deliver the 12 French WATCHMAN FXD Curve™ sheath without the need for exchanges. This system improves procedural efficiency with shorter procedural times and potentially also reduces the risk of air embolism and perforation by decreasing the number of exchanges.

Our Approach

Under fluoroscopic and ultrasound guidance, we obtain two right femoral venous access via 8.5 French sheaths. Left femoral venous access may also be obtained if the right femoral venous anatomy is unsuitable. The ICE catheter is then advanced to the right atrium and is maneuvered until the "home view" is visualized. The IAS and its relationship to the surrounding structures are noted. The ICE is advanced into the right ventricle to visualize the pericardial space, searching for evidence of a preexisting pericardial effusion. This is carefully evaluated in multiple views.

The next step is to advance the transseptal system through the other 8.5 French access site. We use the VersaCross™ transseptal access solution, which includes the 63-cm, 45-degree transseptal sheath with a 67-cm standard curve D0 dilator and the 0.035-inch, 180-cm pigtail RF wire. A 0.035-inch, 180-cm J-tip wire is advanced to the superior vena cava. Over the wire, the transseptal sheath and dilator are advanced into the superior vena cava. Depending on the anatomy of the right atrium as evaluated by ICE, the dilator can be shaped to the desired curve outside the body. TRUform™ shapeable technology helps the dilator maintain the curve as it navigates the venous system. The J-tip wire is then exchanged for the RF wire, which is eventually positioned just proximal to the tip of the transseptal sheath and dilator assembly.

The assembly is then positioned in an appropriate position based on fluoroscopic and ICE guidance. Our preference is a posterior and inferior site on the FO for TSP. This allows for coaxial access to the LAA, making deployment easier. The tip of the RF wire is both radiopaque and echogenic, which helps with understanding the position of the assembly. Once the assembly is well seated in a suitable position on the FO, RF is delivered for 1 second with simultaneous advancement of the RF wire into the left atrium. The unsupported RF wire immediately assumes a pigtail shape with a flexible tip. This can be cushioned against the left atrial wall with a reduced risk of perforation during exchanges.

While maintaining left atrial access with the pigtail, we advance the dilator and the sheath into the left atrium. Using a rotational movement, we advance the assembly back and forth through the FO for an adequate size access to be able to eventually pass the WATCHMAN FXD™ Curve system. With the pigtail in the left atrium, the transseptal sheath and dilator are exchanged for the 15 French WATCHMAN FXD™ Curve system. The 0.035-inch wire provides a sturdy rail for the delivery of the device. Again, the access sheath and dilator are advanced back and forth through the FO. This is done to create enough space on the FO for the eventual advancement of the ICE catheter into the left atrium. The WATCHMAN sheath and dilator system is retracted back to the inferior vena cava with the pigtail maintaining left atrial access. Under fluoroscopic and ICE guidance, the ICE catheter is gently advanced through the same FO puncture site into the left atrium. Once the ICE catheter is positioned in the left atrium, the delivery sheath and dilator are readvanced into the left atrium. The wire and dilator are then removed with the delivery sheath left in place in the left atrium. Figure 8.3 shows our approach to transseptal access for the delivery of the WATCHMAN device. In Table 8.1 we list challenging scenarios with TSP and how to troubleshoot in such situations.

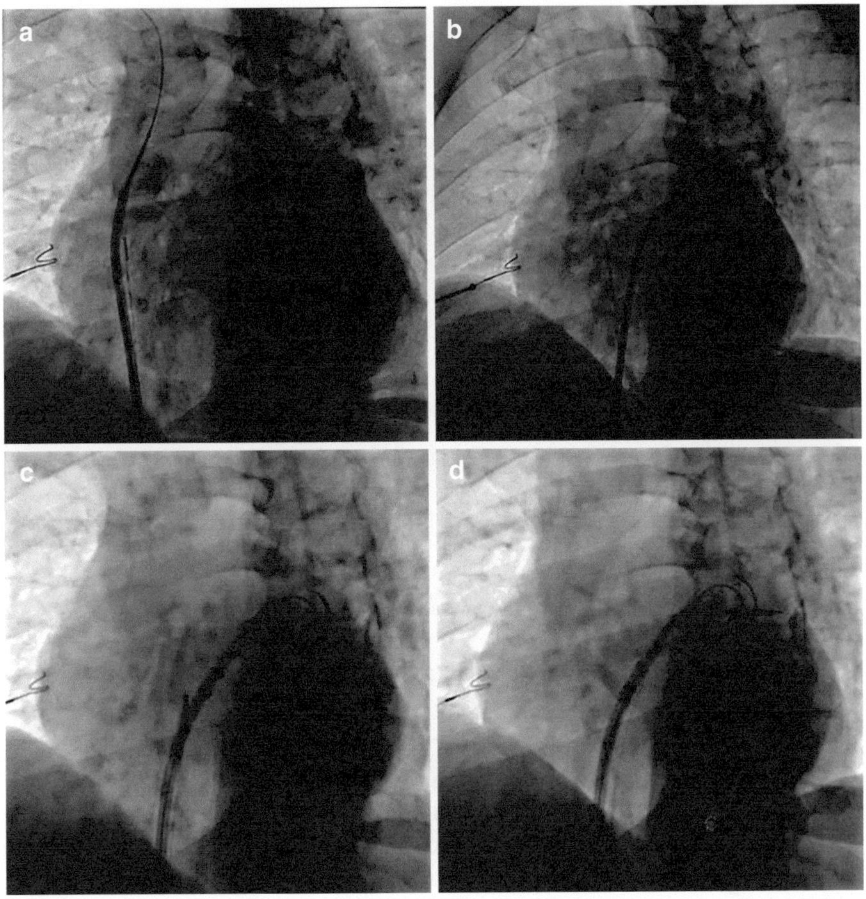

Fig. 8.3 Our approach to transseptal access for the delivery of the WATCHMAN device. (**a**) Over the wire, the transseptal sheath and dilator (VersaCross™ transseptal access) are advanced into the superior vena cava. (**b**) Radiofrequency puncture is performed with simultaneous advancement of the wire into the left atrium, which immediately assumes a pigtail shape with a flexible tip, over which the dilator and sheath are advanced. (**c**) The transseptal system is then exchanged for a 15 French WATCHMAN FXD™ Curve system which is then used to dilate the transseptal access site for eventual delivery of the ICE. (**d**) The ICE catheter is advanced into the left atrium, after which the WATCHMAN FXD™ system is readvanced back in the left atrium

Table 8.1 Problems encountered during transseptal puncture and suggested methods for troubleshooting

Challenging clinical scenarios	Potential solutions
Venous tortuosity	Long access sheaths, alternate venous access site
Inferior vena cava filters	Generally, does not preclude right atrial access
Occluded iliofemoral venous system	Consider transhepatic/internal jugular/subclavian venous access (limited experience confined to case reports and small series)
Difficult to engage fossa ovalis	Large curved transseptal needle and addition of secondary manual curves
Thick and calcified/ aneurysmal interatrial septum	Radiofrequency energy for transseptal access
Prior interatrial septal occluder	Puncture via neighboring native septal tissue Direct trans-occluder puncture is possible via pericardial or Dacron patch but not through Gore-Tex patch
Difficult to advance transseptal apparatus	Guidewire access to the left atrium to facilitate redirecting the apparatus in a safe manner Lower profile sheath-dilator combination (SR0, SL0, etc.) and stepwise dilation of the septum Balloon septostomy

Contraindications and Complications of Transseptal Puncture

The only absolute contraindication for TSP is the presence of a thrombus at the IAS. Relative contraindications include either a thrombus in the atrial cavity or a marked cardiac deformity [3]. The complications of LAAO device deployment are predominantly driven by complications during TSP. Therefore, it is important to promptly identify and appropriately manage complications during TSP. Contemporary registry data suggests an overall low complication rate with WATCHMAN devices of less than 2%, predominantly driven by pericardial effusion requiring intervention in 1.4% of patients [4]. Pericardial effusion and tamponade are generally due to inadvertent cardiac perforation during TSP. The clinical consequences of cardiac perforation depend on several peri-procedural factors including location and size of perforation, coagulation, and hemodynamic status. Prompt recognition, pericardiocentesis, and cardiothoracic surgical backup are the cornerstones of management. It is also reasonable to consider Amplatzer occluders in patients with aortic perforation, as some centers have reported successful closure without the need for open heart surgery.

The reported rates for clinically significant stroke from air or thromboembolism are <0.2% and relate to the presence of equipment in the left atrium. This can be prevented by achieving therapeutic anticoagulation prior to TSP and meticulous deairing of the system, respectively [5]. Iatrogenic atrial septal defects are detected in up to 87% of patients undergoing TSP for LAAO; however, most of them demonstrate left-to-right shunting and resolve within 45 days of the procedure. Rarely in patients with elevated right-sided filling pressures, the atrial septal defects may demonstrate right-to-left shunting, precipitating acute hypoxia. In such circumstances, emergent closure with atrial septal occluder devices may be considered [6].

Conclusion

Transseptal left atrial puncture was described over 60 years ago and has been adapted for a variety of procedures, including left atrial appendage (LAA) closure. Achieving safe transseptal access is crucial for the deployment of LAAO devices. Understanding the anatomy of the IAS combined with the effective use of the available transseptal tools, including echocardiography, various sheaths, and transseptal needles, is a key factor in the safety and effectiveness of LAAO with WATCHMAN devices. It is also important to be able to troubleshoot a challenging transseptal access (e.g., elastic, fibrosed, or aneurysmal septum) and promptly recognize and treat potential complications.

References

1. Ross J, Braunwald E, Morrow AG. Transseptal left atrial puncture: new technique for the measurement of left atrial pressure in man. Am J Cardiol [Internet]. 1959;3(5):653–5. Available from: https://www.sciencedirect.com/science/article/pii/0002914959903479.
2. Faletra FF, Leo LA, Paiocchi VL, Schlossbauer SA, Pedrazzini G, Moccetti T, et al. Revisiting anatomy of the interatrial septum and its adjoining atrioventricular junction using noninvasive imaging techniques. J Am Soc Echocardiogr [Internet]. 2019;32(5):580–92. Available from: https://www.sciencedirect.com/science/article/pii/S0894731719300094.
3. Alkhouli M, Rihal CS, Holmes DR. Transseptal techniques for emerging structural heart interventions. JACC Cardiovasc Interv [Internet]. 2016;9(24):2465–80. Available from: https://www.sciencedirect.com/science/article/pii/S1936879816319082.
4. Freeman JV, Varosy P, Price MJ, Slotwiner D, Kusumoto FM, Rammohan C, et al. The NCDR left atrial appendage occlusion registry. J Am Coll Cardiol [Internet]. 2020;75(13):1503–18. Available from: https://www.sciencedirect.com/science/article/pii/S0735109720300899.
5. Saw J, Holmes DR, Cavalcante JL, Freeman JV, Goldsweig AM, Kavinsky CJ, et al. SCAI/HRS expert consensus statement on transcatheter left atrial appendage closure. J Soc Cardiovasc Angiogr Interv [Internet]. 2023;2(3):100577. Available from: https://doi.org/10.1016/j.jscai.2022.100577.
6. Sunder V, Sabir S, Mark G, Kaddissi G, Peters P, Ragupathi L. Closure of iatrogenic atrial septal defect after placement of left atrial appendage closure device. JACC Case Rep [Internet]. 2022;4(16):1053–5. Available from: https://www.sciencedirect.com/science/article/pii/S266608492200482X.

Chapter 9
Echocardiographic Imaging Guidance for Left Atrial Appendage Closure: Transesophageal Echocardiography (TEE)

Piotr J. Horbal and Mahmoud Houmsse

Abbreviations

CT	Computed tomography
ICE	Intracardiac echocardiography
LAA	Left atrial appendage
LAAC	Left atrial appendage closure
LSPV	Left superior pulmonary vein
TEE	Transesophageal echocardiography
TTE	Transthoracic echocardiography
2D	Two-dimensional
3D	Three-dimensional

Highlights

- Transesophageal echocardiography (TEE) is regarded as the gold standard for visual intra-procedural guidance of left atrial appendage closure (LAAC).
- Multiple views (0, 45, 90, and 135 degrees) using TEE should be obtained both prior to and after device implantation to exclude thrombus, plan the procedure, and assess the device.
- Operators should become familiar with the appearance of different LAAC devices on TEE.
- Immediately post-deployment, final views should be obtained to evaluate for pericardial effusion with comparison made to baseline imaging performed at the beginning of the case.

P. J. Horbal · M. Houmsse (✉)
Division of Cardiology, The Ohio State University Wexner Medical Center, Columbus, OH, USA
e-mail: Mahmoud.Houmsse@osumc.edu

S. J. Filby et al. (eds.), *A Contemporary Manual of Left Atrial Appendage Closure*, https://doi.org/10.1007/978-3-031-68441-8_9

Introduction

Transesophageal echocardiography (TEE) is regarded as the gold standard for visual intra-procedural guidance of left atrial appendage closure (LAAC) [1]. It is imperative to understand the different views and correlations of fluoroscopy throughout the procedure including confirmation of appropriate target site, ruling out exclusion criteria, deployment of the device, and post-deployment monitoring for complications. Covered in other chapters of this book are details as to the various imaging modalities in pre-procedural planning for LAAC and intra-procedural guidance such as the utilization of intracardiac echocardiography (ICE). It should be noted that there have been several studies showing the benefits and accurate correlation of ICE to TEE [1–5]. In this chapter, we review the intra-procedural aspects of TEE-guided LAAC procedure after appropriate pre-procedural evaluation is completed.

General Overview

Following a general anesthesia induction, the TEE probe is inserted to obtain baseline images and perform a general evaluation prior to starting the procedure. This should include a global assessment of the left ventricular systolic function, valvular morphology and evaluation for intracardiac thrombus to confirm no changes to the pre-procedural imaging (TEE, TTE, or CT), along with noting the pericardial space as this can provide a comparison post-deployment of the device, and in chance alterations occur to patient hemodynamics (Fig. 9.1).

The anatomic characteristics of the LAA include the ostium, neck, body/lobar regions, and apex. The ostium is the plane between the left atrium and LAA, oftentimes oval-shaped, with the mitral valve on the inferior and the LSPV on the superior aspects. The neck located between the ostium and body is an important point of anatomy to monitor during deployment, as the left circumflex and sinus node artery lie nearby and may be compressed. The distal aspect of the LAA consists of the body, lobes, and apex, which together form a significant degree of variation (Fig. 9.2); details are covered in the prior chapter. It is crucial to understand the variance as it may play a critical role in deciding device size and deployment maneuver. As an example, cone-shaped appendages with distal narrowing can result in device migration and embolization due to the compressive force pushing the device out towards the atrium. Further, secondary lobes near the ostium may make it difficult to obtain an adequate seal. Finally, although the chicken-wing morphology is one of the most commonly encountered, the early and shallow bend may make the depth assessment and deployment incongruent.

As with pre-procedural planning, the LAA should be re-evaluated to include the assessment of anatomy, morphology, and function and to rule out evidence of thrombus. TEE has a sensitivity and specificity of 92% and 98%, respectively, for the detection of LAA thrombi and is often regarded as the gold standard [6]. To

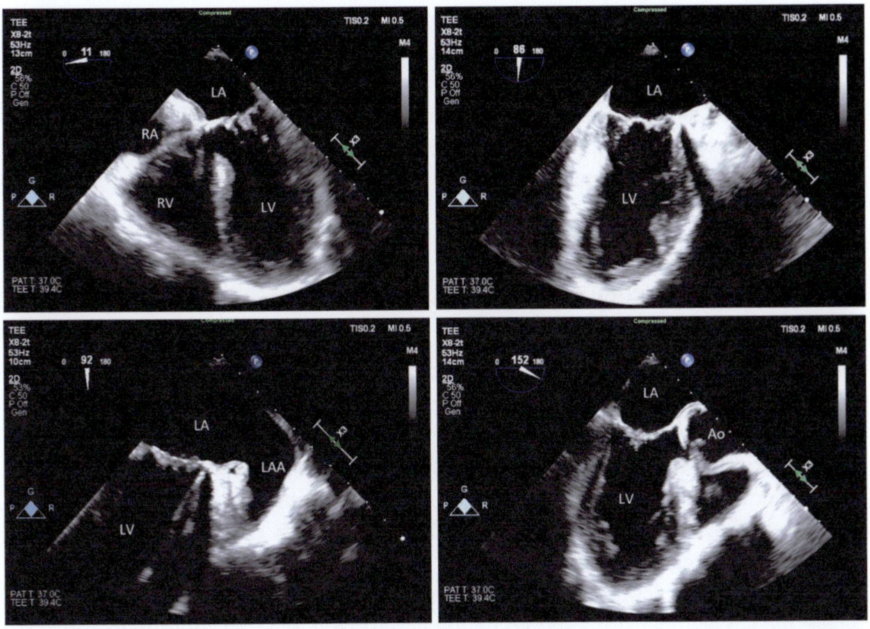

Fig. 9.1 Pre-procedural baseline transesophageal echocardiography images in evaluation of the left ventricular function, mobility of the mitral and aortic valve, pericardial space to rule out significant effusion and confirmation of no evidence of thrombus in the left atrial appendage and intra-cardiac chambers. The panels depict a comprehensive evaluation at different mid-esophageal views along with a magnified examination of the appendage. *LA* left atrium, *LAA* left atrial appendage, *LV* left ventricle, *RA* right atrium, *RV* right ventricle

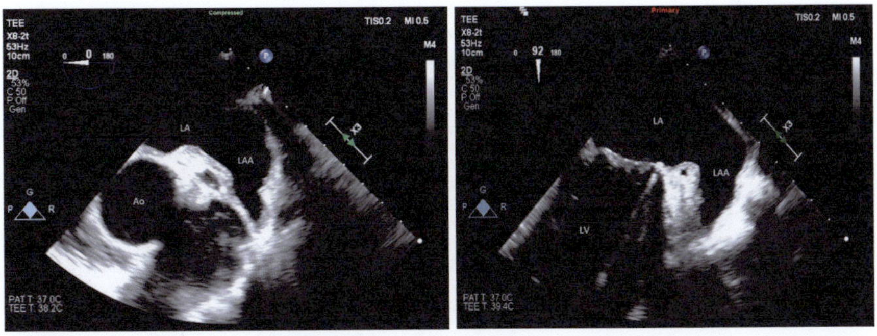

Fig. 9.2 Transesophageal echocardiographic imaging of the left atrial appendage. Baseline evaluation includes ruling out thrombus within the appendage at multiple views (depicted at 0 and 90 degrees). *Ao* aorta, *LA* left atrium, *LAA* left atrial appendage, *LV* left ventricle, *RV* right ventricle

improve visualization of the LAA including the multiple lobes and apex, X-plane (orthogonal 90 degree) views and ultrasound contrast agents may be used. This may be particularly helpful in cases of difficult anatomy or when spontaneous echo contrast is visualized, hindering the degree of certainty in ruling out thrombi. [7]

In addition to visual parameters, quantitative LAA emptying velocity may be obtained. An emptying velocity (obtained via pulsed-wave measurement within 1 cm of the LAA orifice) of <40 cm/s has been shown to correlate with a higher risk of stroke and <20 cm/s associated with thrombus formation. [6, 8] Further, 3D TEE allows for superior thrombus evaluation compared to 2D echo and has been shown to correlate better to CT imaging. [6]

Baseline Intra-Procedure TEE Assessment

Evaluation of the LAA dimensions including the landing zone and depth is critical to improve the outcomes and in limiting complications related to inappropriately sized devices (device migration and embolization, when undersized, and cardiac perforation and effusion, when oversized). These measurements and the experience of the operator may significantly alter the results of cases; as seen in PROTECT AF, there were 5–7% risks of LAAC-related complications due to operator learning curve [9]. To avoid undersizing, the LAA measurements, including that of the landing zone and LAA depth, need to be obtained during the end of ventricular systole, where the LAA dimensions should be the largest (Fig. 9.3). In addition to appropriate timing in cardiac cycle, multiple TEE views need to be obtained due to the previously discussed variety in LAA morphology. These views most often consist of mid-esophageal multiplane views at 0, 45, 90, and 135 degrees, including biplane views (Fig. 9.4), with careful angulation to evaluate all aspects of the LAA body and lobes [10]. Although every patient requires personalized attention to detail, slight

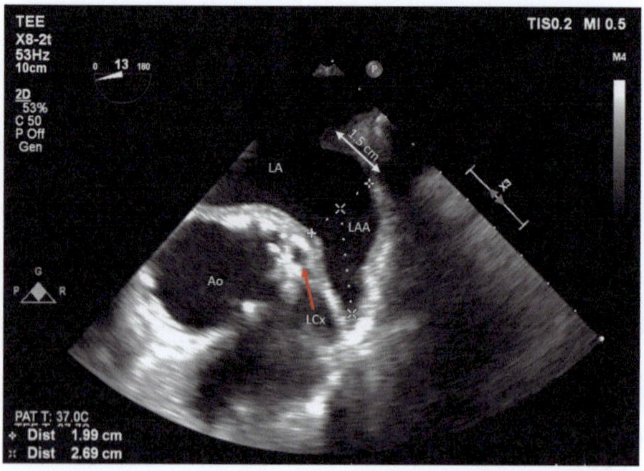

Fig. 9.3 Measurements obtained of the left atrial appendage intra-operatively confirming prior measurements. For the single seal devices (Watchman) the landing zone is measured at the level of the left circumflex artery (red arrow) and 1.5 cm from the Coumadin Ridge, shown here as 1.99 cm. The depth is measured from the landing zone measurement to the apex of the appendage (2.69 cm). *Ao* aorta, *LA* left atrium, *LAA* left atrial appendage, *LCx* left circumflex artery

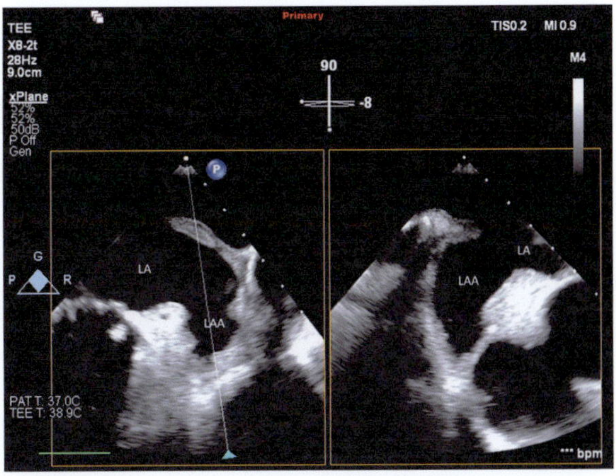

Fig. 9.4 Bi-plane depiction of the left atrial appendage measuring at approximately 0 and 90 degrees. *LA* left atrium, *LAA* left atrial appendage

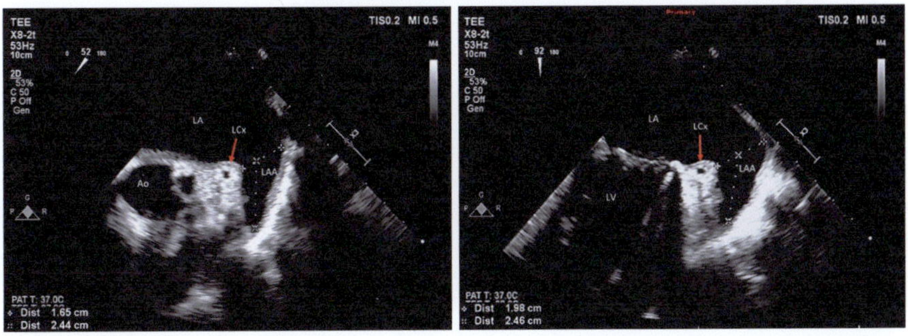

Fig. 9.5 Multiple measurements of the left atrial appendage at approximately 45 degrees and 90 degrees in an attempt to obtain the largest measurement for correct left atrial appendage occlusion sizing. In this depiction, the appendage is located more posteriorly, confirmed with measurements obtained in the 70–90 degree views. Visualized the landing zone in plane with the left circumflex artery and 1.5 cm from the Coumadin ridge. *Ao* aorta, *LA* left atrium, *LAA* left atrial appendage, *LCx* left circumflex artery

adjustment in plane may provide increased optimization. Mid-esophageal 50–70 degrees allows for viewing the LAA in the longest plane and visualizing the mitral annular and circumflex artery medially and the PV ridge and LSPV laterally [6]. If the LAA is located more anteriorly, the long axis may be better visualized at 0–50 degrees, whereas a more lateral LAA can be seen at 70–90 degrees (Fig. 9.5). Short-axis views are best seen at 135 degrees or biplane view at 45 degrees. Similarly to thrombus evaluation, 3D TEE has been shown to more accurately assess the LAA orifice size and depth to similar rates of multiplanar CT, noting that 2D TEE can underestimate size [6, 10] (Fig. 9.6). It should be noted that LAAC procedures have been performed using only TEE guidance and without direct assessment via fluoroscopy. [11] When it comes to comparing TEE views to real-time fluoroscopic imaging, the following general assumptions can be made, as seen in Table 9.1 [12, 13].

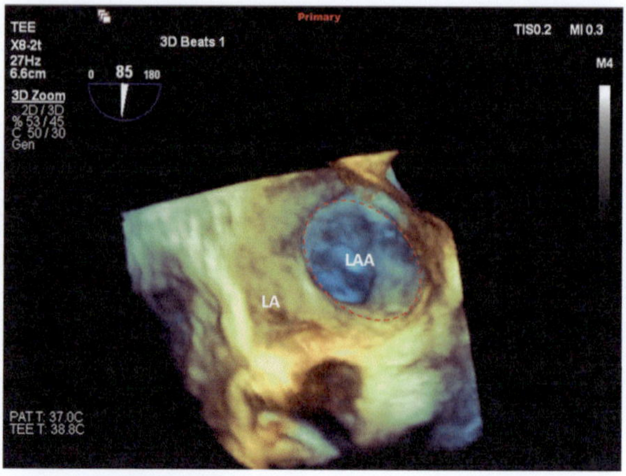

Fig. 9.6 3D representation of the left atrial appendage orifice seen at approximately 90 degrees showing the distinct oblique characterization. *LA* left atrium, *LAA* left atrial appendage

Table 9.1 Comparison between TEE views and real-time fluoroscopic imaging

Approximate correlation between views on TEE and fluoroscopy	
TEE view (degrees)	Fluoroscopy
0	AP
45	RAO 30, cranial 20
90	RAO 30
135	RAO 30, caudal 20

Procedural Specifics

Upon initial confirmation of LAA dimension and agreement on appropriate device size, the transseptal puncture is performed under echocardiographic guidance (see corresponding chap. 8 for details). An extra stiff J-tipped 0.035-inch guide wire is advanced into the LSPV under TEE guidance. The TSP sheath is exchanged over the wire for the LAA occlusion access sheath. A 5F–6F pigtail catheter is advanced into the LAA and carefully manipulated to limit undue pressure in the LAA tip. This may be done under simultaneous TEE (50–90 degrees) and fluoroscopic guidance prior to contrast angiography. In addition, the mean left atrial pressure should be obtained, and in order to limit undersizing, it is recommended that the pressure be >10 mm Hg and resuscitation with IV fluids be performed as needed.

LAAC Device Specifics

The most frequently used LAAC devices can be split into two categories. Single-seal devices, also referred to as plug style, close the appendage via a singular barrier. In the USA, the most commonly utilized single-seal device is the Watchman (Boston Scientific Co., USA). The other category, utilizing a hybrid version of a plug within the body of the appendage and a secondary barrier on the surface, is the double-seal devices such as the Amplatzer Amulet (Abbott Vascular, USA).

Single-Seal Device (Watchman)

The following dimensions are obtained: maximum ostium diameter measured from the circumflex artery to the ridge, and maximum depth measured from the LAA ostium to the tip. The landing zone is measured 1–2 cm inferior to the ridge and at the level of the circumflex artery (Fig. 9.3). The largest LAA landing zone measurement is selected after evaluation at 0, 45, 90, and 135 degrees, and for appropriate fitting, it is recommended to choose a device that is 8–20% oversized [12, 13]. It should be noted that there are certain exclusion criteria, which should be accounted for prior to the procedure: landing zone <14 mm or >31.5 mm; depth is less than the orifice diameter; secondary lobe must be >1 cm away from the orifice; atrial septal aneurysm excursion >15 mm; large interatrial shunt; mobile aortic plaque >4 mm; mitral stenosis with MVA < 1.5 cm^2; and pericardial effusion >2 mm.

When visualizing the LAA under TEE view, fluoroscopic imaging should be adjusted to RAO 20–30 degrees and caudal 20–30 degrees. The Watchman delivery system is inserted and advanced into the LA until the distal markers of the catheter align with the access sheath at the LAA ostium plane (Fig. 9.7). The Watchman device is then deployed, confirming device positioning and compression under dual imaging guidance.

Prior to the final deployment of the Watchman device, confirmation with the PASS criteria needs to be performed: position—correct placement within the LAA with limiting of shoulder protrusion of the device to less than 40–50% of device depth (Fig. 9.8); anchor—under TEE and fluoroscopic guidance, the deployment knob is retracted and released to confirm the device returns to the original position in the LAA (Fig. 9.9); size—under 2D 0, 45, 90, and 135 degrees, the diameter of the

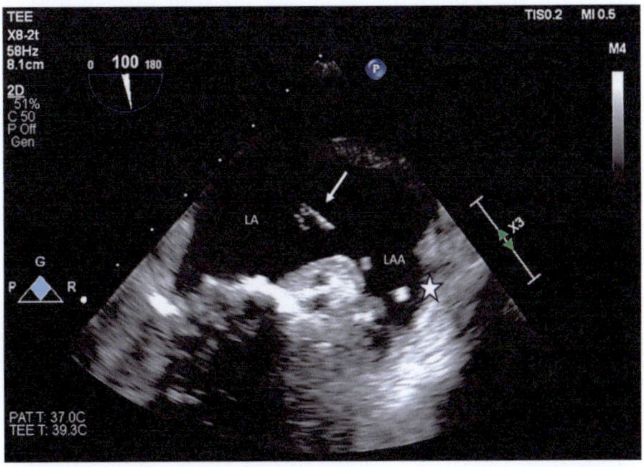

Fig. 9.7 Intraprocedure transesophageal echocardiographic visualization of the left atrial appendage occlusion device system in the left atrium. The deployment sheath (arrow) crosses over from the right atrium (not seen) with a pigtail catheter located within the left atrial appendage (star). *LA* left atrium, *LAA* left atrial appendage

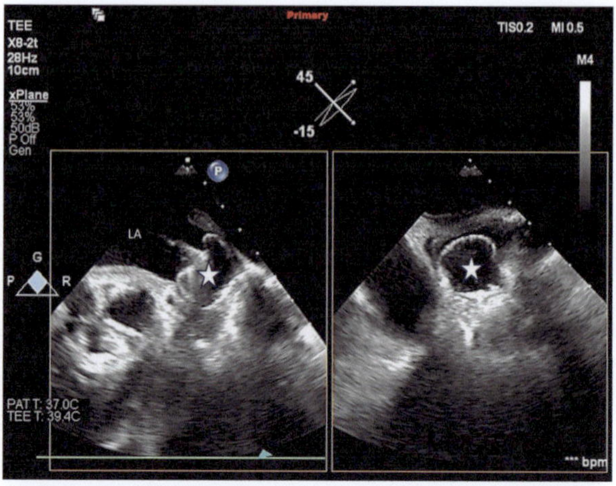

Fig. 9.8 Biplane view assessing the "position" criterion of "PASS" showing the appropriate placement of the device within the left atrial appendage (star) while still not deployed (as seen by the sheath attachment). *LA* left atrium, *LAAO* left atrial appendage occlusion device

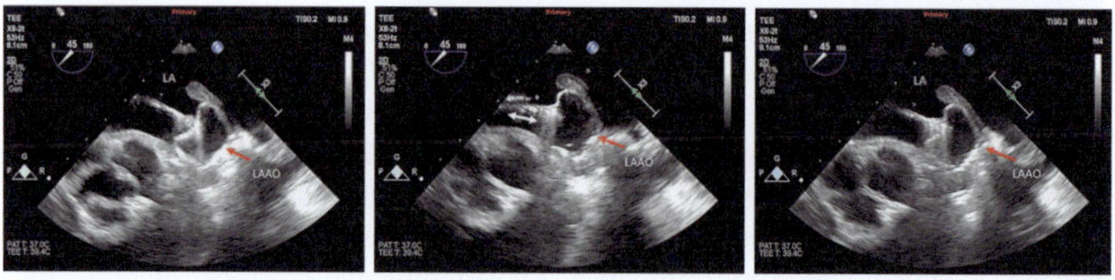

Fig. 9.9 Transesophageal echocardiographic imaging depicting the "Anchor" aspect of the PASS criteria. First panel shows the left atrial appendage occlusion device seated within the left atrial appendage while still attached to the deployment sheath. The second panel shows a "tug test" being performed, visualizing the device face pulling back but no change in device position. This is confirmed in the final panel with no change as compared prior to the performance of the "tug test". *LA* left atrium, *LAAO* left atrial appendage occlusion device

device from shoulder to shoulder, making certain the threaded insert/metal portion is seen, is obtained where compression should be 8–20% (Fig. 9.10); and seal—evaluation for para-device leak under all four angles and using color doppler with low Nyquist limit (20–30 cm/s) to detect low flow and low velocity, and if vena contracta >5 mm, device readjustment should be considered (Fig. 9.11). Further a 3D reconstruction may be obtained to evaluate the LAAC and LAA orifice contact (Fig. 9.12).

Double-Seal Devices (Amulet)

The Amulet has a lobe and disk configuration which slightly changes the deployment maneuver. Also, similar to Watchman, there are certain exclusion criteria: landing zone <14 mm or >32 mm; minimal depth is 10 mm for the 16–22 mm Amulet and 12 mm for the 25–34 mm Amulet; and further similar atrial septal aneurysm size, interatrial shunt, mitral valve stenosis, and pericardial effusion criteria.

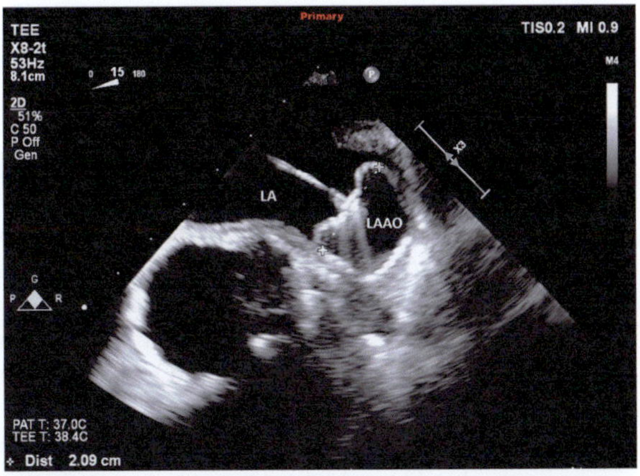

Fig. 9.10 Size is the next aspect of the PASS criteria which is measured as the ratio of compression of the device compared to the landing zone measurement. This should be greater than 8% but less than 20%. Here, the compression comes to 15%. *LA* left atrium, *LAAO* left atrial appendage occlusion device

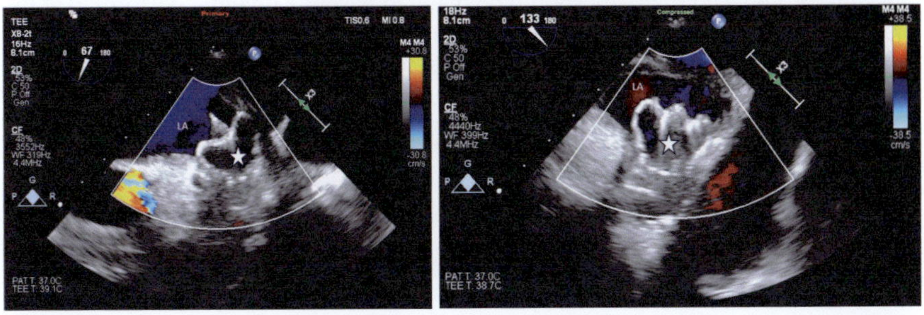

Fig. 9.11 The final criterion for PASS is "seal" which evaluates for peri-device leak using color doppler. The panels listed above show color doppler used two different view points. It is important to visualize that the device outline is directly abutting the appendage wall with no evidence of a leak by color doppler. *LA* left atrium, *star* left atrial appendage occlusion device

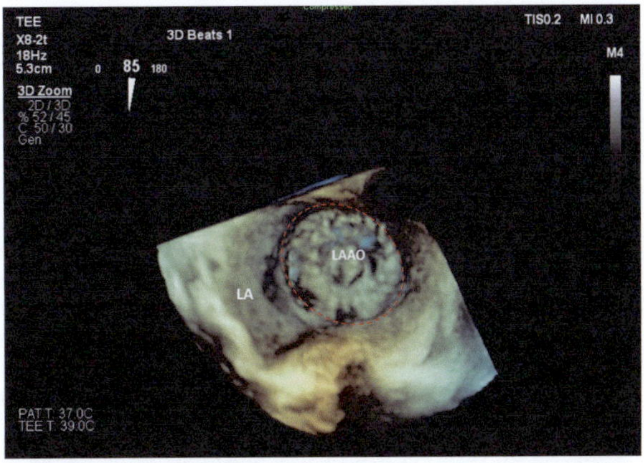

Fig. 9.12 3D reconstruction of the left atrial appendage occlusion device post deployment with adequate positioning within the left atrial appendage as seen from the left atrial view. *LA* left atrium, *LAA* left atrial appendage

Upon similar TSP technique and LA advancement of the delivery sheath, the Amulet sheath is advanced and positioned in the landing zone (10–15 mm distal to the LAA ostium, perpendicular to the LAA neck). Note that the depth is measured from the plane of orifice to the back LAA wall, compared to the plane of orifice to the apex for Watchman devices. The lobe or "ball" is deployed in LA and advanced into the LAA zone. Upon satisfactory positioning, the disk portion is deployed. Five criteria need to be met prior to full release of the device: 1—lobe should be tire-shaped to ensure it is flushed and engaged via stabilizing wires; 2—degree of separation between the lobe and disk that shows a good seal; 3—concave shape of the disk that also confirms seal; 4—perpendicular axis of the lobe to the neck to ensure stability; 5—at least two thirds of the lobe should be adjacent to the circumflex artery, and a tug test may be performed.

Immediately post-deployment, a mid-esophageal four-chamber view and transgastric views should be obtained to evaluate for pericardial effusion and tamponade physiology, and a comparison should be made to baseline imaging performed at the beginning of the case. Further, evaluation for a significant iatrogenic atrial septal defect should be performed as >10 mm may require percutaneous closure [13].

References

1. Akella K, Murtaza G, Turagam M, Sharma S, Madoukh B, Amin A, Gopinathannair R, Lakkireddy D. Evaluating the role of transesophageal echocardiography (TEE) or intracardiac echocardiography (ICE) in left atrial appendage occlusion: a meta-analysis. J Interv Card Electrophysiol. 2021;60(1):41–8. https://doi.org/10.1007/s10840-019-00677-x. Epub 2020 Jan 17.
2. Berti S, Paradossi U, Meucci F, Trianni G, Tzikas A, Rezzaghi M, Stolkova M, Palmieri C, Mori F, Santoro G. Periprocedural intracardiac echocardiography for left atrial appendage closure: a dual-center experience. JACC Cardiovasc Interv. 2014;7(9):1036–44. https://doi.org/10.1016/j.jcin.2014.04.014.
3. Wang DD, Forbes TJ, Lee JC, Eng MH. Echocardiographic imaging for left atrial appendage occlusion: transesophageal echocardiography and Intracardiac echocardiographic imaging. Interv Cardiol Clin. 2018 Apr;7(2):219–28. https://doi.org/10.1016/j.iccl.2018.01.001.
4. Ge J, Chen T, Ma C, Maduray K, Zhong J. Can intracardiac echocardiography completely replace transesophageal echocardiography to guide left atrial appendage closure?-the comparisons of intracardiac echocardiography with transesophageal echocardiography. J Card Surg. 2022;37(9):2766–75. https://doi.org/10.1111/jocs.16695. Epub 2022 Jun 21.
5. He G, Liu H, Huang X, Deng X, Yang G, Luo D, Cai L. Intracardiac versus transesophageal echocardiography for diagnosis of left atrial appendage thrombosis in atrial fibrillation: a meta-analysis. Clin Cardiol. 2021;44(10):1416–21. https://doi.org/10.1002/clc.23698. Epub 2021 Sep 3. PMID: 34480383; PMCID: PMC8495084
6. Gilhofer TS, Saw J. Periprocedural imaging for left atrial appendage closure: computed tomography, transesophageal echocardiography, and Intracardiac echocardiography. Card Electrophysiol Clin. 2020;12(1):55–65. https://doi.org/10.1016/j.ccep.2019.11.007.
7. Bansal M, Kasliwal RR. Echocardiography for left atrial appendage structure and function. Indian Heart J. 2012;64(5):469–75. https://doi.org/10.1016/j.ihj.2012.07.020. Epub 2012 Jul 27. PMID: 23102384; PMCID: PMC3860699.

8. Deegan R, Ellis CR, Bennett JM. The left atrial appendage, including LAA occlusion devices line watchman, amulet, and lariat. Semin Cardiothorac Vasc Anesth. 2019;23(1):70–87. https://doi.org/10.1177/1089253218789159. Epub 2018 Jul 18
9. Reddy VY, Holmes D, Doshi SK, Neuzil P, Kar S. Safety of percutaneous left atrial appendage closure: results from the watchman left atrial appendage system for embolic protection in patients with AF (PROTECT AF) clinical trial and the continued access registry. Circulation. 2011;123(4):417–24. https://doi.org/10.1161/CIRCULATIONAHA.110.976449. Epub 2011 Jan 17.
10. Wunderlich NC, Beigel R, Swaans MJ, Ho SY, Siegel RJ. Percutaneous interventions for left atrial appendage exclusion: options, assessment, and imaging using 2D and 3D echocardiography. JACC Cardiovasc Imaging. 2015;8(4):472–88. https://doi.org/10.1016/j.jcmg.2015.02.002.
11. Huang H, Chen L, Liu J, Wang W, Cao Y, Yuan B, Tao E, Fang Q, Tang L, Wang F, Wan L. Clinical application of percutaneous left atrial appendage occlusion guided only by transesophageal echocardiography without fluoroscopy and angiography in the patients with nonvalvular atrial fibrillation. J Card Surg. 2022;37(6):1479–85. https://doi.org/10.1111/jocs.16463. Epub 2022 Mar 30.
12. Sanchez CE, Yakubov SJ, Amin A, Arshi A. Left atrial appendage closure: technical considerations of endocardial closure. Card Electrophysiol Clin. 2020;12(1):47–54. https://doi.org/10.1016/j.ccep.2019.11.002.
13. Vainrib AF, Harb SC, Jaber W, Benenstein RJ, Aizer A, Chinitz LA, Saric M. Left atrial appendage occlusion/exclusion: procedural image guidance with transesophageal echocardiography. J Am Soc Echocardiogr. 2018;31(4):454–74. https://doi.org/10.1016/j.echo.2017.09.014. Epub 2017 Nov 20.

Chapter 10
Echocardiographic Imaging Guidance for Left Atrial Appendage Closure: Intracardiac Echocardiography

Esseim Sharma and Mauricio Arruda

Highlights

- 2D ICE allows for greater procedural control, efficiency, and flexibility compared to historical imaging with TEE.
- Key ICE benefits include avoiding general anesthesia, streamlining workflows, leveraging existing skills from related procedures, and controlling imaging acquisition.
- Step-by-step guidance and instructions on obtaining the four key LA views are described to ensure appropriate device alignment and fit.
- Advancements in ICE imaging with 3D and 4D capabilities are discussed, along with their potential impact.

Introduction

Transesophageal echocardiography (TEE) has traditionally been the standard modality for imaging during left atrial appendage closure (LAAC). While TEE is a reliable and comprehensive imaging modality during LAAC, it also presents some practical challenges regarding availability, the need for general anesthesia, and the potential need for an additional cardiac imager during the case to provide TEE imaging. Intracardiac echocardiography (ICE) has emerged as an efficacious alternative that offers unique advantages.

ICE-guided LAAC has become increasingly popular due to its potential to increase lab efficiency and to obviate the need for general anesthesia, and numerous studies have

E. Sharma (✉) · M. Arruda
Division of Cardiology, Harrington Heart & Vascular Institute, University Hospitals Cleveland Medical Center, Cleveland, OH, USA
e-mail: Esseim.Sharma@uhhospitals.org

S. J. Filby et al. (eds.), *A Contemporary Manual of Left Atrial Appendage Closure*, https://doi.org/10.1007/978-3-031-68441-8_10

now demonstrated that ICE is a safe imaging platform for LAAC across varying operator experience and equivalent to TEE in terms of efficacy [1, 2]. This chapter will review the benefits of ICE versus TEE, best practices for performing procedures under ICE guidance, areas that warrant special attention, important follow-up considerations, and key references for those wishing to adopt ICE-guided workflows. We will also briefly discuss newer technologies such as three-dimensional and four-dimensional ICE which improve on some of the limitations of traditional 2D ICE-guided LAAC.

Comparative Advantages and Limitations of ICE vs. TEE Guidance

While TEE is the standard of care for real-time visualization during LAAC, drawbacks such as throughput, personnel needs, and procedural risks exist. Comparatively, ICE solves many of the limitations of TEE, but also comes with its own downsides, such as single-plane orientation. Understanding the inherent differences in these imaging modalities can help operators in their pre-procedural planning.

Benefits of ICE over TEE

Several tangible benefits exist for ICE over TEE during LAAC procedures. The most fundamental is placing imaging control in the hands of the operator. Eliminating the communication between a separate echocardiographer and the operator permits faster reactions to subtle visual cues that may prompt adjustments in device positioning and deployment. By avoiding TEE, ICE also precludes the need for general anesthesia, as ICE-guided LAAC can be performed under conscious, moderate sedation. This not only helps to eliminate the risks of general anesthesia and TEE to the patient in this relatively frail population, which can include delirium and esophageal injury, but also limits the infectious risks of aerosolized procedures [3]. Additionally, it eliminates significant bottlenecks associated with anesthesiology services and post-anesthesia care bed availability as procedural volumes rise. By eliminating these constraints, ICE-guided LAAC can boost laboratory throughput to meet growing LAAC demand. Finally, many LAAC operators have developed an extensive ICE skillset during atrial fibrillation ablation or atrial septal defect closures, and this skillset is directly transferable to ICE-guided LAAC.

Limitations Relative to ICE

The improved logistic efficiency of ICE comes with some imaging tradeoffs. As a single physical transducer, manipulation of catheter positioning and angle is necessary to obtain complementary views. Additionally, the farther an object is from the ultrasound crystal in the ICE catheter, the worse the resolution. This is compounded when there are structures between the ultrasound crystal and the structure of interest. Thus, optimal visualization of the left atrial appendage with ICE requires crossing into the left atrium with the ICE catheter. This can pose difficulty in some patients with a difficult-to-traverse interatrial septum, and it can also be technically challenging. 3D TEE also better defines LAA depth and selects device size, while ICE must be combined with pre-procedural imaging and fluoroscopy during the case. Hence, a learning curve exists for proficiency with ICE catheter handling and advancement across the interatrial septum to visualize all left atrial anatomy adequately.

Furthermore, ICE requires additional venous access and intracardiac placement with its attendant risks. However, modern catheters have flexible designs and hydrophilic coatings to minimize this downside. The ICE catheter can also increase costs of performing the procedure, though this is usually offset by the elimination of anesthesia, TEE, and lab efficiency [4]. Finally, despite its widespread adoption, the use of ICE during LAAC, particularly for the Watchman FLX, currently remains off-label in the United States at the time of this writing [5].

Procedural Steps for ICE-Guided LAAC

Familiarity with necessary steps will facilitate successful ICE-guided LAAC deployment. The following represents a general step-by-step guide, with required patient-specific procedural alterations expected.

Pre-procedural Planning

Appropriate patient selection and imaging remain imperative prior to the procedure date. Imaging of the left atrial appendage must be performed before the procedure to ensure optimal device sizing, as well as to exclude the presence of a left atrial appendage thrombus. This can be done with either cardiac CT with delayed imaging protocols to opacify the LAA or 3D TEE, based on operator preference.

Access and Transseptal Puncture

After standard sterile preparation and draping, moderate sedation is administered for patient comfort. Two femoral venous access sites area obtained, allowing for the insertion of both the intracardiac ultrasound catheter and LAAC delivery sheath. These can be obtained either unilaterally or bilaterally, depending on operator preference [6]. Therapeutic heparin bolus follows successful femoral venous sheath insertion. Visualization of the heart then begins from the mid-right atrium to identify anatomical landmarks, assess for pericardial effusion, and guide transseptal catheterization (Figs. 10.1c and 10.2a). The ICE catheter can then be advanced into the right ventricle and clocked until the left ventricle comes into view, to ensure that there is no pericardial effusion around the left ventricle (Figs. 10.1a, b). If necessary, the catheter can be further clocked and advanced until it reaches the RVOT, where the left atrial appendage can be visualized preliminarily to confirm there is no thrombus.

The ICE catheter is then retracted back to the right atrium and clocked until the interatrial septum is in view. Transseptal puncture can then be performed per the operator's preference, either with the aid of fluoroscopy and ICE or with ICE-only guidance (Figs. 10.1c, d). Typically, a low and posterior puncture site on the fossa ovalis is recommended, though some operators prefer a slightly more central or even anterior approach, especially in the case of a "reverse chicken-wing" or posterior bending of the left atrial appendage [6, 7].

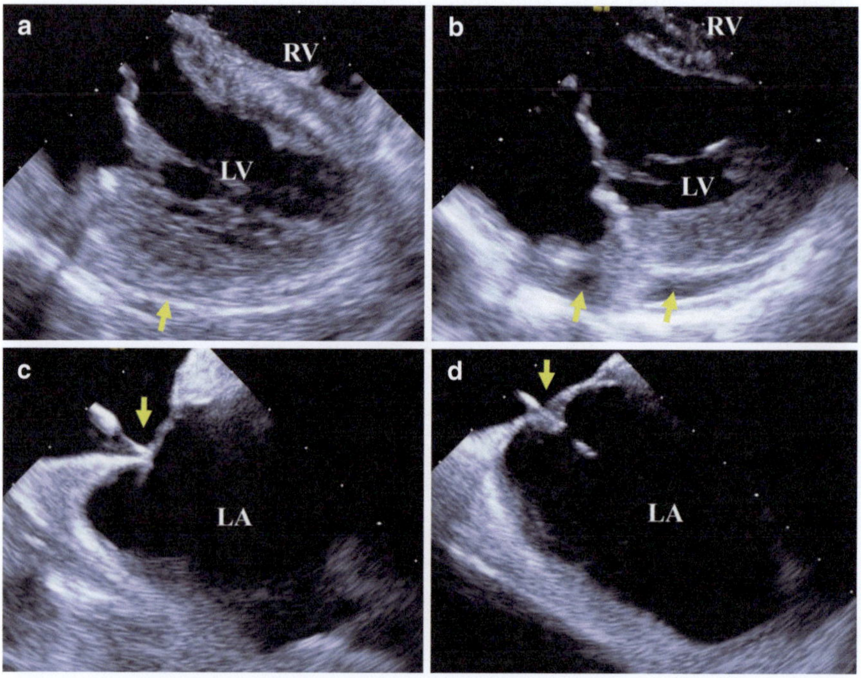

Fig. 10.1 **Panel A** shows the ICE view of the left ventricle (LV), the right ventricle (RV), and the pericardial space (arrow) with trivial pericardial effusion. In **panel B**, the ICE probe was withdrawn, exhibiting a preexisting small posterobasal pericardial effusion (arrow). **Panel C** shows ICE image of the left atrium (LA) during transseptal puncture. Note the tenting of the interatrial septum at the infero-posterior aspect of the fossa ovalis. **Panel D** shows the loss of tenting following the puncture

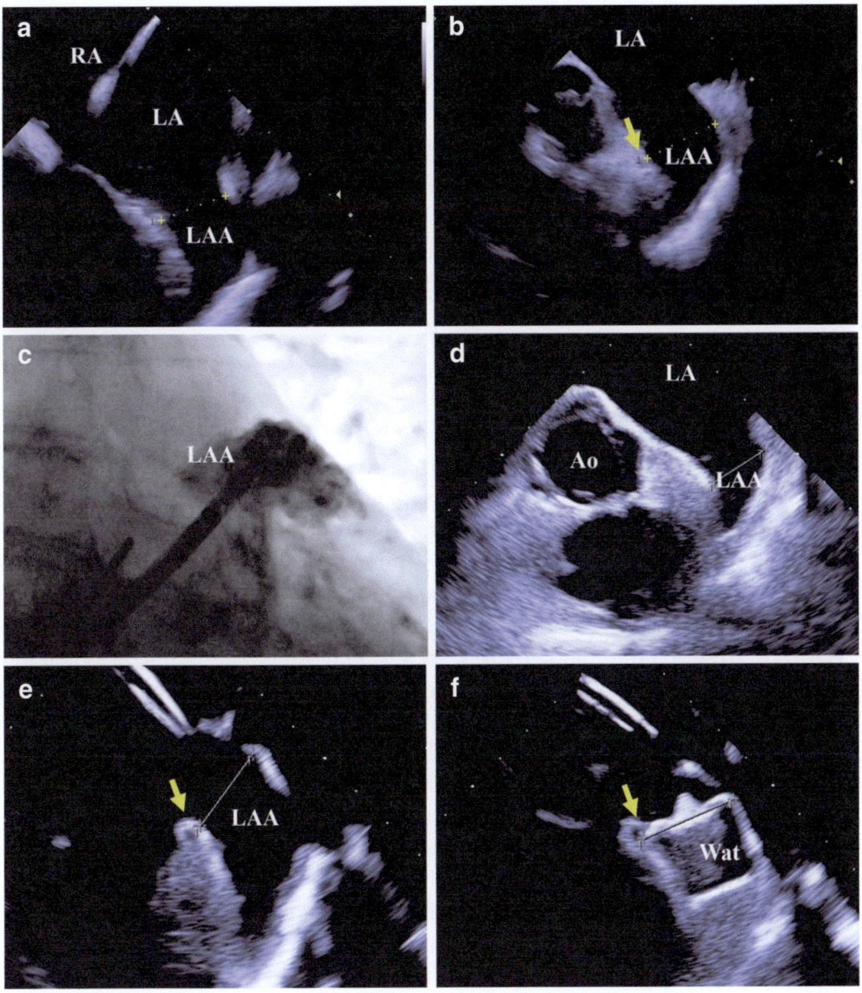

Fig. 10.2 **Panel A** shows ICE imaging of the LA and left atrial appendage (LAA) with the probe still in the right atrium (RA). In **Panel B**, the LAA is imaged from the LA (LAA AV view). The arrow is pointing to the left circumflex coronary artery. **Panel C** shows LAA angiography. **Panel D** again shows the LAA AV view, with the short-axis of the aortic valve (Ao) now visible. **Panel E** shows the LAA AV view in another patient, with the arrow pointing to the left circumflex coronary artery. Note the Watchman (Wat) device at an ideal deployment site with measurments at the level of the left circumflex coronary artery

Advancing ICE into the Left Atrium

After transseptal puncture, the ICE catheter must now be advanced into the left atrium itself. First, the LAAC sheath is advanced into the left atrium over a stiff guidewire placed in the left pulmonary veins, as per the usual LAAC implantation technique. This allows for adequate dilation of the interatrial septum. Next, the

LAAC sheath is pulled back into the right atrium while maintaining the wire in the pulmonary vein. The ICE catheter is then advanced through the interatrial septum into the left atrium by aligning the catheter with the wire based on fluoroscopy and images from the ICE catheter itself. Sometimes, orthogonal fluoroscopic views are necessary to align the ICE catheter with the wire. Once the ICE catheter is in the left atrium, the LAAC sheath is then advanced back over the wire into the left atrium. Thus, the ICE catheter and the LAAC sheath are advanced into the left atrium through the same transseptal puncture [8].

Left Atrial ICE Views

The ICE catheter should now be maneuvered into the LAA mitral valve (MV) view, also known as the "home view" (Fig. 10.3b), which is roughly analogous to the 45–90° view on TEE. This is achieved by rotating the ICE catheter until the mitral valve and LAA are both in view. A slight rightward and especially posterior tilt toward the right superior pulmonary vein is often needed to fully bring both the left atrial appendage and mitral valve into view. This posterior tilt helps to bring the ICE catheter away from the anterior left atrium, giving a better view directly into the LAA (Fig. 10.4c). From the LAA MV view, initial ostial measurements of the left atrial appendage can be made. Measurements should only be made where the left circumflex coronary artery ostium (Fig. 10.2f) os is also in view as a landmark. Furthermore, clockwise rotation of the ICE catheter will reveal any posterior lobes, and counterclockwise rotation will reveal any anterior lobes, which will be useful when assessing LAA depth. After contrast injection of the LAA with a pigtail catheter (Fig. 10.2c), measurements of the ostia and depth of the appendage can also be made fluoroscopically and compared against ICE measurements.

The second view of the LAA is typically taken from the left superior pulmonary veins and is known as the aortic valve (AV) view as the aortic valve is visible in this view. This view is especially useful when the full LAA depth cannot be appreciated. The ICE catheter can be advanced into the left superior pulmonary vein (LSPV) by bringing the LSPV into view and slowly advancing, rotating the ICE catheter anteriorly to visualize the full depth of the LAA (Figs. 10.3c, d, e). As with any manipulation with the ICE catheter, care should be taken to only advance the ICE catheter when blood, which appears echolucent or black on ultrasound, is visible, to avoid advancing into the cardiac wall and inadvertently causing damage or perforation. The ICE catheter should never be advanced into an echodense structure. If any resistance is met, catheter advancement should be halted, and the ICE catheter should be retracted and redirected before advancing again. Successful advancement into the LSPV is confirmed by identifying the lateral border of the Coumadin ridge. Rightward tilt from the LSPV approximates the 0° view on TEE, while leftward tilt approximates the 90° view. Counterclockwise rotation of the ICE catheter anteriorly from this view can help visualize anterior lobes and help insertion of the sheath over the pigtail catheter. The LAA AV view can also be taken from the LA itself rather than the LSPV, which may be advantageous in certain cases (Fig. 10.2d).

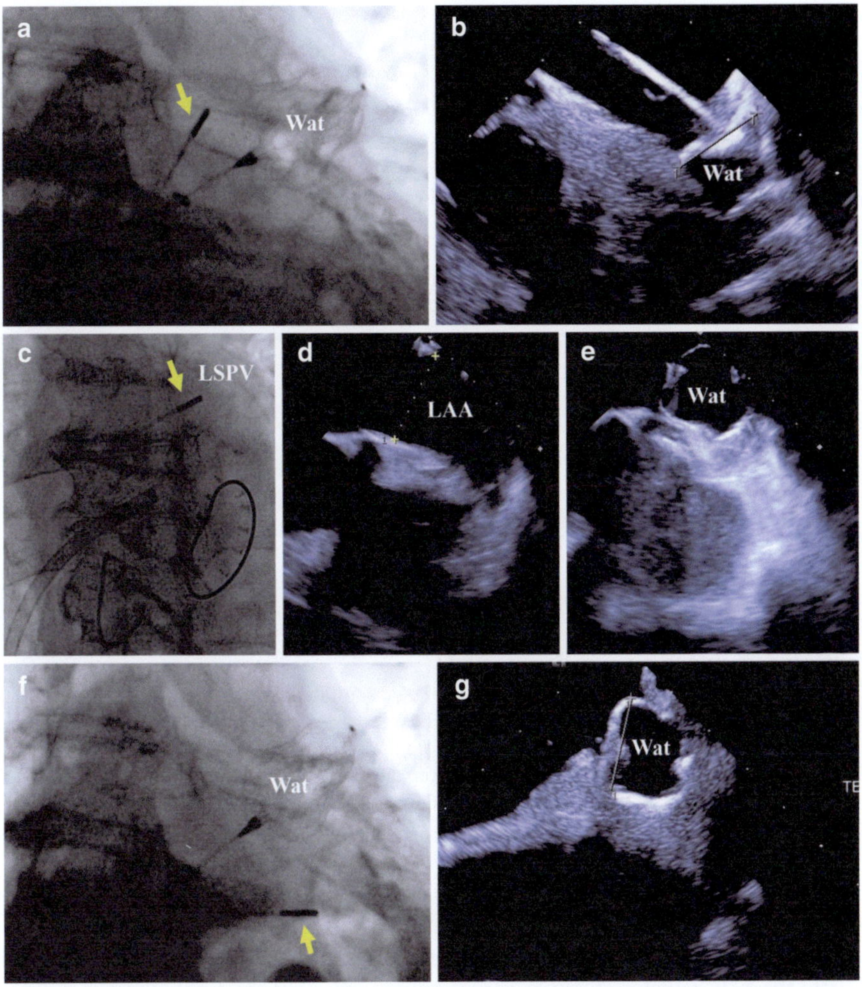

Fig. 10.3 **Panel A**: fluoroscopic view showing the ICE probe position in the LA and the Watchman device in the LAA, which is also seen by ICE in **panel B**. In **panels C**, **D**, and **E**, the ICE probe is positioned in the left superior pulmonary vein (LSPV) (arrow). Note the ICE images of the LAA and the Watchman device. **Panel F** shows the ICE probe is deflected toward the mitral valve underneath the Watchman device which is visualized by ICE in **panel G (the "PA view")**

The final view on ICE is the pulmonary artery (PA) view and is the most technically challenging to obtain. It is called the PA view as the short-axis of the pulmonary artery is also seen in this view. This view best approximates the 135° view on TEE, where the ICE catheter will be across the valve looking "up" at the left atrial appendage (Figs. 10.3f, g and 10.4a, b). The traditional way to obtain this view is by first ante-flexing the ICE catheter down toward the mitral valve and then applying counterclockwise rotation until it is in the left ventricle. At this point, the inferior wall of the left ventricle will be in view. Flexion is then relaxed, and the catheter is

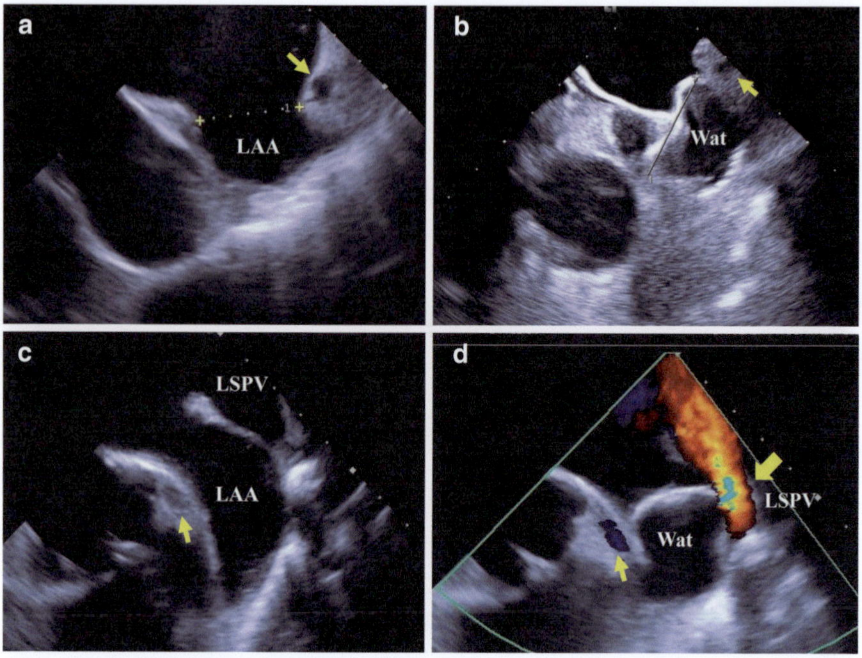

Fig. 10.4 **Panels A** and **B**—ICE image of the LAA and the Watchman device from the mitral view. The arrows in all panels indicate the left circumflex coronary artery. **Panel C** shows the LAA and its close proximity to the LSPV imaging from the LA home view. **Panel D**—color Doppler from the same view showing LSPV blood flow (bold arrow). Importantly there is no flow around the Watchman device, confirming excellent circumferential opposition with the LAA without peri-device leaks

rotated until the LAA is in view. The ICE catheter will now be appropriately positioned toward the valve, and only minimal rightward or leftward tilt is needed to get the LAA into view appropriately. An alternative method of obtaining this view is to rotate the ICE catheter clockwise from home view until the right superior pulmonary vein (RSPV) is in view. Once the RSPV is in view, the catheter can gently be posteriorly flexed and advanced toward the mitral valve. This view can also be quite helpful in assessing the depth of the LAA and can be very useful in addition to standard fluoroscopic views during the deployment of the device to ensure that the sheath and device are coaxial to the LAA.

Final Intraprocedural Assessment

After deployment of the LAAC device, color Doppler should be used in all of the above views to assess for any leaks (Fig. 10.4d). It is vital to lower the Nyquist limit to adequately assess for any leaks, as most machines default to a higher Nyquist limit for ICE catheters. Typically, a Nyquist limit of around 0.2–0.25 meters per second is used [2]. Contrast injection under fluoroscopy should also be used to confirm device position and further evaluate for any peri-device leak. The device should also be evaluated for stability with a tug test. Compression of the device should be measured to ensure adequate compression of 10–30% in multiple views. Finally, the device "shoulders" should be examined to ensure there is no interference with the left superior pulmonary vein or mitral valve.

Once satisfactory positioning of the device is achieved, the ICE catheter is withdrawn into the right atrium, and then advanced into the right ventricle to again check for pericardial effusion, before being removed from the body.

A Look to the Future

Three-dimensional and four-dimensional ICE are new technologies that are slowly becoming incorporated into LAAC procedures. Three-dimensional ICE refers to the ability of newer ICE catheters to reconstruct 3D images via multiplanar reconstruction (MPR), similar to TEE. This allows for more extensive and accurate sizing and imaging of the LAA. Four-dimensional ICE refers to the addition of volumetric imaging to 3D ICE, allowing for a rigorous assessment of device placement and leaks within the left atrial appendage [9]. Previous 4D ICE catheters had a limited field of view, but newer models now have expanded 90° × 90° fields of view. This mitigates the need to physically manipulate the ICE catheter into multiple views and allows for direct visualization of anatomy and flow from a single location, greatly simplifying the procedure [10]. In some cases, the entire procedure can be performed with the ICE catheter in the right atrium. While more studies will be needed to determine the reliability and cost-effectiveness of these newer ICE catheters moving forward, based on the utility of MPR and 3D imaging with TEE, these advancements in ICE imaging are quite promising.

Conclusion

In just over a decade, intracardiac echocardiographic guidance for left atrial appendage closure has transformed from a novel concept to the standard of care in many high-volume institutions. ICE offers unique advantages over historical imaging with TEE in regard to safety, efficiency, and cost. Growing evidence demonstrates comparable effectiveness as well. This chapter reviewed the considerations in choosing ICE versus TEE guidance, technical details on the performance of ICE-guided LAAC, and a look to the future of ICE imaging during LAAC.

References

1. Alkhouli M, Chaker Z, Alqahtani F, Raslan S, Raybuck B. Outcomes of routine intracardiac echocardiography to guide left atrial appendage occlusion. JACC Clin Electrophysiol. 2020;6(4):393–400.
2. Nielsen-Kudsk JE, Berti S, Caprioglio F, Ronco F, Arzamendi D, Betts T, et al. Intracardiac echocardiography to guide watchman FLX implantation: The ICE LAA study. JACC Cardiovasc Interv. 2023;16(6):643–51.
3. Freitas-Ferraz AB, Bernier M, Vaillancourt R, Ugalde PA, Nicodeme F, Paradis JM, et al. Safety of transesophageal echocardiography to guide structural cardiac interventions. J Am Coll Cardiol. 2020;75(25):3164–73.
4. Hemam ME, Kuroki K, Schurmann PA, Dave AS, Rodriguez DA, Saenz LC, et al. Left atrial appendage closure with the watchman device using intracardiac vs transesophageal echocardiography: procedural and cost considerations. Heart Rhythm. 2019;16(3):334–42.
5. Alkhouli M, The ICE. LAA study: another proof of concept or a PASS to the future? JACC Cardiovasc Interv. 2023;16(6):652–4.
6. Patel A, Venkataraman R, Schurmann P, Dave A, Valderrabano M. Left atrial appendage occlusion using intracardiac echocardiography. Heart Rhythm. 2021;18(2):313–7.
7. Fukutomi M, Fuchs A, Bieliauskas G, Wong I, Kofoed KF, Sondergaard L, et al. Computed tomography-based selection of transseptal puncture site for percutaneous left atrial appendage closure. EuroIntervention. 2022;17(17):e1435–e44.
8. Paiva LV, Costa MP, Barra SC, Goncalves L. Intracardiac echography for left atrial appendage closure: a step-by-step tutorial. Catheter Cardiovasc Interv. 2019;93(5):E302–E10.
9. Khalili H, Patton M, Taii HA, Bansal P, Brady M, Taylor J, et al. 4D volume intracardiac echocardiography for intraprocedural guidance of transcatheter left atrial appendage closure. J Atr Fibrillation. 2019;12(4):2200.
10. Sharma A, Bertog S, Tholakanahalli V, Mbai M, Chandrashekhar YS. 4D intracardiac echocardiography-guided LA appendage closure under conscious sedation: initial experience and procedural technique. JACC Cardiovasc Imaging. 2021;14(11):2254–9.

Chapter 11
Computed Tomography-Fluoroscopy Fusion Guidance for Left Atrial Appendage Closure

Herman Carneiro, Luis Augusto Palma Dallan, Juliana Knezevich, Imran Rashid, and Steven J. Filby

Abbreviations

CPR	Cardiopulmonary resuscitation
CT	Computed tomography
CCTA	Cardiac computed tomography angiography
DAP	Dose area product
ICE	Intracardiac echocardiography
LA	Left atrium
LAA	Left atrial appendage
LAAC	Left atrial appendage closure
3D	Three-dimensional
PACS	Picture archive and communication system
ROI	Region of interest
SVC	Superior vena cava
TEE	Transesophageal echocardiography

Highlights

- Fusion imaging leverages the advantages of complementary imaging modalities by combining fluoroscopy with its high temporal resolution and CT with its good soft tissue resolution for real-time percutaneous left atrial appendage closure guidance.

H. Carneiro
Division of Cardiology, Department of Medicine, Northwestern University, Chicago, IL, USA

L. A. P. Dallan · J. Knezevich · I. Rashid (✉) · S. J. Filby
Division of Cardiology, Harrington Heart & Vascular Institute, University Hospitals Cleveland Medical Center, Cleveland, OH, USA
e-mail: Imran.rashid@uhhospitals.org

S. J. Filby et al. (eds.), *A Contemporary Manual of Left Atrial Appendage Closure*, https://doi.org/10.1007/978-3-031-68441-8_11

- CT-fluoroscopy fusion can lower procedure times, fluoroscopy times, radiation exposure, and contrast volume used.
- CT-fluoroscopy fusion offers more successful first-time transseptal punctures, first-pass device deployment, and complete left atrial appendage seals.

Introduction

As technology advances, the number and complexity of percutaneous procedures in interventional cardiology continue to grow. Multimodality imaging is essential for the planning and execution of many of these procedures. With respect to left atrial appendage closure (LAAC) procedures, pre-procedural imaging with transesophageal echocardiography (TEE) and computed tomography (CT) is used to assess the anatomy of the left atrial appendage (LAA) and to size the closure device. Fluoroscopy, which is the workhorse of percutaneous procedures, has good temporal resolution but poor soft tissue resolution. Imaging modalities with good soft tissue resolution, such as TEE and intracardiac echocardiography (ICE), are, therefore, used in combination with fluoroscopy for procedural guidance. These imaging modalities are used separately during the procedure, and focus shifts between them at different points within the procedure.

Fusion imaging leverages the advantages of these complementary imaging modalities by combining fluoroscopy and one of the imaging modalities with good soft tissue resolution for procedural guidance. The basic concept of fusion imaging is to project a three-dimensional (3D) image of an anatomical structure outlined in TEE, CT, or magnetic resonance imaging (MRI), among others, onto the fluoroscopy screen for real-time guidance of percutaneous procedures. In the case of LAAC procedures, the LAA is traced and projected on the fluoroscopy screen. The projected 3D image of the LAA rotates with the fluoroscopy unit to match the desired viewing angles. TEE and CT are the imaging modalities used most often in fusion imaging for LAAC procedures. The goal of fusion imaging is to increase the safety, efficacy, and efficiency of interventional procedures.

This chapter focuses on how to create and use CT-fluoroscopy fusion imaging in LAAC cases and discusses the current evidence on the use of fusion imaging in the published literature.

Pre-procedural Imaging

Newer facilities may have hydrid OR-CT suites under the auspices of cardiology (Fig. 11.1). Patients can be scheduled to have a CT scan prior to their procedure, making same-day procedure protocols possible. Cardiac CT angiography (CCTA) images can be interpreted by cardiologists who specialize in cardiac imaging.

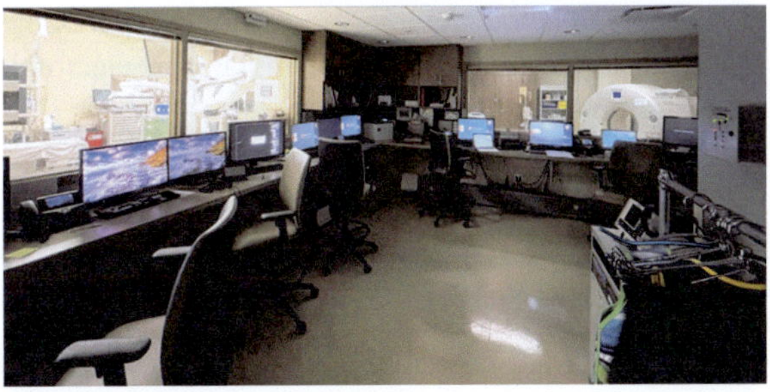

Fig. 11.1 A hybrid OR-CT suite which can be used for left atrial appendage occlusion pre-procedural imaging, image interpretation, LAAC planning, and the LAAC procedure

Computed Tomography Acquisition

Pre-procedural imaging with CCTA offers high-quality multiplanar and 3D-reconstructed images for procedural planning and intraprocedural guidance. CCTA scanning techniques have been covered elsewhere in detail (Chap. 5). However, there are special considerations when it comes to CT-fluoroscopy fusion for LAAC. For CT-fluoroscopy fusion to be viable, CCTA image acquisition should be carried out with patients scanned in the same position as they would be on the procedure table. This allows for the same lie of the organs and heart during CCTA image acquisition and the procedure. To that end, image acquisition techniques have been developed to achieve the highest possible success of CT-fluoroscopy fusion.

CT scanner tables are curved, whereas procedure tables are flat. Scanning patients on a curved table leads to a difference in the lie of the organs during CCTA and the procedure. To overcome this, a hard, radiolucent board can be placed under the patient's chest during CT image acquisition. A cardiopulmonary resuscitation (CPR) backboard, which is available on most CPR carts in radiology suites, is ideal for this use.

It is also conventional practice to perform CCTA with the patient holding their arms above their heads [1]. This is done to reduce radiation exposure and artifact from suboptimal arm position. For CT-fluoroscopy fusion, patients should be scanned with their arms down by their side to match their position on the procedure table. This technique also allows for the same lie of the organs during CTA and during the implant procedure.

Neutralizing the respiratory cycle during image acquisition also enables the organs to have the same lie as they would for image co-registration of the CCTA and baseline fluoroscopy images for CT-fluoroscopy fusion. Image acquisition should be done with the patient doing a breath hold in end-expiration. This neutralizes intrathoracic pressure, allowing organs to settle in a baseline position for the CT angiogram. This, in turn, makes image co-registration for CT-fluoroscopy fusion more accurate.

The standard cardiac CT acquisition window is restrained to the area just outside the cardiac silhouette to reduce radiation exposure. In CT-fluoroscopy fusion, image co-registration is improved by increasing the number of anatomical landmarks for image co-registration. To that end, the image acquisition window is expanded from the clavicle to below the inferior cardiac border. Doing so maximizes the bony and soft tissue landmarks and cardiac implantable electronic devices that can be used for image co-registration.

Baseline Fluoroscopy Images

Image co-registration requires CCTA and baseline fluoroscopy images. Patients should be placed on the fluoroscopy table in a position that they will be in for the duration of their procedure. Baseline anteroposterior and left lateral fluoroscopic images of the patient should be taken in end-expiration for image co-registration. The CT-fluoroscopy fusion software requires two fluoroscopy images at least 30 degrees apart for image co-registration.

Creation and Integration of Fusion Images

Imaging software from different vendors differ in their interfaces, but the general principles of CT-fluoroscopy fusion are the same. CCTA images are transferred from the CT image storage software, such as the picture archive and communication system (PACs), to the fusion software package.

A 3D reconstruction of the thorax is rendered. The next step is to select the anatomy to be removed from the image volume, which is most of the soft tissue. The region of interest (ROI) tool is used to select nonessential soft tissue and subtract it from the image volume.

The CCTA images are then used to trace around the LAA in the axial, coronal, and sagittal views (Fig. 11.2). The LAA orifice is traced at the level of the left atrium-LAA junction and the left superior pulmonary vein ridge. The fusion software then uses these tracings to project a 3D shell of the LAA onto the 3D reconstruction of the chest (Fig. 11.3).

The next step is co-registration of the CCTA reconstruction with the LAA shell and the baseline fluoroscopy images. Co-registration can either be done manually or by using automated co-registration. The automated algorithm lines up the bony lands and soft tissue landmarks to co-register the CCTA and fluoroscopy images. Manual co-registration allows more freedom and control in image co-registration; it allows more landmarks to be used in image co-registration. Bony landmarks, such as the clavicle, ribs, sternum, and vertebrae, as well as soft tissue landmarks, such as the trachea and cardiac silhouette, are used to line up the 3D reconstruction of the thorax from the CCTA and the baseline fluoroscopy images for co-registration. Cardiac implantable electronic devices, such as implantable loop recorders, pacemakers and defibrillators, and their leads, can also be used to align the 3D-reconstructed CCTA images and baseline fluoroscopy images for image co-registration.

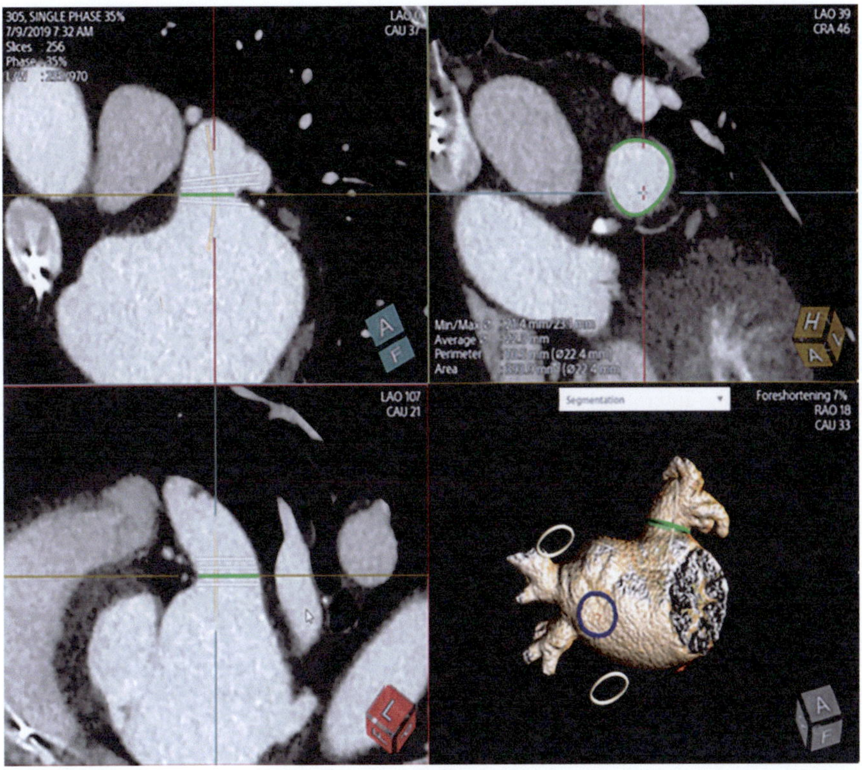

Fig. 11.2 Outlining the left atrial appendage (LAA) in the axial, coronal, and sagittal views to build a three-dimensional shell of the LAA for computed tomography-fluoroscopy fusion

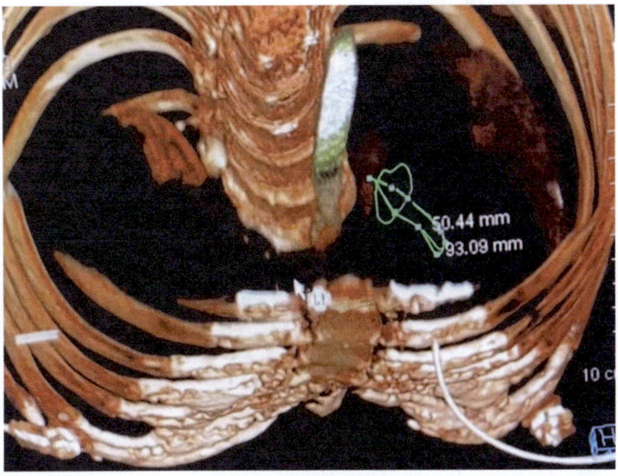

Fig. 11.3 Three-dimensional (3D) reconstruction of the thorax with the soft tissue subtracted from the image volume with a projection of the left atrial appendage to be used in CT-fluoroscopy fusion image co-registration

The fused images, with a 3D LAA projected on the live fluoroscopy screen, are then ready for the proceduralist to use during the procedure. The CT-fluoroscopy fusion images can be captured and stored along with other fluoroscopy images in the imaging storage system (Fig. 11.4).

It should be noted that CT-fluoroscopy fusion can also be used to guide transseptal puncture. The ideal transseptal puncture site is one with a co-axial approach to the LAA landing zone for device implantation. Once this site has been identified, the interatrial septum can be examined on the CCTA for the ideal transseptal puncture site and marked. Ideally, the fossa ovalis and the transseptal site within the fossa ovalis should be traced. This outline is co-registered at the same time as the LAA is co-registered. A 3D transseptal puncture site is projected onto the real-time fluoroscopy screen for the operator to use. This technique does not identify the thinnest part of the interatrial septum for transseptal puncture, but it generally orients the proceduralist in the anterior-posterior and superior-inferior locations on fluoroscopy. The ideal transseptal puncture location can be further fine-tuned using TEE or ICE.

Procedural Workflow Using CT-Fluoroscopy Fusion

The procedural details are covered in more detail elsewhere and can vary on the chosen LAAC device. Essentially, the LAAC procedure is done via common femoral access. The transseptal system and device are typically delivered via the right common femoral vein. Echocardiography guidance is either by TEE or ICE based on operator skill and preference. Echocardiography should be used to rule out pericardial effusion prior to transseptal puncture and to examine the interatrial septum for the ideal transseptal site. A transseptal system is then brought up into the superior vena cava (SVC) and brought down and maneuvered into the fossa ovalis.

If the transseptal puncture site was traced and co-registered during CT-fluoroscopy fusion, the transseptal system can be moved to the desired transseptal puncture site

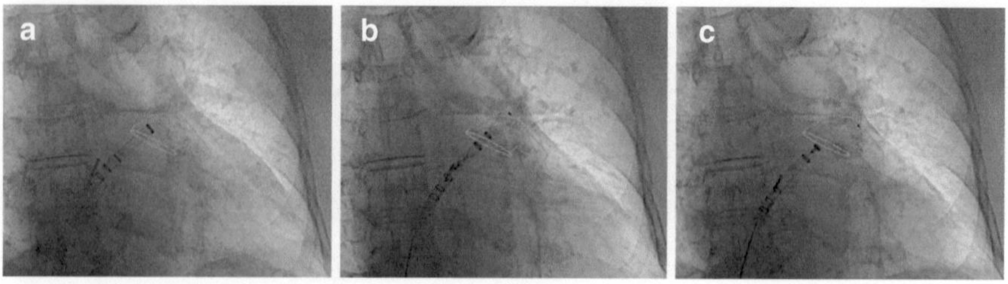

Fig. 11.4 Computed tomography-fluoroscopy fusion showing a projection of the three-dimensional left atrial appendage shell on the fluoroscopy screen for procedural guidance, an ICE catheter, and a Watchman FLX delivery sheath. *Panel A*. Device delivery sheath inserted into LAA. *Panel B*. Formation of flex ball and device guided to the desired deployment location. *Panel C*. Watchman FLX deployment

on the real-time fluoroscopy screen. Again, the thinnest part of the septum in the target location, which is ideal for transseptal puncture, is best appreciated on echocardiography. Immediately after transseptal puncture, echocardiography should be used to rule out a pericardial effusion.

When the sheath is across the septum in the left atrium (LA), the dilator is exchanged for a pigtail catheter. The real-time CT-fluoroscopy fusion image can be used to guide the pigtail catheter towards and into the LAA. With the pigtail catheter in the LAA, a contrast injection is done to opacify the LAA. The precise location of the LAA can then be compared to the location of the marked LAA on the fluoroscopy screen to determine how accurately the actual LAA lines up with the LAA outlined with CT-fluoroscopy fusion. If the location of the fused LAA image and the contrast-opacified image line up well, the fused CT-fluoroscopy image, in combination with ICE or TEE, can be used to position and deploy the LAAC device (Fig. 11.4, Video 1). If the CT-fluoroscopy fusion image and LAA are not adequately aligned, TEE, ICE, and fluoroscopy can be used to guide device implantation. Currently, there is no data on what offset between the contrast-opacified LAA and the fused LAA tracing on the CT-fluoroscopy image is acceptable for device positioning and deployment.

Once the device is deployed, rigorous evaluation of the implant with ICE, TEE, and angiography to assess the site of deployment, compression, device stability, and peri-device leak should be undertaken.

Current Clinical Evidence

Transcatheter procedures using fluoroscopy fusion technology are increasingly used for congenital and structural interventions. Pre-procedural imaging is paramount to the safety and success of these procedures. Currently, TEE is the gold standard in pre-procedural imaging, but cardiac CT offers high-quality multiplanar and 3D-reconstructed images. Cardiac CT provides not only extensive anatomical information about the LAA but also valuable information on surrounding structures that can be used in CT-fluoroscopy fusion image co-registration. Furthermore, the LAA anatomy can be complex with many lobes, which may not be seen on TEE or ICE. The lie of the LAA may be better appreciated on CT when there are acute angles of the neck of the LAA. While TEE is used in fluoroscopy fusion, cardiac CT, with its extra imaging information, is likely better for fluoroscopy fusion. There are few studies on TEE- and CT-fluoroscopy fusion in the published literature, and studies comparing these two modalities are lacking.

CT-fluoroscopy fusion potentially improves the safety, efficacy, and efficiency of percutaneous LAAC procedures. Specifically, some studies showed lower procedure times, contrast volume used, fluoroscopy times, total radiation used, and redo transseptal punctures. There was also evidence of a higher rate of successful first-time device deployment. However, the results are mixed with three positive studies and one negative study.

Roy et al. compared clinical and procedural parameters in patients undergoing percutaneous LAAC with and without CT-fluoroscopy fusion [2]. A total of 57 patients were included in the study, with 16 patients in the CT-fluoroscopy fusion group. Both the Watchman™ (Boston Scientific, MA, US) and Amplatzer Amulet™ (St. Jude Medical, St. Paul, MN) devices were implanted. They found significant reductions in contrast volume, procedure time, and fluoroscopy time. They also reported complete sealing of the LAA orifices and successful device deployment in all CT-fluoroscopy fusion cases.

Chen et al. also conducted an observational study of clinical and procedural parameters in patients undergoing percutaneous LAAC with and without CT-fluoroscopy fusion [3]. The Watchman™ LAA plug device was implanted in this study. Included in the study were 82 patients, with 41 patients in the control and intervention arms. They reported significant reductions in procedural time, total radiation dose, dose area product (DAP), and contrast volume used. Both groups had one patient with incomplete LAA sealing (>3 mm).

Mo et al. did a randomized control study in which 117 patients were randomized in a 1:2 fashion to undergo Watchman™ implantation with and without CT-fluoroscopy fusion [4]. This was the only study in which CT-fluoroscopy fusion was used to guide transseptal puncture as well. The patients undergoing device implantation with CT-fluoroscopy fusion guidance had significantly higher successful deployment rates and a lower number of device recaptures and devices used per patient. Patients in the CT-fluoroscopy group all had successful first-time transseptal punctures, while five in the control group required redo transseptal punctures. At the 45-day follow-up, there was no peri-device leak in either group.

In contrast to the studies above, Carneiro et al. reported a negative study. They conducted a single-center, prospective, single-blinded, randomized control trial [5]. Included in the trial were 59 patients, with 33 patients in the CT-fluoroscopy fusion group and 26 patients in the control group. The Watchman FLX™ device (Boston Scientific, MA, USA) was implanted for LAAC. They found no significant difference between the two groups in procedure time, contrast volume used, fluoroscopy time, radiation dose, and radiation DAP. There was no peri-device leak in either group in the immediate 1-month post-procedure follow-up period.

It should be noted that the number of participants in the study by Carneiro et al. was small, which could have contributed to the lack of significant differences between the interventional and control groups.

Alternate Study Protocols

Currently, the conventional protocol for LAAC procedures is pre-procedural imaging with TEE days in the days leading up to the procedure and selection of the appropriate device and size for the procedure for the patient. The procedure itself is done under general anesthesia with TEE for intraprocedural guidance.

These LAAC procedures can also be done under moderate sedation and, depending on the skill and comfort of the operator and their preference, using ICE for procedural guidance. There are several advantages of doing the procedure under moderator sedation using ICE guidance. First and foremost, the patient is spared an invasive procedure with potentially serious side effects. Furthermore, no additional personnel are required for the procedure. If no cardiac anesthetists are available, the procedure requires two additional physicians for the procedure: an anesthetist for general anesthesia and a cardiologist to perform TEE. This makes scheduling procedures easier, and from the hospital's point of view, these other health professionals can render their services elsewhere.

In the studies discussed in the prior section, there were significant differences in the study protocols. The three positive studies all had pre-procedural imaging with TEE, and the LAAC procedures were done under general anesthesia with TEE for intraoperative procedural guidance. Carneiro et al. used a same-day protocol where patients would undergo CCTA on the morning of their procedure. The procedures were done under moderate sedation with ICE guidance. The venotomy sides were closed with a vascular closure device, Vascade® (Haemonetics Corporation, Boston, USA), and patients were discharged home the same day. Utilizing this protocol, additional personnel such as anesthetists and echocardiographers were not required for these procedures. In addition, the LAA plug device used in the positive studies was the first-generation Watchman™ device, whereas Carneiro et al. implanted the newer Watchman FLX™ device. The protocol used by Carneiro et al. may have been streamlined to the point that the use of CT-fluoroscopy fusion was not able to improve the study metrics any further.

CT-Fluoroscopy Fusion Process Challenges

Currently, the main issue with CT-fluoroscopy fusion is the image co-registration process. There are often differences in the position of the organs on the CCTA images when compared to the fluoroscopy images, making it difficult to line up the anatomy on the different imaging modalities accurately. CCTA image acquisition protocols can be modified to alleviate this issue by scanning patients with a hard board under their chests and with their arms down by their sides. Image acquisition should also be done during a breath hold in end-expiration to neutralize intrathoracic pressures to allow organs to settle at their baseline.

Another issue with image co-registration encountered with some fusion software packages is that the imported CCTA images are magnified when compared to baseline fluoroscopy images. One approach to overcome this is to expand the image acquisition window to include as much anatomy as possible to increase the number of landmarks that can be lined up when co-registering CCTA and fluoroscopy images. Bony landmarks such as the ribs, sternum, vertebrae, and clavicles and soft tissue landmarks such as the trachea, bronchi, and cardiac silhouette can be used to align the baseline CCTA and baseline fluoroscopy images. Pacemakers, defibrillators, and their leads can also be used to align the images during co-registration.

Some fusion software packages have automated image co-registration algorithms that will do the co-registration for the user. These algorithms are often inaccurate. For the best results, manual co-registration is recommended. Users can undergo training from the fusion software companies to make them more adept at image co-registration. Having one or two dedicated users who specialize in fusion imaging is recommended to allow users to hone their skills in CT-fluoroscopy fusion.

Future Directions

Percutaneous LAAC procedures with real-time CT-fluoroscopy fusion have the potential to make percutaneous LAAC procedures safer for patients, increase the procedural success, and reduce the time it takes to such procedures. However, the issues with image co-registration have limited its use. More research and technological developments are needed to improve CT and fluoroscopy image co-registration.

One exciting prospect is the development of artificial intelligence (AI) algorithms for automated image co-registration. Deep learning is an AI technique that learns how to recognize objects in pictures. It is currently being used in radiology to teach machines to interpret images from a variety of imaging modalities and potentially appreciate nuances that are not readily perceived by the human eye.

Large datasets are required for neural networks to learn to recognize patterns. Conceivably, AI algorithms can create a high-density 3D LAA with associated relevant thoracic anatomy from CCTA scans and accurately co-register those images with baseline fluoroscopy images to create CT-fluoroscopy fusion images that can be used to guide LAAC procedures. The majority of the LAAC procedure could rely on AI-supported CT-fluoroscopy fusion, including transseptal puncture and device siting and deployment. This would make procedures faster and safer for patients and staff.

Conclusions

CT-fluoroscopy fusion for real-time guidance of percutaneous LAAC procedures offers many benefits including lowering procedure times, fluoroscopy times and radiation exposure, and contrast volume used. In addition, it offers more successful first-time transseptal punctures, first-pass device deployment, and complete LAA seals. Further development of this technology is required for it to achieve its potential.

References

1. Korsholm K, Berti S, Iriart X, Saw J, Wang DD, Cochet H, et al. Expert recommendations on cardiac computed tomography for planning transcatheter left atrial appendage occlusion. JACC Cardiovasc Interv. 2020;13(3):277–92.
2. Roy AK, Horvilleur J, Cormier B, Cazalas M, Fernandez L, Patane M, et al. Novel integrated 3D multidetector computed tomography and fluoroscopy fusion for left atrial appendage occlusion procedures. Catheter Cardiovasc Interv. 2018;91(2):322–9.
3. Chen T, Liu G, Mu Y, Xu WH, Guo YT, Guo J, et al. Application of cardiac computed tomographic imaging and fluoroscopy fusion for guiding left atrial appendage occlusion. Int J Cardiol. 2021;331:289–95.
4. Mo BF, Wan Y, Alimu A, Sun J, Zhang PP, Yu Y, et al. Image fusion of integrating fluoroscopy into 3D computed tomography in guidance of left atrial appendage closure. Eur Heart J Cardiovasc Imaging. 2021;22(1):92–101.
5. Carneiro HA, Dallan LAP, Yoon SH, Arora S, Knezevich J, Wass S, et al. Efficacy of 3D-multidetector computed tomography and fluoroscopy fusion for percutaneous left atrial appendage occlusion procedures. J Cardiovasc Electrophysiol. 2023;34(10):2076–83.

Chapter 12
The Watchman Left Atrial Appendage Closure Device: Technical Considerations and Procedural Approach

Mohammad Atif Rana, Luis Augusto Palma Dallan, Hamza Ali Lodhi, Kara J. Quan, and Steven J. Filby

Abbreviations

AF	Atrial fibrillation
CTA	Computed tomography angiography
DRT	Device-related thrombus
ICE	Intracardiac echocardiography
LA	Left atrium
LAA	Left atrial appendage
LAAC	Left atrial appendage closure
LAO	Left anterior oblique
LPV	Left pulmonary vein
LUPV	Left upper pulmonary vein
LVEF	Left ventricular ejection fraction
LZ	Landing zone
OAC	Oral anticoagulation
PDL	Peri-device leak
RAO	Right anterior oblique
TEE	Transesophageal echocardiogram
3D	Three-dimensional

M. A. Rana · L. A. P. Dallan · H. A. Lodhi · K. J. Quan (✉) · S. J. Filby
Division of Cardiology, Harrington Heart & Vascular Institute, University Hospitals Cleveland Medical Center, Cleveland, OH, USA
e-mail: KARA.QUAN@UHhospitals.org

S. J. Filby et al. (eds.), *A Contemporary Manual of Left Atrial Appendage Closure*, https://doi.org/10.1007/978-3-031-68441-8_12

Highlights

- Detailed explanation of the optimal procedural steps for the Watchman FLX device implantation and complication management.
- Comparative anatomy, clinical indications, and unique considerations for the LAAC with Watchman FLX device.
- Unique characteristics and additional advantages of the Watchman FLX Pro device.

Introduction

Percutaneous left atrial appendage closure (LAAC) with the WATCHMAN™ FLX device (Boston Scientific Co.) is a US Food and Drug Administration (FDA)-approved procedure for stroke prevention in patients with nonvalvular atrial fibrillation (AF) who have an appropriate rationale to seek an alternative to oral anticoagulation.

The size and shape of the left atrial appendage (LAA) vary widely among individuals. Imaging guidance for the LAAC procedure is of utmost importance for procedural success, as it helps guide the choice and size of the device. Successful LAAC depends on appropriate interaction and apposition of the Watchman device with the LAA walls, ensuring adequate compression of the device and complete exclusion of all LAA lobes. LAAC is affected by various factors including LAA ostial diameter, LAA depth, morphology ("chicken-wing," "cauliflower," "cactus," "windsock," etc.), septations, trabeculations, number of lobes, and orientation of the LAA body. Failure in device sizing or inadequate device positioning may result in peri-device leakage or even in device embolization.

Characteristics of the Watchman FLX Device

Figure 12.1 shows the details of the Watchman FLX device. Table 12.1 shows the evolutionary changes in Watchman FLX over its predecessor Watchman 2.5 devices.

Description of the Device

The Watchman FLX device is built on a nitinol frame with dual-row precision anchors and a permeable polyethylene terephthalate fabric skirt facing the appendage wall. The nitinol frame provides radial expansion and engagement and has an 18-strut frame, providing 80% more contact points than the Watchman 2.5 platform. There are 18 "J" shaped anchors arranged in 2 rows—proximal and distal—for stabilization of the device.

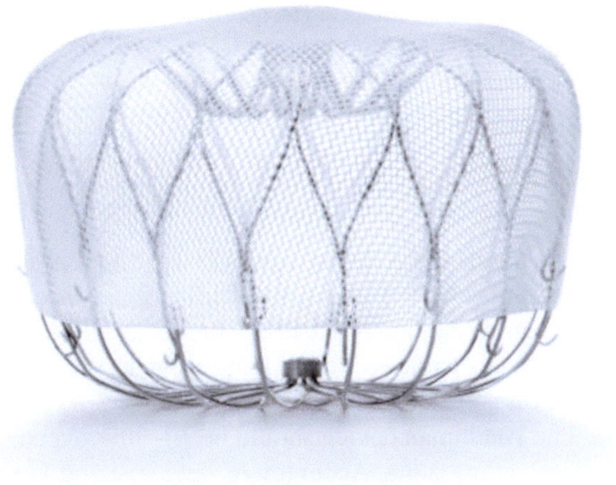

Fig. 12.1 Watchman FLX device. (Image provided courtesy of Boston Scientific.)

Table 12.1 Evolutionary changes in Watchman FLX over its predecessor Watchman 2.5 devices

Improved implant success and safety
Larger size range and shorter device
Distal tines folded back
Greater number of struts
Dual rows of anchors
Increased fabric coverage
Reduced complications

The Watchman FLX device is 10% shorter than the previous generation Watchman and has a closed end which makes its utilization possible in shallower as well as more complex anatomies. Watchman FLX™ also allows for "ball-shaped" fully rounded, atraumatic configuration which facilitates safe navigation and advancement within the LAA for precise placement. The device comes with complete recapturing and redeployment capabilities which are excellent tools for repositioning of the device, if needed. The updated design has shown a more successful and safer procedure with less peri-device leaks and device-related thrombus as compared to Watchman 2.5.

Indications and Contraindications

The Watchman™ FLX device is FDA approved for patients with an increased CHA_2DS_2-VASc score ≥2 and an indication to avoid long-term systemic OAC (class IIa recommendation per 2023 ACC/AHA/ACCP/HRS guidelines). Contraindications include active infective endocarditis or systemic infection, incompatible anatomy, hypersensitivity to device material, inability to tolerate post-procedure antiplatelet therapy, inability to safely undergo the procedure steps including sedation, vascular access, and intraprocedural anticoagulation. Relative contraindications include intracardiac thrombus or the presence of ASD or PFO closure device.

Device Sizing

The Watchman FLX device comes in five different sizes (20, 24, 27, 31, and 35 mm). It can be implanted in a LAA landing zone (neck) diameter ranging from 14 to 31.5 mm in width, considering the accepted 10–30% compression range post-deployment. Compressions slightly outside of this range may be acceptable in select cases.

The Watchman device should be 10–30% oversized to allow lobe compression at the landing zone. Accuracy of device sizing is consequential for a successful procedure. On one hand, undersized devices can lead to device migration and incomplete closure, and on the other, oversized devices can cause device embolization, tissue erosion, and appendage injury. The sizing of the device depends on two main factors: the size of the ostium, which corresponds to the most proximal landing zone for the device, and the depth of the appendage, which corresponds to the accommodation of the distalmost part of the device. The ostium of the appendage is measured 10–20 mm from the limbus of the Coumadin ridge to the left circumflex artery.

Multiple modalities can be used to accurately measure the LAA size for optimal device selection. Traditionally, transesophageal echocardiography (TEE) has been used for the assessment of the appendage and device sizing. It continues to remain the most frequently used modality. Typically, the LAA sizing is done on a dedicated TEE done prior to the procedure on a separate occasion to ensure feasibility of percutaneous LAAC. Multiple TEE views (0°, 45°, 90°, 135°) are used to confirm the size and shape of the appendage. Due to very low screen failure rates using the FLX, many centers have moved to performing the pre-LAAC TEE on the day of the procedure. When using TEE intraoperatively, common practice is to recheck LAA measurements after volume load and confirming mean LA pressure >10–12 mm Hg, if the opening LA pressure is below this threshold as measured by the TSP catheter.

Cardiac computed tomography assessment (CCTA) has been increasingly adopted for preprocedural planning. CCTA provides superior spatial resolution and facilitates 3D reconstruction. Studies show that CCTA provides larger LAA dimensions and more accurate device sizes which increases procedure efficiency. Multiple purpose-built software such as TruPlan™ (Circle CVI), FEops™ HEARTguide (FEops, Belgium), 3mensio LAA (Pie Medical Imaging, Maastricht, the Netherlands), etc. are available which make LAA assessment and device sizing (Fig. 12.2) more convenient.

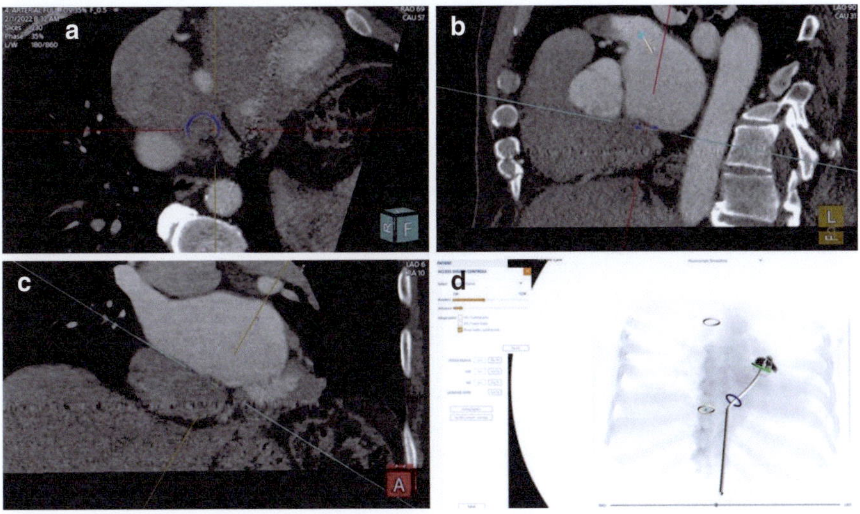

Fig. 12.2 Example of simulation of the transseptal puncture preplanning using the TruPlan™ software workstation for LAAC with the WATCHMAN™ device. **Panel A:** axial view. **Panel B:** sagittal view. **Panel C:** coronal view. **Panel D:** angiography simulation

Step-by-Step Implant

It is of utmost importance to have a systematic and consistent procedural workflow for the Watchman implantation. The Cath lab team should be familiarized with a well-established, structured protocol so that all the steps can be followed diligently, minimizing any chances of misinformation or lack of data before, during, or after the procedure. With a comprehensive commitment and involvement of a multidisciplinary team, the chances of a successful procedure are higher. An example of LAAC procedural workflow is shown in Table 12.2.

Before Puncture

The procedure can be done under general anesthesia or conscious sedation. If TEE is used, general anesthesia is usually utilized. In the case of ICE, conscious sedation is sufficient. As with other general anesthesia cases, continuous arterial pressure monitoring is warranted when performed under TEE guidance. However, when ICE is utilized along with conscious sedation, most centers use noninvasive hemodynamic monitoring.

Table 12.2 Example of LAAC procedural workflow

Example LAAC procedural workflow	1. Cardiac CTA imaging pre-planning
	2. Pre-procedure antibiotics
	3. Conscious sedation
	4. Common femoral vein access × 2 (a. ICE probe; b. Transseptal sheath)
	5. IV heparin
	6. Single transseptal puncture (Baylis/VersaCross) with ICE guidance
	7. Delivery sheath exchange
	8. LAA angiography with pigtail catheter
	9. 3 ICE views (mitral, aortic, and pulmonic views)
	10. Device delivery and release after P.A.S.S. Criteria satisfied
	11. Hemostasis with Perclose × 1(delivery sheath), Vascade × 1 (ICE sheath), and protamine

If there are no contraindications like elevated baseline left ventricular end diastolic and left atrial pressures, severe mitral insufficiency, etc., we recommend volume loading the patient with ≥500 ccs of intravenous fluid to achieve left atrial pressures of ≥10–12 mm Hg, which helps with accurate LAA measurements. This method is utilized if TEE-based sizing was performed as part of the planning or in borderline situation in case of CTA-based sizing.

Sterile precautions are maintained throughout the procedure. Intravenous prophylactic antibiotics can be administered prior to and after the procedure, as per facility protocol.

Intraprocedural Imaging

TEE is the most used modality worldwide for procedural guidance. Images are first obtained to rule out LAA thrombus and identify pericardial effusion. Subsequently, baseline LAA measurements at 0°, 45°, 90°, and 135° are obtained to determine the maximum and minimum diameters of the landing zone at the ostium. Real-time 3D TEE can also be utilized for intraprocedural imaging, and several studies have demonstrated that compared to 2D TEE, real-time 3D TEE shows improved spatial resolution and accuracy in measurements of LAA orifice. Studies show a higher successful implantations rate, lesser need for utilization of more than one device, and decreased procedural time when additional CCTA preprocedural planning is utilized along with TEE compared to standalone TEE.

Alternatively, intracardiac echocardiography (ICE) can also be used to guide device implantation. ICE is typically performed under local anesthesia and conscious sedation, thus avoiding the need for an anesthesiologist or echosonographer. The ICE catheter is inserted through the femoral vein and positioned throughout the heart (right atrium, left atrium, main/left pulmonary artery, or coronary sinus) to obtain the various views for the transseptal puncture and device placement. For device deployment, the catheter must be placed in the left atrium and multiple views obtained ("mitral," "aortic," and "pulmonic" views). In case of ICE utilization, pre-procedural imaging is mandatory, and CTA is strongly recommended.

Access and Transseptal Approach

We consider ultrasound-guided venous access and micropuncture technique to be best practice for LAAC. Ultrasound-guided vascular access can be obtained through either common femoral vein (CFV), though the right CFV is more commonly used as it is more proximate for the operator. If ICE guidance is used, separate access should be obtained in the CFV and may be obtained on the same vessel. Care must be taken to keep sufficient separation between the two access sites to avoid sheath interaction and to avoid creating a single large venotomy after sheath insertion, which may make post-procedure access site closure challenging. We routinely reserve the lower of the two accesses for ICE catheter sheath and place a 23 cm 8 French sheath to support a 2D 8 French ICE catheter. At procedure completion we typically use Perclose (Abbott Medical Laboratories, IL, USA) for the large venotomy (15 Fr) which houses the Watchman sheath and Vascade (Haemonetics, Boston, USA) for the smaller venotomy (8 Fr) used for ICE catheter.

The transseptal device sheath can be advanced directly through the primary site, or alternatively a long 12 Fr venous sheath may be used to overcome venous tortuosity and facilitate transseptal access and delivery sheath manipulation.

Accurate site-specific transseptal puncture allows optimal orientation of the delivery sheath in relation to the LAA anatomy and is essential for a successful procedure. Transseptal puncture may be performed using a variety of catheter systems: SL-1, SL-0 sheath with BRK-1 needle (Abbott Vascular), Baylis NRG needle (Baylis Medical), or VersaCross RF needle system (Baylis Medical). As compared to mechanical transseptal systems, RF system can improve the TSP time and may be associated with better overall success of TSP. Typically, a posterior and inferior site in the atrial septum is preferred in most cases. In select cases, like a reverse chicken-wing anatomy, a more anterior puncture may be needed. To achieve this, TEE biplane short axis with bicaval view is ideal to simultaneously assess anterior-posterior and superior-inferior location. When using ICE, the transseptal sheath dilator is descended under fluoroscopic and ICE guidance on the septum with SVC on the superior aspect of the ICE septal view and IVC inferiorly. Then clockwise (posterior) or counterclockwise (anterior) rotation is used to optimize the location of transseptal sheath dilator tip. The short axis of the aorta indicates too anterior location, and the descending aorta may indicate too posterior of a location. Acceptable locations show LAA or pulmonary vein in the far field. The ideal TSP site should be carefully identified before needle advancement or RF energy application.

The deployment of the Watchman device can be attempted when the patient has a PFO or an existing ASD. However, in these circumstances, the recommended approach is to use a traditional transseptal approach and not attempt going through a PFO or ASD which may be too anterior and superior for coaxial sheath position in the LAA. Prior TSP procedures with excessive scarring of the IAS, thickened IAS and lipomatous hypertrophy, and prior surgical ASD/PFO patch repair can all pose challenges. Significant tortuosity of the IVC or the presence of an IVC filter can also pose a challenge, though it may be overcome with the use of a long sheath (e.g., 45 cm).

Intravenous heparin is administered to maintain an activated clotting time (ACT) of over 250–300 seconds to prevent thrombotic complications. The initial recommended dose to achieve therapeutic levels is 100 U/kg, and further additional doses are administered if required based on ACT readings. A full dose of heparin at the beginning of the procedure or a half-dose before and half-dose after transseptal puncture strategy can be employed for procedural anticoagulation. Routine measures, like frequent flushing of the catheters and scheduled intermittent ACT checks, are recommended for additional heparin administration.

Planning for Transseptal Puncture

Pre-procedure TEE or CTA imaging allows detailed transseptal puncture planning, as depicted in Fig. 12.2. For this, the interatrial septum is first aligned in two of three planes with one plane axis across the septum and the other through the appendage. In this way, the interatrial septum may be surveyed allowing for the most ideal puncture site to be chosen for coaxial device delivery. The correct orientation of the catheter should be coplanar with the axis of the principal LAA lobe, and generally, an inferior and posterior transseptal puncture is best for LAAC. However, the interatrial septum may not have ideal thickness at this location. In addition, some LAA anatomies are suitable for mid-septal or even anterior puncture. By selective image processing, it is possible to simulate multiple sites of transseptal punctures, to understand the optimal site where that catheter should cross the interatrial septum, and even to select the ideal delivery catheter for a given LAA anatomy.

Delivery Sheath Positioning

Following transseptal puncture, a long stiff exchange wire with a soft tip or a stiff body spiral wire is placed in the LUPV. RUPV may also be used for wire placement in some cases. Rarely the spiral wire can be cautiously kept in the LA itself, particularly if the septum is thin and dilated easily. Afterwards, the Watchman delivery sheath is advanced carefully under fluoroscopic and echocardiographic guidance. The wire and the delivery sheath dilator are always kept away from the LAA to avoid perforation. As the dilator and the wire are removed, the position of the sheath is optimized. The delivery sheath comes in various shapes which includes single curve, anterior curve, double curve, and the most recently fixed curve. In our center the fixed curve 15F sheath is exclusively used. Next, a 5–6 Fr angled pigtail catheter is advanced in the LAA, over which the sheath is positioned at the ostium of the LAA to facilitate angiographic evaluation. We do not recommend advancing the sheath over a wire, as the wire may cause injury to the appendage. In most cases, the RAO 30°–cranial 20° view reasonably shows the ostium and the neck of the appendage, whereas the RAO 30°–caudal 20° view reasonably depicts the mid-distal LAA anatomy in its widest axis. The RAO 30°/cranial 20° and RAO 30°/caudal 20° perspectives typically align with the 45° and 135° TEE views, respectively. In reality, the optimum fluoroscopic projection differs in each case and can be easily and accurately determined by CT. Baseline CT also helps in case of difficult anatomies. Appendage angiography can be performed using hand injection of 7–10 cc of contrast and allows for further anatomic understanding of the LAA. Using a still frame of a full opacified appendage, a dry erase marker can delineate the appendage and demarcate a landing zone on the monitor screen to assist with device deployment.

Device Preparation and Deployment

Device preparation is performed based on the step-by-step instructions available online at abbottmentor.com. The core purpose is to de-air the system properly. Device preparation is performed after the Watchman delivery sheath has been positioned, pigtail angiography has been performed, and device size has been finalized. As the pigtail is removed, the delivery sheath position is further optimized to be placed minimally beyond the LAA ostium. The device is prepared to remove the air from the system. This may be performed by flushing the device with a 60 cc syringe while keeping the distal tip of the device submerged in saline. However, we find continuous flushing from a high-pressure saline bag to be more effective. For this method, the tip of the Watchman delivery catheter is covered with a fingertip, the hemostatic valve at the back of the catheter is loosened, and the core wire is withdrawn to first back-flush the device. Then the hemostatic valve is tightened, and a needle driver or a Kelly forceps is used to tap the whole delivery catheter to ensure de-airing of the whole system with continuous saline flush running. Air bubbles may adhere to the delivery cable or harbor within the plastic connector system. The core wire is then advanced to align with the radio-opaque delivery sheath marker. Once prepared, the device is carefully introduced into the sheath in a wet-to-wet manner opposing back-flow bleeding from the delivery sheath and forward flush through the device loader. Once inside, the hemostatic valve is tightened, and the flush is stopped. As the device is advanced, one should avoid counterclockwise rotation of the delivery cable to prevent the device from disconnecting inside the delivery sheath. Upon the device reaching the right atrium, a brief fluoroscopic check is advised to ensure there is no air inside the sheath.

The device is advanced until the radio-opaque marker bands of the inner and outer sheaths align, and the outer sheath is pulled back to securely lock onto the delivery catheter with a "snap." This married system is then slowly unsheathed back over a fixed core wire to form a "ball" device configuration in which the ball diameter is roughly twice the delivery sheath diameter. In ball configuration, the system may be safely advanced as a unit or even rotated within the LAA to achieve an ideal position. Once positioned, the Watchman device is deployed most often by a combination of unsheathing the device and advancing the core wire to maintain the desired position. Caution must be taken not to push the device aggressively against the back wall to prevent appendage injury (Fig. 12.3a, b).

Before the device release, the following "PASS" criteria have been defined to ensure adequate deployment:

1. "P"—"Position"
2. "A"—"Anchoring"
3. "S"—"Sizing"
4. "S"—"Sealing".

Position includes whether the device is not too proximal to have a significant shoulder on echocardiography or too deep that it misses a proximal lobe.

Anchor assessment involves testing that the device will maintain its position due to appropriately engaged anchors. This is confirmed by performing a "tug test," where under fluoro/cine and echo visualization, the core wire is gently tugged upon. The tug both tests device stability and helps to engage the anchors. There should be a gentle pull on the device in which the face of the device everts slightly and snaps back to position. A too strong of a tug can overpower the anchors, move the device

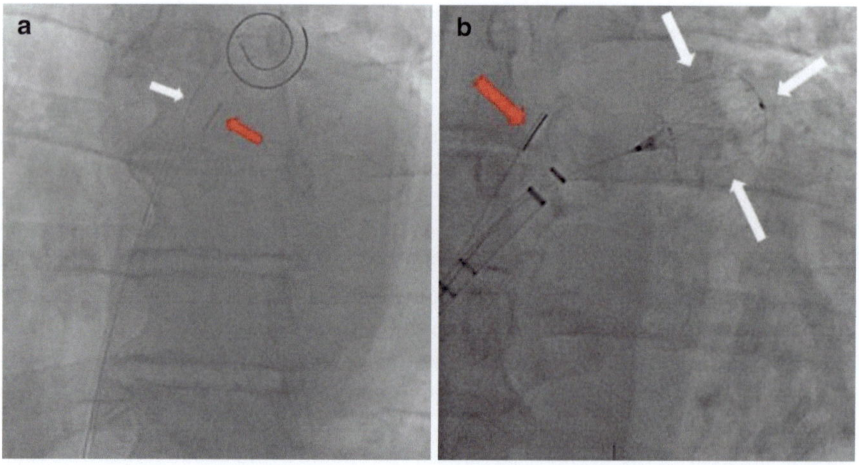

Fig. 12.3 Example of deployment of the Watchman FLX device. **Panel A:** both Baylis wire (white arrow) and ICE catheter (red arrow) in the left atrium. **Panel B:** white arrows showing the final position of the device. Red arrow showing the ICE catheter for assessment of "PASS" criteria

proximally, and potentially damage the LAA. A well-anchored device will maintain its original position after the tug test.

Sizing entails that the device has appropriate compression between the 10% and 30% range, confirmed in at least two echocardiographic views. At our center we target compression at 15–25%.

Seal implies that there is no significant flow around the device into the appendage. This is determined by color Doppler flow imaging of the device and contrast injection through the sheath. At times, there might be a shallow flow between the tissue and the sealing fabric of the device, a "gutter," which is different from a leak that extends all the way beyond the sealing fabric. In some centers, very small leaks (<3 mm) have been considered acceptable, but recent data has shown that any leak may increase the risk of future thromboembolic events. Thus, attention is paid to make sure that no leak is present prior to device release. Our practice is to ensure zero leak prior to device release, and this is almost always achievable with the FLX design.

Once satisfied the device is released with three to five counterclockwise turns on the core wire. Once released the core wire is quickly pulled back into the sheath to avoid injury to LA with the core wire tip and engagement of the core wire with the fabric on the face of the device. It is of utmost importance that the pericardial space be assessed before the end of the procedure by ICE or TEE. The final images should be compared to the initial images. In addition, many operators opt for a final limited transthoracic echocardiogram before the patient is discharged home for the assessment of pericardial effusion. At the end of the procedure, the sheaths and delivery system are removed, and hemostasis is obtained for the femoral vein via manual compression, closing with vascular closure device (Perclose), or via figure-of-eight suturing. For smaller sheaths such as the 8Fr sheath site used for ICE, hemostasis can be obtained using manual compression or Vascade (Haemonetics, Boston, MA). In addition, we also administer 50 mg of protamine sulfate at case completion.

Device Recapture

In difficult anatomies, several device deployments may be necessary to achieve an acceptable position. For this, a partial or full device recapture is often necessary. Device recapture is achieved by anchoring the core wire with the right hand and advancing the sheath forward over the device. Resheathing to ball (partial recapture) is often sufficient, but if there is concern about anchor engagement, a full recapture is achieved by completely advancing the sheath over the device. In this scenario, the same protocol of device deployment is repeated. Care should be undertaken not to allow the core wire to be counterclockwise rotated during recapture, as this can lead to inadvertent device separation. If there is concern for this, a gentle 20° clockwise rotation of the core wire can test the system connectivity. If more than three recaptures are required, exchanging for a new device may be advisable.

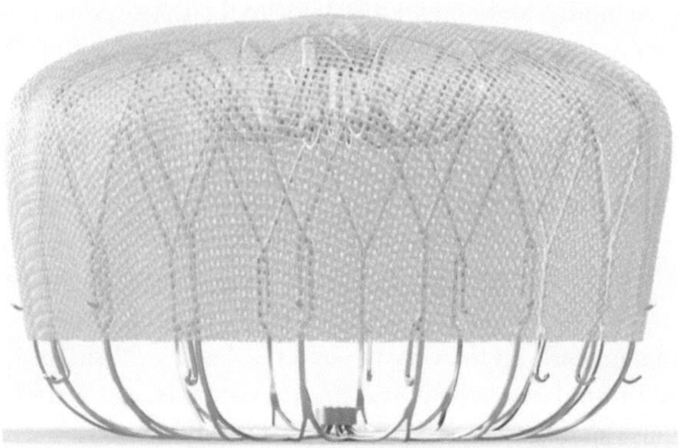

Fig. 12.4 Watchman FLX Pro device. (Image provided courtesy of Boston Scientific. © 2024 Boston Scientific Corporation or its affiliates. All rights reserved)

Future Perspectives: Watchman FLX Pro Device

Watchman FLX Pro device is now available (Fig. 12.4). It has an option of a 40 mm size (along with 20 mm, 24 mm, 27 mm, 31 mm, and 35 mm sizes), hemocoat technology (hemocompatible material coat to facilitate rapid and complete endothelialization), and three new radio-opaque markers for accurate device positioning and to aid in confirmation of stable position during the tug test. The Watchman FLX Pro device has shown decreased thrombogenicity (device-related thrombus (DRT)) in preclinical studies done on canine model as well as increased albumin binding which decreases platelet activation, reduces inflammation, and enhances endothelialization.

Conclusions

The Watchman™ FLX device offers significant improvements compared to its predecessor, Watchman™ 2.5, and demonstrates improved safety and procedural success with a wider variety of appendage anatomies. The Watchman FLX Pro device continues the evolution of the Watchman device through advancements in device coating, marker design, and larger size offering.

References and Suggested Readings

1. Agasthi P, Arsanjani R. Catheter management of left atrial appendage closure devices. [Updated 2023 Jun 12]. In: StatPearls [Internet]. Treasure Island (FL): StatPearls Publishing; 2023. Available from: https://www.ncbi.nlm.nih.gov/books/NBK557458/.
2. Dallan LAP, Bezerra HG, Cochet A, Kobayashi A, Attizzani GF, Rashid I, Rajagopalan S, Simon DI, Shishehbor MH, Arruda M, Filby SJ. Safety, efficacy, and cost-effectiveness of same-day discharge for left atrial appendage occlusion. J Invasive Cardiol. 2022;34(2):E124–31.

3. Dallan LAP, Arruda M, Yoon SH, Rana MA, Mogalapalli A, Carneiro HA, Reed J, Rashid I, Rajagopalan S, Filby SJ. Novel computed tomography angiography-based sizing methodology for WATCHMAN FLX device in left atrial appendage closure. J Cardiovasc Electrophysiol. 2022;33(8):1781–7.
4. De Backer O, Iriart X, Kefer J, et al. Impact of computational modeling on transcatheter left atrial appendage closure efficiency and outcomes. J Am Coll Cardiol Intv. 2023;16(6):655–66.
5. Enriquez A, Saenz LC, Rosso R, Silvestry FE, Callans D, Marchlinski FE, Garcia F. Use of Intracardiac echocardiography in interventional cardiology: working with the anatomy rather than fighting it. Circulation. 2018;137(21):2278–94. https://doi.org/10.1161/CIRCULATIONAHA.117.031343.
6. Filby SJ, Dallan LAP, Cochet A, et al. Left atrial appendage occlusion using cardiac CT angiography and Intracardiac echocardiography: a prospective. Single-Center Study J Invasive Cardiol. 2021;33(11):E851–6.
7. Freitas-Ferraz AB, Bernier M, Vaillancourt R, et al. Safety of transesophageal echocardiography to guide structural cardiac interventions. J Am Coll Cardiol. 2020;75:3164–73.
8. Lopez-Minguez JR, Gonzalez-Fernandez R, Fernandez-Vegas C, Millan-Nunez V, Fuentes-Canamero ME, Nogales-Asensio JM, Doncel-Vecino J, Yuste Dominguez M, Garcia Serrano L, Sanchez Quintana D. Comparison of imaging techniques to assess appendage anatomy and measurements for left atrial appendage closure device selection. J Invasive Cardiol. 2014;26:462–7.
9. Nadeem F, Igwe C, Stoycos S, et al. A new WATCHMAN sizing algorithm utilizing cardiac CTA. Cardiovasc Revasc Med. 2021;33:13–9. https://doi.org/10.1016/j.carrev.2021.01.009.
10. Naksuk N, Padmanabhan D, Yogeswaran V, Asirvatham SJ. Left atrial appendage: embryology, anatomy, physiology, arrhythmia and therapeutic intervention. JACC Clin Electrophysiol. 2016;2(4):403–12. https://doi.org/10.1016/j.jacep.2016.06.006. Epub 2016 Aug 15.
11. Ribeiro J, Teixeira R, Puga L, et al. Comparison of intracardiac and transesophageal echocardiography for guidance of percutaneous left atrial appendage occlusion: a meta-analysis. Echocardiography. 2019;00:1–8.
12. Saw J, Lopes JP, Reisman M, et al. Cardiac computed tomography angiography for left atrial appendage closure. Can J Cardiol. 2016;32:1033.e1–9.
13. Saw J, Fahmy P, Spencer R, et al. Comparing measurements of CT angiography, TEE, and fluoroscopy of the left atrial appendage for percutaneous closure. J Cardiovasc Electrophysiol. 2016;27:414–22.
14. Saw J, Holmes DR, Cavalcante JL, et al. SCAI/HRS expert consensus statement on Transcatheter left atrial appendage closure. J Soc Cardiovasc Angiogr Interv. 2023;2:100577. https://doi.org/10.1016/j.jscai.2022.100577.
15. Wang DD, Eng M, Kupsky D, et al. Application of 3-dimensional computed tomographic image guidance to Watchman implantation and impact on early operator learning curve: single-center experience. JACC Cardiovasc Interv. 2016;9:2329–40.

Chapter 13
The AMULET Left Atrial Appendage Closure Device: Technical Considerations and Procedural Approach

Tuna Ustunkaya and Christopher R. Ellis

Abbreviations

ACP	Amplatzer Cardiac Plug
ACT	Activated clotting time
ASD	Atrial septal defect
DRT	Device-related thrombus
ICE	Intracardiac echocardiography
LA	Left atrium
LAA	Left atrial appendage
LAAO	Left atrial appendage occlusion
LAO	Left anterior oblique
LPV	Left pulmonary vein
LUPV	Left upper pulmonary vein
LVEF	Left ventricular ejection fraction
LZ	Landing zone
OAC	Oral anticoagulation
PDL	Peri-device leak
PFO	Patent foramen ovale
RAO	Right anterior oblique
TEE	Transesophageal echocardiogram

Highlights
- In-depth look at the Amulet LAAO device design.
- Comparative anatomy, clinical indications, unique considerations.
- Detailed discussion on optimal procedural steps for device implantation and complication management.

T. Ustunkaya · C. R. Ellis (✉)
Division of Cardiovascular Medicine, Vanderbilt Heart and Vascular Institute, Vanderbilt University Medical Center, Nashville, TN, USA
e-mail: christopher.ellis@vumc.org

S. J. Filby et al. (eds.), *A Contemporary Manual of Left Atrial Appendage Closure*, https://doi.org/10.1007/978-3-031-68441-8_13

Introduction

The Amplatzer™ Amulet™ Left Atrial Appendage (LAA) Occluder (Abbott Medical, Inc.) is a percutaneous device designed to lower the risk of thrombus embolization from the LAA in patients with nonvalvular atrial fibrillation (AF) [1]. Amulet retains the core framework of the index Amplatzer Cardiac Plug™ (ACP) while aiming to enhance operational efficiency and bolster safety aspects, resulting in improvements in sealing and stability. The Amplatzer™ Amulet™ device consists of a self-expanding nitinol mesh anchoring lobe inserted into the LAA with paired stabilizing wires connected to a covering disc that seals the LAA ostium. The lobe and disc of the Amulet are connected by a central waist and contain a polyester fabric layer to facilitate tissue ingrowth.

In comparison to ACP, the Amulet disc diameter is wider, measuring 6–7 mm greater than the distal lobe diameter. Furthermore, the distal lobe is thicker, by 2–3 mm more than the ACP (7.5 mm tall in 16–22 mm device, 10 mm tall in 25–34 mm device). The stabilizing wires are stiffer and more numerous, increasing from 6 pairs in the ACP to up to 10 pairs in the Amulet. The waist length is longer, ranging from 5.5 mm to 8 mm depending on the device's size. Additionally, the Amulet incorporates an inverted attaching screw on the proximal disc (see Fig. 13.1).

ACP/AMULET DESIGN FEATURE COMPARISON

Feature	ACP								Amulet							
Sizes (mm)	16	18	20	22	24	26	28	30	16	18	20	22	25	28	31	34
Disc Ø	Lobe + 4mm				Lobe + 6mm				Lobe + 6mm				Lobe + 7mm			
Lobe Length	6.5mm								7.5mm				10mm			
Waist Length	4mm								5.5mm				8mm			
# SW Pairs	6								6		8			10		
Oversizing	1.5-3.0mm								3-5mm				3-6mm			
Sheath (Fr)	9	10			13				12 or 14 (w/adapter)					14		
Disc End Screw	Protruding								Recessed							
PKG	Partially pre-loaded								Fully pre-loaded							

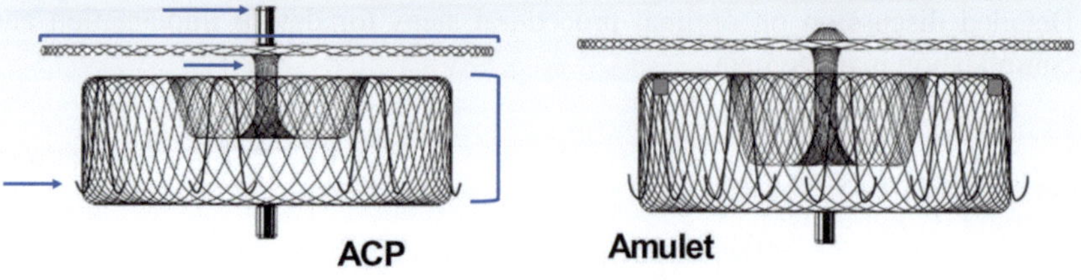

Fig. 13.1 ACP and Amulet LAAO device differences. Blue arrows and brackets highlight the components of ACP that were changed to the current Amulet LAAO device. (Courtesy of Abbott Medical, Inc.)

The Amulet IDE trial demonstrated the non-inferiority of the Amulet™ LAA Occluder device to the Watchman 2.5 device (Boston Scientific, Inc.) in 1878 patients who were randomized either to Watchman or Amulet. In the trial, 98.8% of the patients achieved the primary mechanism of action endpoint (<5 mm of residual jet around the device) in the Amulet arm compared to 96.8% in the Watchman arm, which met the non-inferiority margin and garnered FDA approval for Amulet device in 2021 [2]. The 3-year outcomes from the Amulet IDE study demonstrated that there are no significant differences in ischemic stroke or systemic embolism (5.0% vs. 4.6%), all-cause mortality (11.1% vs. 12.7%), or major bleeding (16.1% vs. 14.7%) between Amulet and Watchman recipients, respectively. Ischemic stroke preceded by DRT or PDL was numerically lower in the Amulet group (5 events vs. 20 events in the Watchman group) [3].

Patients with Watchman had more peri-device leaks (PDL) >3 mm at 12 months follow-up compared to Amulet (22% vs 9%). Patients with a PDL >3 mm had a higher composite stroke, systemic embolism, or CV death (8.1% vs 4.7%) at the 18-month follow-up timepoint compared to patients with no significant PDL 0–2 mm (HR 1.75, CI 10.8–2.83) [4]. Complications from implant were higher in the Amulet group including device embolization (6 with Amulet, 2 with Watchman) and pericardial effusions (22 with Amulet, 11 with Watchman), with a unique issue of delayed pericardial effusion >2 days post-implant in the Amulet group. Avoidance of these complications, optimal patient anatomy selection, and details of implant technique will be discussed further.

Patient Selection

The Amplatzer™ Amulet™ LAA Occluder device is FDA approved for patients with increased CHA_2DS_2-VASc scores of 3–9 and an indication to avoid long-term systemic OAC. The presence of active LAA thrombi at the time of the implant procedure is a relative contraindication and in specific situations, and ad hoc LAAO procedure might be considered appropriate. LAAO is contraindicated when there is active endocarditis or other systemic infections until adequately treated. Additionally, rare circumstances involving extreme LAA dimensions may also preclude LAAO placement (< 11 mm LAA landing zone (LZ), <12 mm implant depth, > 31 mm LZ measurement). Attempted LAAO in the setting of a mechanical ASD closure or PFO closure device or IVC filter is relatively contraindicated [5].

Anatomical LAA Features that Are Advantageous for Amulet

The Amulet device overall sits more proximally than Watchman and as such can provide adequate LAA closure (LAAC) in situations where large mid-cavitary pectinates may push a LAAC device forward. Cases with an extremely elliptical LAA orifice with extensive pits along the LPV–LAA ridge, which may remain uncovered by Watchman FLX, also may be appropriate to select Amulet upfront. Amulet devices are especially preferred when the co-axial implant depth is <15 mm as the uncompressed lobe height is only 7.5 mm with 16–22 mm devices and 1 cm with larger 25–34 mm devices. The chicken wing LAA anatomy and the Swan LAA anatomy are often preferable to start with Amulet first as distal retraction and shift of Watchman FLX may pull the FLX device deep leaving a PDL, and, when too proximal, flow can persist under or around the fabric cap. The Amulet lobe can be positioned in the proximal bend of the Swan LAA, and the disc can sit on the ostium proper supported by angulation of the device from the PV ridge to MV annulus (See Fig. 13.2). Additionally, consideration of pericardial effusion or pulmonary artery injury risk based on the location of lobe and stabilizing wires may advise avoiding Amulet LAAO in certain cases ("cuddling" lobe). Thickness of the LAA tissue <2 mm, lack of space in transverse sinus between PA and LAA in 135 TEE view, and oversized Amulet device may increase pericardial effusion risk [6, 7].

Medical Characteristics that Are Advantageous for Amulet

There are certain scenarios where patients' comorbidities can lead to preferential selection of Amulet over Watchman. One such is CAD with recent stent placement. As these patients are on DAPT regardless, placement of Amulet does not change the anticoagulation management compared to Watchman FLX (though DAPT label with Watchman FLX is now deemed suitable). Similarly, patients with a prior history of intracranial hemorrhage may benefit from refraining from any OAC regimen; hence Amulet may be preferred given the somewhat lower reported rates of

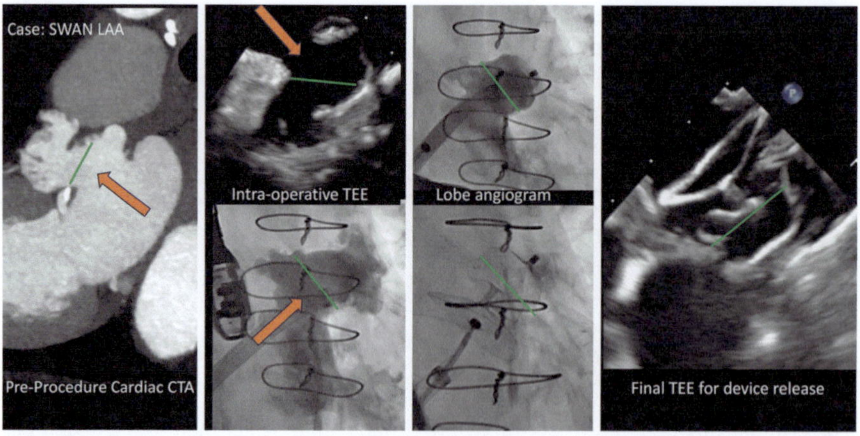

Fig. 13.2 Swan LAA example with Amulet. Green line = LZ. Orange arrows denote LAA orifice for disc position. Note complex trabeculae on PV ridge

device-related thrombus (DRT). On the other hand, Amulet placement tends to require more contrast, longer procedure, and fluoroscopy time, and hence frail patients and those with renal failure may benefit from Watchman FLX placement over Amulet.

Device Sizing

The Amulet LAAC device comes in eight different sizes (16, 18, 20, 22, 25, 28, 31, and 34 mm). The Amulet can be implanted in an LAA LZ (neck) diameter ranging from 11 to 31 mm and requires an LAA depth of at least 12 mm. Amulet sizes ranging from 16 to 22 mm possess a lobe length of 7.5 mm, a waist length of 5.5 mm, and six pairs of stabilizing wires [8]. Contrarily, sizes from 25 to 34 mm feature a lobe length of 10 mm, a waist length of 8 mm, and eight or 10 pairs of stabilizing wires. Furthermore, for 16–22 mm devices, the disc is 6 mm larger than the lobe; for 25–34 mm devices, the disc is 7 mm larger than the lobe. It is imperative to appreciate that subtle changes in the measurement angle or dimension may quickly affect the optimal device size to implant. Figure 13.3 shows the optimal TEE LZ and disc orifice measurement for sizing in contrast to the location of the ostial Watchman LAAO.

Amulet needs to be oversized to allow lobe compression at the LZ. A tighter range of LZ measurement should be adhered to avoid significant "low" compression (embolization risk, incomplete LAA closure) or "over" compression (potential for

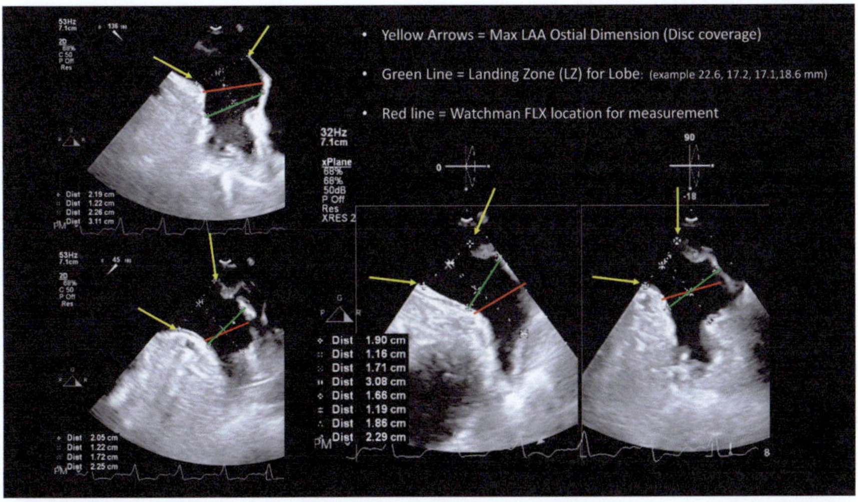

Fig. 13.3 TEE measurement of target LZ, LAA ostium, and implant orientation in comparison to Watchman FLX. Green line = Amulet LZ. Red line = Watchman measurement location. Yellow arrows denote LAA orifice

erosion or reduced anchor engagement). Device sizing with CT angiography has excellent spatial resolution and 3D abilities and when done under adequate loading conditions, whereas TEE and ICE have the advantage of providing real-time evaluation during the procedure. Factors such as contractility and LAA dimension change with volume load, or LAA stretch with device placement may alter final device selection. There is usually strong agreement (i.e., <2 mm difference) between the imaging modality at corresponding positions. When significant disparity arises, it's crucial to appreciate differences in static versus dynamic or live images (typically CTA provides a larger estimation of LZ and final device size used versus TEE).

LZ/neck diameter is the primary factor in sizing provided the disc is large enough to cover the ostium. The ostial measurement spans the tip of the LPV–LAA ridge ideally to the LAA edge at the mitral annular aspect; from this line, a second measurement is made 10–12 mm into the LAA, coaxial to the neck, for LZ measurement (see Fig. 13.3). For sizing, a standard recommendation is to upsize the Amulet by 3–6 mm. The official Amplatzer™ Amulet™ LAA Occluder sizing chart refers to the maximum LAA landing zone width using 2D imaging modalities which most operators typically use (see Fig. 13.4) [5–8].

There are scenarios where over- or under-sizing even further than recommended may be helpful. One such scenario is oval/elliptical LAA anatomies. When the LZ is quite elliptical (>2:1 long to short axis), the largest width should be considered as the Amulet device size, and operators should be cautious for oversizing as excessive

IMAGING AND SIZING

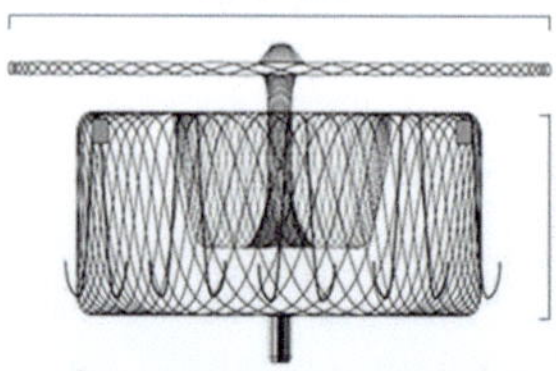

Device Selection

MAXIMUM LANDING ZONE WIDTH (mm)	AMULET™ DEVICE SIZE	LOBE LENGTH (mm)	MINIMUM LAA DEPTH (mm)	DISC DIAMETER (mm)	SHEATH DIAMETER
11.0 - 13.0	16	7.5	≥10	22	12 F or 14 F (with adaptor)
13.0 - 15.0	18	7.5	≥10	24	
15.0 - 17.0	20	7.5	≥10	26	
17.0 - 19.0	22	7.5	≥10	28	
19.0 - 22.0	25	10	≥12	32	
22.0 - 25.0	28	10	≥12	35	14 F
25.0 - 28.0	31	10	≥12	38	
28.0 - 31.0	34	10	≥12	41	

Fig. 13.4 Amulet sizing chart (courtesy of Abbott Medical, Inc.)

oversizing may lead to an over-compressed device. Similarly, a slight increase in size (around 1–2 mm beyond the sizing chart recommendation) might be contemplated when employing a smaller Amulet or in patients with prior sternotomy. An additional reason to oversize could be high LAA ostium/neck ratio, where a larger device disc might be necessary for proper coverage of the LAA ostium, provided space to deploy the corresponding lobe exists. Lastly, the larger lobes are more compliant and softer hence a wider size range for suitable compression.

Step by Step Implant

Before Puncture

General anesthesia or conscious sedation is employed during the procedure, primarily to alleviate the discomfort associated with the use of intraprocedural TEE. Considering potential risks of cardiac tamponade and anesthesia complications, invasive (femoral or radial) arterial pressure monitoring could help early management of hemodynamic instability, but most centers avoid arterial access.

Depending on the patient's clinical condition and volume status (LVEF, mitral regurgitation, and pulmonary pressures), administering 500–1000 cc of intravenous fluids can be helpful before TEE measurements to elevate mean left atrial pressure to >10 mmHg. This aims to ensure adequate LAA filling, reducing chances of device under-sizing and subsequent embolization. Esmolol or IV Metoprolol can transiently reduce contractility and heart rate allowing improved stability during Amulet deployment. Intravenous prophylactic antibiotics are typically given before and after the procedure, per institution protocol. Sterile patient preparation at the site of the venous access and procedure table for device preparation are essential [5, 9, 10].

Intraprocedural Imaging

Regarding intraprocedural imaging, TEE is the go-to for most operators. TEE is performed to rule out thrombus, identify pericardial effusion before the procedure, and assess the mitral valve function and the patency of the LUPV. This is followed by baseline LAA measurements. Scanning the LAA from 0° to 135°, TEE should carefully determine the maximum and minimum diameters of the ostium and LZ.

While not mandatory, real-time 3D TEE is beneficial for improved spatial visualization of the anatomy. Comparative studies between 2D and real-time 3D TEE have demonstrated the greater accuracy and reproducibility of real-time 3D TEE in assessing the LAA orifice size. During the final steps of the procedure, 3D TEE aids in assessing the disc's relationship with surrounding structures within the left atrium, notably mitral valve and PV ridge.

An alternative to TEE is intracardiac echocardiography (ICE), which can eliminate general anesthesia. The ICE catheter can be inserted through the femoral vein and positioned in the right atrium, LA, main or left pulmonary artery, or coronary sinus at baseline. 2D ICE presently lacks the ability to capture images from multiple angles at a single ICE probe location. ICE may appear to over accentuate the presence of "smoke" or spontaneous echo contrast (SEC) and sludge affecting the ability to exclude thrombus. ICE for LAAC deployment should be placed in the LA (LPV, mid-LA, sub-mitral view) [9, 10].

Access and Transseptal Approach

After baseline imaging, ultrasound-guided vascular access is obtained through the right femoral vein. A 3–4 mm skin incision and subcutaneous separation of the access site can be performed to ease advancement of the transseptal and delivery sheath. Use of a 16–18 Fr long central venous sheath (20–40 cm long Cook Medical Check-Flow, or Gore Medical Dry-Seal) can facilitate transseptal and delivery sheath manipulation and overcome proximal venous tortuosity. This is particularly useful in obese patients, or those with significant scoliosis, or potentially in cases (off-label) when an IVC filter is present. The sheath should be hooked to a continuous flush line to avoid thrombus formation within the long sheath.

Transseptal puncture is conducted using standard methodology employing an SL-1, SL-0 sheath with BRK-1 needle (Abbott Vascular), Baylis NRG needle (Boston Scientific Inc.), or now preferably with the Versa-cross RF needle system (Boston Scientific, Inc.). Precise placement of the transseptal puncture is pivotal for a successful procedure to properly orient the delivery sheath in relation to LAA ostium. The mid-inferior site in the atrial septum is considered optimal in most cases. To achieve this, TEE biplane short axis with bicaval view is ideal to simultaneously assess anterior-posterior and superior-inferior location. Ideal site will show needle tenting toward the LAA or LPV ridge. Needle advancement or RF energy should not be applied until the ideal location is identified with stable needle position. ICE orientation may differ, and a view in which the ostium of the LAA is a visible target while the inferior limbus of the atrial septum is in view is ideal.

A more anterior puncture may be needed in reverse chicken wing anatomy with a more anterior ostium. If the patient has a PFO or an existing ASD, deployment of an Amulet device may still be attempted; however, a traditional transseptal approach should always be pursued (do not attempt through a PFO). Lipomatous hypertrophy, multiple prior TSP access procedures (i.e., AF ablations), and prior surgical ASD/PFO patch repair can lead to a challenging transeptal puncture.

To avoid thrombus formation on wires, sheaths, or the device within the potentially fibrillating environment of the LA or LAA, intravenous heparin is administered to maintain an activated clotting time (ACT) of over 250–300 s. Initial recommended dose to achieve therapeutic levels are 100–120 IU/kg. Depending on the operator preference and anticipated difficulty of transseptal puncture, either a full dose upfront or half-dose before and half-dose after transseptal puncture strategy can be employed. Frequent flushing of the catheter is advised, and if the procedure lasts >30 min, repeat heparin should be administered as necessary to maintain the ACT in range [5, 9, 10].

Fluoroscopic Calibration

Following transseptal puncture, a long stiff exchange wire in the LUPV, or a spiral wire in the LA, is used to cautiously exchange to the Torque View 45–45 12Fr or 14Fr Amulet delivery sheath. The tip of the Torque View sheath is then placed at the level of LAA ostium with a 5–6 Fr pigtail catheter in the LAA to obtain sheath injection LAA. The RAO 30°/cranial 20° view shows the ostium and the neck of the appendage, whereas the RAO 30°/caudal 20° view depicts better the mid-distal LAA anatomy in its widest axis. The RAO 30°/cranial 20° and RAO 30°/caudal 20° perspectives typically align with the 45° and 135° TEE views, respectively. Baseline CT also helps in case of difficult anatomy and is essential when performing an ICE-guided procedure. Use of CTA pre-procedure for Amulet has been shown to increase the chances of a single device deployment potentially shortening procedure times and reducing complications [5–7, 11].

Delivery Sheath Positioning

The selection of the delivery sheath size (either 12 or 14F) relies on the device size and is determined by the sizing chart (16–25 mm devices through the 12 Fr sheath, 28–34 mm devices through 14 Fr sheath). The conventional method of engaging the delivery sheath within the LAA is with a pigtail catheter, similar to Watchman implantation. However, more recently, a preferred approach involves the extrusion of the Amulet lobe as a "ball" shape in the left atrium, followed by meticulous insertion into the LAA under TEE guidance. Once the "ball" is formed, the system can be advanced or withdrawn relatively safely within the proximal LAA to achieve optimal lobe position, advancing cable through the "triangle" position to the fully deployed lobe (see Fig. 13.5). A bare sheath should not be advanced without a pigtail leading or the Amulet in the ball position [9, 10].

Device Preparation and Deployment

Device preparation is performed based on the step-by-step instructions available online at abbottmentor.com. Device preparation typically occurs following the transseptal procedure and prior to the placement of the Torque Vue sheath in the

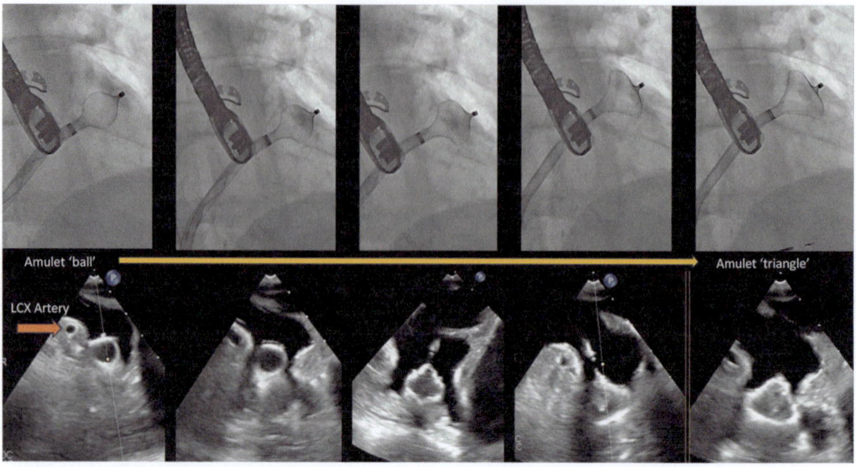

Fig. 13.5 Sequential deployment of the Amulet lobe from ball to triangle with simultaneous X-Ray and TEE view. Matched panels from left to right show gradual deployment with advancement of device cable while maintaining position in TEE biplane 45 and 135 degree view

LAA neck. The device introducer is carefully connected to the delivery sheath in a wet-to-wet manner opposing back-flow bleeding from the delivery sheath and forward flush through the device loader. Avoid counterclockwise rotation of the delivery cable to prevent the device from disconnecting inside the delivery sheath. Upon the device reaching the right atrium, a brief fluoroscopic check is advised to ensure there is no air inside the sheath.

RAO-cranial or RAO-caudal view visualizing and marking the LZ the best is the view of choice for device deployment. The delivery catheter is slowly unsheathed to expose the distal portion of the device to form the so-called "ball" with radiopaque markers aligned with the tip of the delivery sheath. To ensure proper alignment with the LAA LZ, a counterclockwise rotation of the sheath is typically necessary once the device is in place. Following the stable and optimal positioning of the sheath, the delivery cable is advanced without unsheathing to complete the deployment of the distal lobe. Failure to push the cable while continuing to unsheathe could lead to the emergence of the lobe in a more proximal position, potentially missing the LZ. The deployment of the proximal disc is then achieved by gently advancing the delivery cable while unsheathing the disc. Use of a steerable delivery sheath may allow more detailed positioning of the disc in relation to the PV ridge and provide better alignment of the cable to disc attachment, reducing any cable bias (Fig. 13.5).

Before device release, the following 5 "CLOSE" criteria have been defined to ensure adequate deployment:

1. "C" An adequate compression of the distal lobe to LAA wall
2. "L" Lobe position at least two-thirds distal to the left circumflex artery on TEE/ICE
3. "O" Orientation of the distal lobe in the axis of LAA neck axis (LZ)

4. "S" Separation between the proximal disc and the distal lobe
5. "E" Elliptical/concave shape of the disc for good seal.

After device is deployed, device stability is ensured placing the disc in tension (shaping it like an olive or football) by pulling away from the anchored lobe. After holding for at least 20–30 s, the tension on the delivery cable is released, allowing the device to return to its initial position. Heart contractions influence the device's placement, so providing a few minutes for the device to stabilize in its ultimate position is ideal before releasing it [5, 8].

After device deployment but before release, TEE (with lowered Nyquist limit at 50 cm/s) verification of the absence of peri-device leak is performed. TEE is also useful to exclude any interference with the surrounding structures (MV annulus, LPV). Once the operator confirms an optimal device position, imaging confirms adequate sealing, the "CLOSE" signs are re-verified, and the device is released by performing counterclockwise rotations (8–10 typically) of the delivery cable. TEE should then evaluate for pericardial effusion and iatrogenic ASD features.

At the end of the procedure, sheaths and delivery system are removed and hemostasis is obtained for the femoral vein via manual compression, pre-closing with a vascular closure device (Perclose) or via figure-of-eight suturing.

Repositioning/Recapturing the Device

Several scenarios can lead to suboptimal closure of the LAA, prompting the operator to consider repositioning the device. These scenarios include, but are not limited to:

- Excessive compression and deep positioning of the device lobe, which engages the entire distal LAA structure, avoid release if the lobe is 2× longer than the width of the lobe on X-Ray (see Fig. 13.6).
- An unstable or overly proximal lobe position after tension testing or disc placement.
- Inadequate compression in the lobe.
- Identification of a significant PDL (>3 mm) by Doppler US or contrast angiography around the lobe.
- Compression of the pulmonary vein or contact of the disc with the mitral valve annulus.
- The disc lying flat and contacting the lobe, or forming a very acute angle (<45 degrees) to the PV ridge which may increase risk of DRT (see Fig. 13.7).

During recapture to ball, the device can be repositioned and deployed in a new location. Should the device be entirely removed, the manufacturer advises replacing the delivery sheath before advancing a new device. However, in many cases, the original sheath can be used provided the tip is not damaged. If a new device is chosen, the reused sheath must accommodate its size [12, 13].

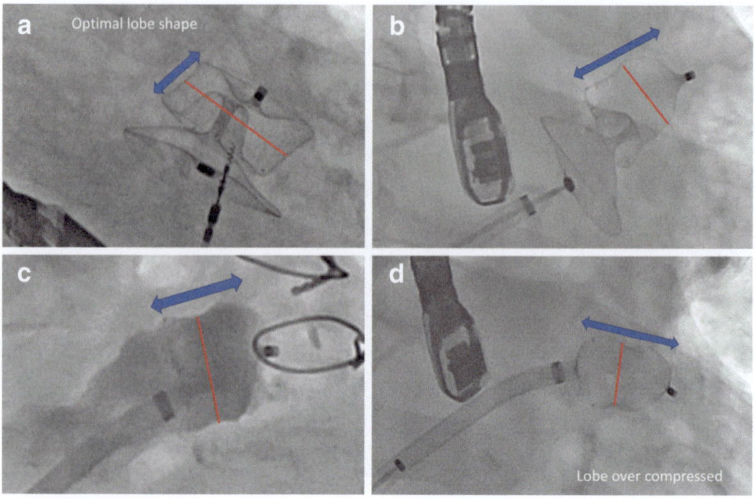

Fig. 13.6 Typical Amulet lobe compression, and assuring length (blue arrow) of the lobe does not exceed the lobe width (red line) by >2:1

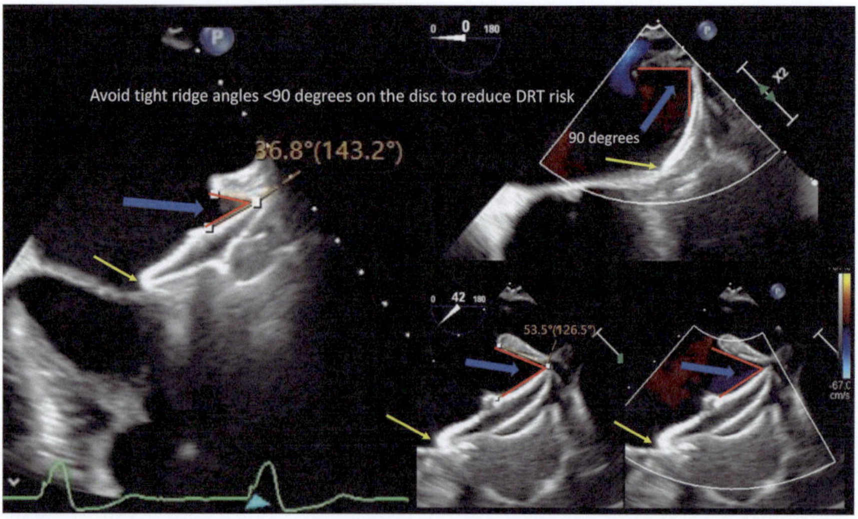

Fig. 13.7 Disc position that could warrant repositioning due to increased risk for DRT

Acute Complications and Management

Procedure-related complications occurred in 4.5% of the patients in the Amulet arm of the Amulet IDE trial. Primary drivers for the higher rate of procedure-related complications in the Amulet group were device embolization (DE) and pericardial effusion (PE). Thus, management of DE and PE are essential skills for implanters.

Most of the pericardial effusion in the IDE trial happened within the first 2 days (55%) and should be managed by pericardiocentesis and drain placement. Managing an acute effusion by reversing anticoagulation and placing a drainage system must be performed rapidly. It is also advisable to have on-site cardiothoracic surgery available at Amulet implant centers, primarily for the rare occurrence of Amulet embolization into the left ventricle, or ascending aorta, or in the setting of uncontrolled bleeding after pericardiocentesis [14, 15].

Device embolization occurred in 6 patients (0.6%) of the patients randomized in the Amulet trial largely due to proximal, under-compressed devices. In case of device embolization, the retrieval of an Amulet using a combination of a large bore (14Fr +) sheath in the left atrium (LA) with a gooseneck snare and GI Raptor grasping device (Steris Medical, Dublin, Ireland) through an AGILIS steerable 8Fr (Abbott Medical, Inc) is a feasible approach. As mentioned, if the former fails, patients may need emergent surgical evaluation (see Fig. 13.8) [5].

Fortunately, complications associated with airway or TEE are rare. To prevent complications, it is essential to pay careful attention to vascular access technique and transeptal access location, follow the "CLOSE" signs, exercise caution when moving sheaths and the device in the LA–LAA, and ensure proper device size and positioning.

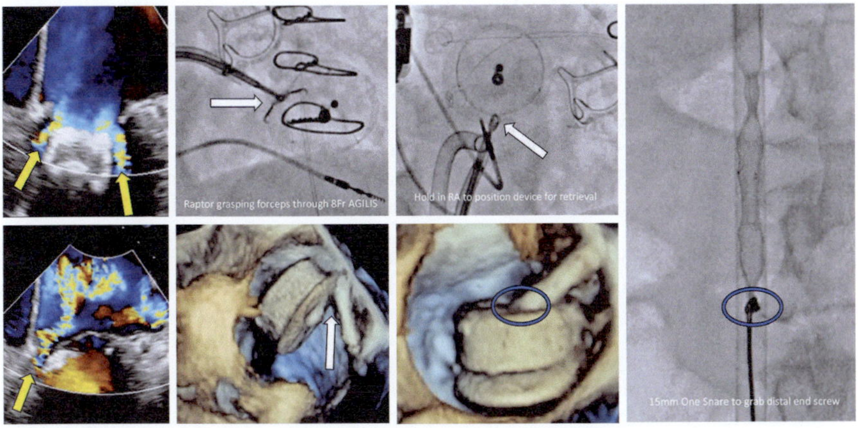

Fig. 13.8 Embolized Amulet LAAO device in the LV, retrieved with GI Raptor forceps, and One Snare due to acute mitral valve regurgitation. Yellow arrow = acute severe MR and flail leaflet. White arrows = GI Raptor grasping forceps (Steris Medical). Blue circle = site of gooseneck snare retrieval on distal end screw

Conclusion

The Amplatzer™ Amulet™ Left Atrial Appendage (LAA) Occluder device offers significant improvements compared to its predecessor ACP and provides another option for LAAO to the Watchman FLX (and now Watchman FLX PRO). The Amulet device has advantages in certain patient populations and LAA anatomies. Although a similar implant procedure to Watchman, the two-stage disc and lobe deployment, longer stabilizing wires, complex sizing grid, and more proximal location offer unique challenges to the operators who will implant these devices.

References[1]

1. January CT, Wann LS, Calkins H, Chen LY, Cigarroa JE, Cleveland JC Jr, Ellinor PT, Ezekowitz MD, Field ME, Furie KL, Heidenreich PA, Murray KT, Shea JB, Tracy CM, Yancy CW. AHA/ACC/HRS focused update of the 2014 AHA/ACC/HRS guideline for the management of patients with atrial fibrillation: a report of the American College of Cardiology/American Heart Association Task Force on Clinical Practice Guidelines and the Heart Rhythm Society. J Am Coll Cardiol. 2019;74(1):104–32. https://doi.org/10.1016/j.jacc.2019.01.011. Epub 2019 Jan 28. Erratum in: J Am Coll Cardiol. 2019 Jul 30;74(4):599. PMID: 30703431
2. Lakkireddy D, Thaler D, Ellis CR, Swarup V, Sondergaard L, Carroll J, Gold MR, Hermiller J, Diener HC, Schmidt B, MacDonald L, Mansour M, Maini B, O'Brien L, Windecker S. Amplatzer Amulet left atrial appendage occluder versus watchman device for stroke prophylaxis (Amulet IDE): A randomized, controlled trial. Circulation. 2021;144(19):1543–52. https://doi.org/10.1161/CIRCULATIONAHA.121.057063. Epub 2021 Aug 30. PMID: 34459659; PMCID: PMC8570346.
3. Lakkireddy D, Thaler D, Ellis CR, Swarup V, Gambhir A, Hermiller J, Nielsen-Kudsk JE, Worthley S, Nair D, Schmidt B, Horton R, Gupta N, Anderson JA, Gage R, Alkhouli M, Windecker S. 3-year outcomes from the Amplatzer Amulet left atrial appendage Occluder randomized controlled trial (Amulet IDE). JACC Cardiovasc Interv. 2023;16(15):1902–13. https://doi.org/10.1016/j.jcin.2023.06.022. PMID: 37587599
4. Price MJ, Ellis CR, Nielsen-Kudsk JE, Thaler D, Gupta N, Koulogiannis K, Anderson JA, Gage R, Lakkireddy D. Peridevice leak after Transcatheter left atrial appendage occlusion: an analysis of the Amulet IDE trial. JACC Cardiovasc Interv. 2022;15(21):2127–38. https://doi.org/10.1016/j.jcin.2022.09.001. PMID: 36357016
5. Ellis CR. Amplatzer Amulet™ left atrial appendage occluder: a step-by-step guide to device implantation. J Cardiovasc Electrophysiol 2022 33(8):1881–87. https://doi.org/10.1111/jce.15420. Epub 2022 Feb 28. PMID: 35175683.
6. Tzikas A, Gafoor S, Meerkin D, Freixa X, Cruz-Gonzalez I, Lewalter T, Saw J, Berti S, Nielsen-Kudsk JE, Ibrahim R, Lakkireddy D, Paul V, Arzamendi D, Nietlispach F, Worthley SG, Hildick-Smith D, Thambo JB, Tondo C, Aminian A, Kalarus Z, Schmidt B, Sondergaard L, Kefer J, Meier B, Park JW, Sievert H, Omran H. Left atrial appendage occlusion with the AMPLATZER Amulet device: an expert consensus step-by-step approach. EuroIntervention. 2016;11(13):1512–21. https://doi.org/10.4244/EIJV11I13A292. PMID: 27107315

[1] 5 key references are in BOLD.

7. Messas N, Ibrahim R. The Amplatzer Amulet device: technical considerations and procedural approach. Interv Cardiol Clin. 2018;7(2):213–8. https://doi.org/10.1016/j.iccl.2017.12.012. PMID: 29526289
8. Amplatzer Amulet Left Atrial Appendage Occluder IFU.
9. Clinical Cases in LAA Occlusion, Springer, 2018, Martin W. Bergmann, Apostolos Tzikas, Nina C. Wunderlich.
10. Saw J, Kar S, Price MJ. Left atrial appendage closure: mechanical approaches to stroke prevention in atrial fibrillation. Cham: Springer; 2016.
11. De Backer O, Iriart X, Kefer J, Nielsen-Kudsk JE, Aminian A, Rosseel L, Kofoed KF, Odenstedt J, Berti S, Saw J, Søndergaard L, Garot P. Impact of Computational modeling on transcatheter left atrial appendage closure efficiency and outcomes .JACC Cardiovasc Interv 2023 16(6):655–666. https://doi.org/10.1016/j.jcin.2023.01.008. Epub 2023 Feb 22.PMID: 36990554 Clinical Trial.
12. Lakkireddy D, Nielsen-Kudsk JE, Windecker S, Thaler D, Price MJ, Gambhir A, Gupta N, Koulogiannis K, Marcoff L, Mediratta A, Anderson JA, Gage R, Ellis CR. Mechanisms, predictors, and evolution of severe peri-device leaks with two different left atrial appendage occluders. Europace 2023 25(9):euad237. https://doi.org/10.1093/europace/euad237. PMID: 37584233.
13. Schmidt B, Nielsen-Kudsk JE, Ellis CR, Thaler D, Sabir SA, Gambhir A, Landmesser U, Shah N, Gray W, Swarup V, Lim DS, Koulogiannis K, Anderson JA, Gage R, Lakkireddy D. Incidence, predictors, and clinical outcomes of device-related thrombus in the Amulet IDE trial. JACC Clin Electrophysiol 2023 Jan;9(1):96–107. https://doi.org/10.1016/j.jacep.2022.07.014. Epub 2022 Sep 28. PMID: 36697204.
14. Simard T, Jung RG, Lehenbauer K, Piayda K, Pracoń R, Jackson GG, Flores-Umanzor E, Faroux L, Korsholm K, Chun JKR, Chen S, Maarse M, Montrella K, Chaker Z, Spoon JN, Pastormerlo LE, Meincke F, Sawant AC, Moldovan CM, Qintar M, Aktas MK, Branca L, Radinovic A, Ram P, El-Zein RS, Flautt T, Ding WY, Sayegh B, Benito-González T, Lee OH, Badejoko SO, Paitazoglou C, Karim N, Zaghloul AM, Agrawal H, Kaplan RM, Alli O, Ahmed A, Suradi HS, Knight BP, Alla VM, Panaich SS, Wong T, Bergmann MW, Chothia R, Kim JS, Pérez de Prado A, Bazaz R, Gupta D, Valderrabano M, Sanchez CE, El Chami MF, Mazzone P, Adamo M, Ling F, Wang DD, O'Neill W, Wojakowski W, Pershad A, Berti S, Spoon D, Kawsara A, Jabbour G, Boersma LVA, Schmidt B, Nielsen-Kudsk JE, Rodés-Cabau J, Freixa X, Ellis CR, Fauchier L, Demkow M, Sievert H, Main ML, Hibbert B, Holmes DR Jr, Alkhouli M. Predictors of Device-related thrombus following percutaneous left atrial appendage occlusion. J Am Coll Cardiol. 2021;78(4):297–313. https://doi.org/10.1016/j.jacc.2021.04.098. PMID: 34294267
15. Pracoń R, De Backer O, Konka M, Kępka C, Kruk M, Trochimiuk P, Dębski M, Dzielińska Z, Søndergaard L, Demkow M. Imaging risk features for device related pulmonary artery injury after left atrial appendage closure with Amplatzer™ Amulet™ device. Catheter Cardiovasc Inter. 2021;98(3):E420–6. https://doi.org/10.1002/ccd.29393. Epub 2020 Nov 21. PMID: 33220011

Chapter 14
Novel Percutaneous Left Atrial Appendage Closure Devices

Timothy Petrie, Shashank Jain, and Mauricio Arruda

Highlights Atrial fibrillation (AF) increases the risk of stroke and peripheral embolism-related deaths.

- Left atrial appendage occlusion (LAAO) is a IIa recommendation for non-valvular AF patients with high thromboembolic risk and contraindication for oral anticoagulation.
- The role of LAAO in stroke prevention and bleeding risk as compared to oral anticoagulation.
- Endocardial percutaneous transcatheter closure remains the most widely used and clinically tested method for LAAO.
- The Watchman and Amulet devices are currently the only two devices approved by the US Food and Drug Administration for clinical use. The ATRICLIP has been used for epicardial surgical LAA closure. Several newer devices are currently undergoing further investigation.

Introduction

Atrial fibrillation is one of the most common cardiac arrhythmias with an estimated 12 million patients in the United States by 2050 and an estimated prevalence of 18 million patients in Europe by 2060 [1]. This arrhythmia carries significant healthcare costs as well as an increased risk for stroke compared to the general population. Atrial fibrillation is estimated to be responsible for 25% of strokes that occur in the United States on an annual basis [2]. Patients with atrial fibrillation are asked to take

T. Petrie (✉)
Department of Electrophysiology, Southwest General Hospital, Middleburg Heights, OH, USA

S. Jain · M. Arruda
Department of Electrophysiology, University Hospitals Cleveland Medical Center, Cleveland, OH, USA

S. J. Filby et al. (eds.), *A Contemporary Manual of Left Atrial Appendage Closure*, https://doi.org/10.1007/978-3-031-68441-8_14

anticoagulation long term to prevent stroke. An estimated one-third of patients on newer direct oral anticoagulants for atrial fibrillation are said to be non-adherent at 2 years [2]. The newer anticoagulants can also carry a high burden of cost for patients. In addition, a significant population of patients cannot tolerate long-term anticoagulation because of bleeding, anemia, frequent falls, and other factors.

Novel Percutaneous Left Atrial Appendage Closure Devices

Mechanical occlusion of the LAA has emerged as an alternative to anticoagulation for stroke prevention in select patients [1]. The LAA is an attractive target for occlusion devices because more than 90% of thrombi originates from the appendage [2]. Multiple devices have been developed over the years for transcatheter LAA closure (Fig. 14.1). The Watchman Flx from Boston Scientific and Amplatzer Amulet from Abbott Vascular are currently the only two endocardial devices that have been approved by the US Food and Drug Administration (FDA) for clinical use [4]. Several other devices are in clinical trials or being actively used in Europe or China, as seen in Fig. 14.1.

Endocardial transcatheter closure remains the most widely used and clinically tested method for LAA closure [5]. The Watchman device from Boston Scientific was approved by the FDA in 2015 [1]. The Watchman is a parachute-shaped, self-expanding nitinol device with active fixation barbs and a permeable polyester membrane fabric in five sizes, ranging in diameter from 21 to 33 mm [1]. The sizes accommodate left atrial appendage ostia of 17 to 31 mm [1]. Device size is based on the maximum LAA ostium diameter, and oversizing by 10–20% is recommended [1]. The Watchman Flx device, an evolution of the original concept, has a 10–20% shorter length, eighteen struts versus the original ten, J-shaped anchors, and a closed distal end to minimize the risk for perforation during device placement [1]. The Flx device comes in five different sizes (from 20 to 35 mm) for LAA ostia measuring from 14 to 32 mm [1]. Polyethylene terephthalate membrane fabric extends distally on the device to reduce leaks and create a better seal [4]. The Watchman device currently remains the most studied of the LAA closure systems [4].

The Amplatzer Cardiac Plug from Abbott Vascular is a self-expanding nitinol device with a distal lobe and proximal disc, connected by a short central waist [1]. During implantation, the distal lobe looks around its circumference and anchors the device in the appendage, while the proximal disc occludes the ostium of the LAA [5]. The Amplatzer Amulet device is its successor [1]. The Amulet is available in eight different sizes (16–34 mm) fitting LAA sizes from 11 to 31 mm [1]. The distal lobe and device waist were lengthened to make the placement easier and more stable [5]. Polyester patches were sewn into the lobe and disc to aid with appendage occlusion [4]. Sizing is determined by the maximum landing zone at 10–12 mm from the ostium with oversizing recommended by 2–4 mm [1].

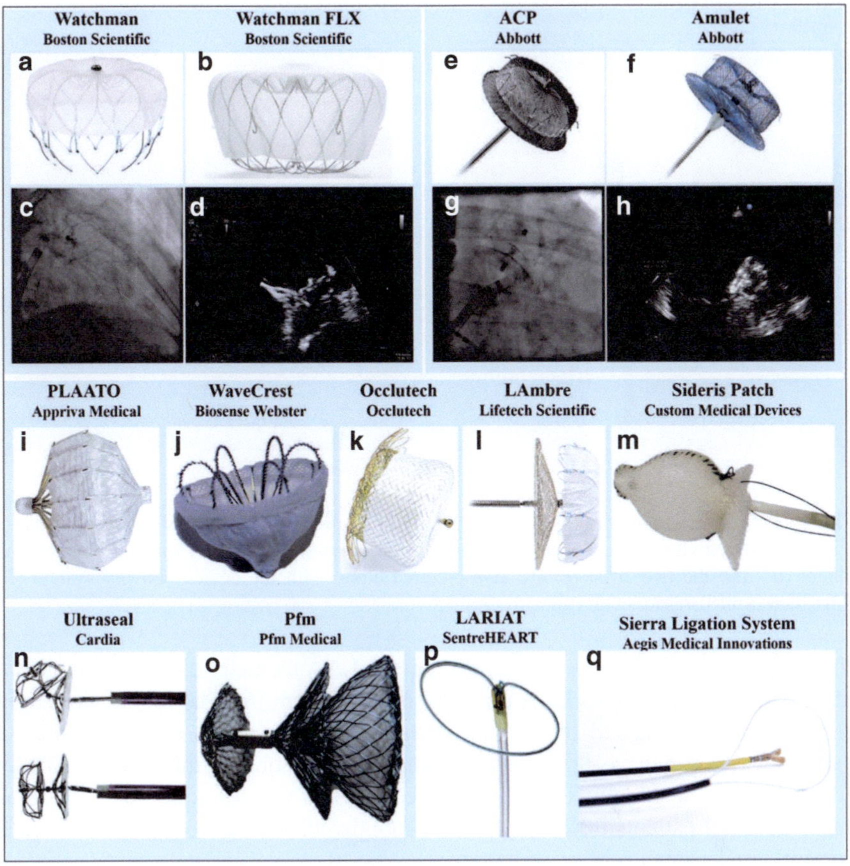

Fig. 14.1 Left atrial appendage occlusion devices. The Watchman (**a**) and Watchman FLX (**b**) are pictured with fluoroscopic (**c**) and echocardiographic (**d**) images of the devices. The Cardiac Plug (**e**) and Amulet (**f**) devices are pictured with fluoroscopic (**g**) and echocardiographic (**h**) views of the Cardiac Plug device. The PLAATO device (**i**), WaveCrest (**j**), Occlutech occluder (**k**), LAmbre (**l**), Sideris Patch (**m**), Ultraseal (**n**), Pfm (**o**), LARIAT (**p**), and Sierra ligation system (**q**) are also pictured. (Modified from Asmarats et al. [3])

A newer device in development is the conformal left atrial appendage seal (CLAAS) (Fig. 14.2). This LAA occlusion device is foam-based and self-expanding with a cylindrical nitinol endoskeleton covered by a conformable, porous, polyurethane-carbonate matrix foam cup [4]. Compression of the foam in one dimension causes expansion in the perpendicular dimension to achieve a better fit in the appendage than other devices [6]. The foam cup also acts as an atraumatic distal tip for implantation [6]. This device is highly conformable and promotes tissue ingrowth with an endothelial layer eventually growing over the implant site [6]. The endoskeleton has two rows of anchors for stability, and the device is available in two

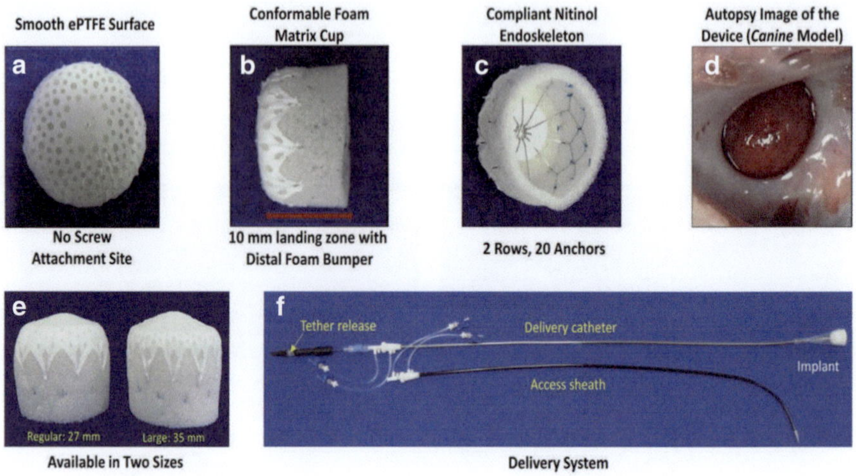

Fig. 14.2 Left atrial appendage closure with a foam-based device. The left atrial face has a polytetrafluoroethylene cover (**a**). A side view (**b**), inside view (**c**), autopsy image from a canine model (**d**), and the two sizes (**e**) are also pictured along with the device delivery system (**f**). (Modified from Turagam et al. [6])

sizes [6]. There is a 27 mm version for a mean LAA diameter of 13–25 mm and a 35 mm version for a mean LAA diameter of 20–32 mm [6]. The first device study was in canines, followed by human patients [4]. The success rate in 15 human patients was reported as 100% with no complications requiring intervention [6]. An adequate LAA seal, defined as a device leak of less than or equal to 5 mm, was achieved in all patients followed up to 12 months with imaging [6]. The device is currently undergoing further evaluation.

The Laminar left atrial appendage exclusion (LAAX) system uses a different mechanism than the other occlusion devices to seal the appendage. Left atrial appendages are often oval instead of round, which can cause suboptimal device placement with occlusion devices that try to fit inside the appendage itself [7]. This device has an integrated ball with a lock that excludes and eliminates the appendage pouch while still using a transcatheter-based approach (Fig. 14.3). The ball rotates, closes the left atrial appendage ostium with its own native tissue, and then locks it closed so that the appendage is excluded [7]. The Laminar system uses a self-expanding nitinol ball to engage the LAA tissue, and the lock is flower shaped with six "petals" that interlock with the ball for tissue compression [7]. The ball is unsheathed, directed, and advanced into the center of the LAA ostium before touching the back wall of the appendage [7]. The ball is then rotated counterclockwise to engage appendage tissue, which is brought together and wrapped around a spindle between the ball and the lock [7]. The device lock is then advanced to the ball, under fluoroscopy and transesophageal echocardiography, to compress the appendage tissue and exclude it [7]. The steps are reversible up until the final release step [7]. Both 12 mm and 16 mm ball diameters were used in human implant cases [7].

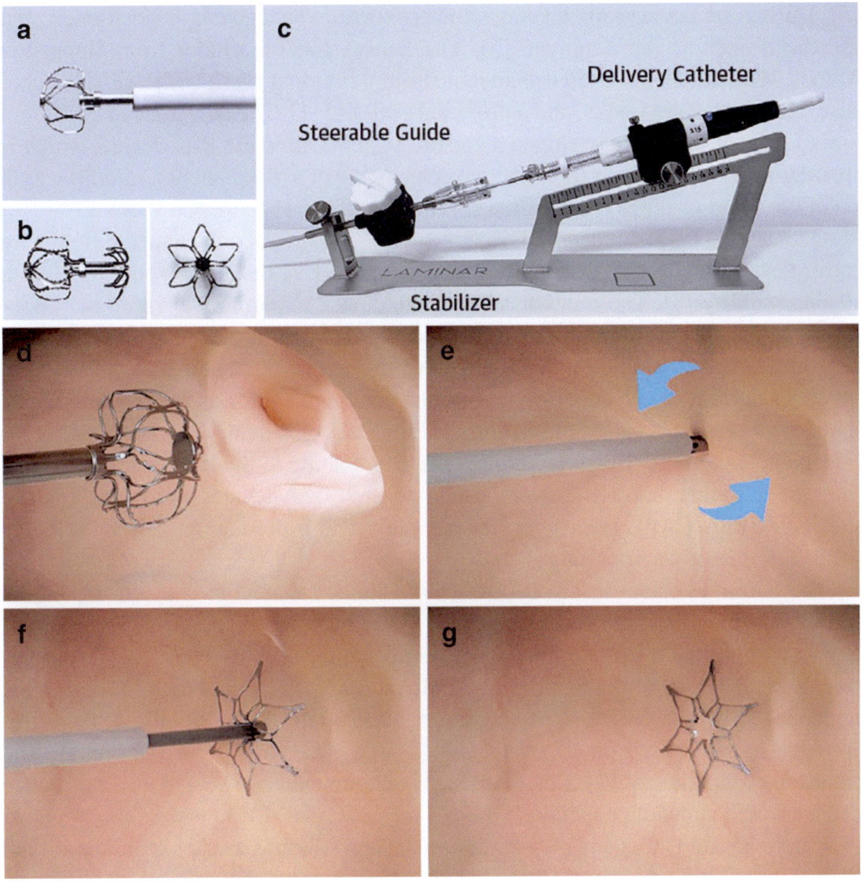

Fig. 14.3 Transcatheter left atrial appendage exclusion with the Laminar system. The Laminar device uses rotational closure and elimination to exclude the left atrial appendage. The Laminar ball (12 mm) is unsheathed from the delivery catheter (**a**). The 16 mm Laminar implant is also pictured (**b**). The system (**c**) features a steerable guide, stabilizer, and delivery catheter. (**d**) shows the implant ball unsheathed and advanced into the appendage, then rotated (**e**). After the appendage is rotated closed (**f**), the lock is deployed, and the delivery system is removed (**g**). (Modified from Wong et al. [7])

Implantation in 15 human patients demonstrated procedural success in all patients with no procedural safety events up to 12 months post-implant and no leaks over 5 mm [7]. This is the first transcatheter device to use rotational closure and elimination as its primary mechanism of appendage closure [7].

There are several devices in development or in active use outside of the United States which fit into and occlude the appendage. The WaveCrest left atrial appendage occlusion system by Biosense Webster is a nitinol single-lobe device in three different sizes (22, 27, and 32 mm) covered by expanded polytetrafluoroethylene (PET) with 20 anchoring points [1]. The device will fit LAA ostia from 14 to 32 mm

[1]. During the device implant stage, the proximal expanded cap is positioned, and the distal anchors are deployed [5]. The SeaLA LAA occluder from Hangzhou Valued Medtech Co. is a self-expandable nitinol braiding mesh with a distal anchor disc, nine anchoring hooks, and a proximal seal disc [1]. The device has 11 different sizes [1]. Pfm Medical developed a closure system called the Pfm device, which is made from nitinol and has three sections consisting of a distal anchor, middle-length connector, and proximal disc with a secondary anchor [1].

Occlutech's LAA occlusion device is a self-expanding, cone-shaped nitinol wire mesh that adapts to the shape of the appendage [8]. A distal loop rim helps with device stability [8]. The outer surface of the device is partially covered by a non-woven, biostable poly-urethane layer, and the device's larger proximal diameter seals the ostium [8]. The original version of the device was available in sizes from 18 to 33 mm [1, 8]. Oversizing by 2–4 mm for implantation is recommended [1]. The newer version is called the Occlutech Plus LAA closure device. The Plus device added anchors to the design to help ensure safe fixation to the left atrial appendage, and the polymer surface was modified to improve device ingrowth [8]. The Occlutech Plus LAA closure device was studied in a porcine model, and clinical trials in humans were pending [8].

The LAmbre LAA closure system from Lifetech Scientific is a self-expanding nitinol device with a proximal cover of PET, a distal umbrella featuring eight hooks, and an additional PET membrane cover connected by a central waist [1]. The proximal cover is larger in diameter than the distal umbrella, which aids in sealing the appendage [4]. The device sizes range from 16 to 36 mm [1]. Two different designs were developed based on the cover-to-umbrella ratio to address both single and multilobed appendages [1]. Device sizing is recommended to be 4–8 mm larger than the measured appendage ostium [1].

Cardia has an Ultraseal LAA occlusion device, which is a self-expanding nitinol device with a lobe and disc design [1]. The device has a distal bulb, 12 hooks for stabilization, and a proximal multilayered sail of three leaflets connected by an articulating joint for multidirectional movement of the device [1]. The sail is larger in diameter than the bulb to ensure the sealing of the appendage [4]. There are ten sizes (16–32 mm) with sizing determined by the maximum measured landing zone, and 10–20% oversizing is recommended [4]. The second generation of the device has a lower radial force, and the overall length of the device was reduced by changing the length of the articulating joint [4].

Pulse Scientific's Leftear occlusion device (Fig. 14.4) is a disc-like, self-expanding, nitinol-based device with a fixed umbrella and blocking disc connected by a central waist [9]. The distal umbrella has eight claws with stable hooks and a polyethylene terephthalate membrane on the distal surface and proximal disc [9]. The distal umbrella is released into the left atrial appendage on implantation, and then the sheath is withdrawn to expose the proximal disc, so it can seal the LAA ostium [9]. This device has 16 diameter sizes (referring to the size of the umbrella) from 15 to 33 mm [9]. An oversize of 4–8 mm more than the ostial diameter was used in human clinical trials in China [9]. The immediate success rate of occlusion was 100% (defined as less than or equal to a 3 mm peri-device leak), and 98.3% of

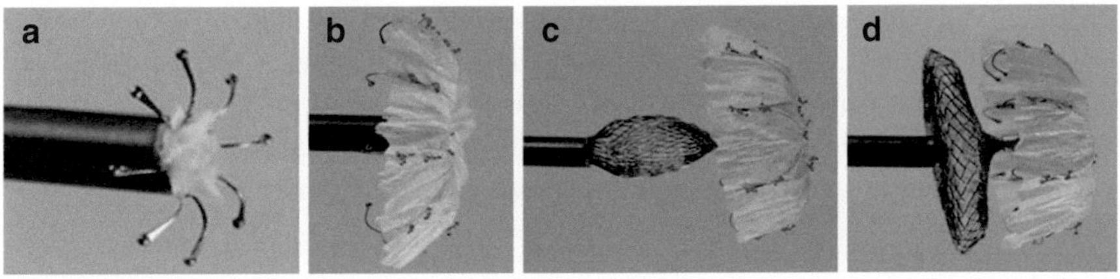

Fig. 14.4 The Leftear disc-like left atrial appendage closure system. (**a**) to (**d**) shows the device in the stages of being released. (Modified from Zhang et al. [9])

patients had appendages that were successfully occluded at 12-month follow-up [9].

Epicardial approaches for LAA closure have also been developed. The LARIAT suture delivery device performs LAA ligation and requires both transseptal and pericardial access [5]. After the transseptal puncture, a magnetic wire is placed at the LAA apex with balloon identification of the ostium, and a second magnetic wire is advanced from an epicardial approach [1]. Once the magnetic wires connect and form a rail, a lasso-like suture is advanced and cinched around the left atrial appendage to close it [1]. The LARIAT system may be considered when the appendage is too large for the use of an endocardial device, but the LAA ostium has to be less than 40 mm for the procedure to work effectively [5].

The ATRICLIP by Atricure uses an epicardial approach. The device is an epicardial clip made of two parallel titanium tubes with elastic nitinol springs covered by a polyester sheath [5]. During open cardiac surgery, the device is placed epicardially at the base of the left atrial appendage to close the appendage [5]. Safety and efficacy were demonstrated for left atrial appendage occlusion in patients undergoing concomitant cardiac surgery [5]. During short-term follow-up, CT imaging and transesophageal echocardiography found complete exclusion of the LAA in 98.4% of the study patients [5].

The Sierra ligation system from Aegis Medical Innovations has an electrocardiography-guided LAA ligation system that uses an epicardial-only approach [1]. An appendage grasper and jaws with mounted electrodes enable electrocardiographic identification and capture of the LAA [1]. A hollow suture loop is advanced over the grasper and then looped around the LAA for closure [1].

Conclusions

Left atrial appendage occlusion has emerged as a valid alternative for stroke prevention in non-valvular atrial fibrillation patients with contraindications to anticoagulation [1]. Safety and efficacy data are growing for the current LAA occlusion devices on the market. Several newer devices, as mentioned in this section, are currently undergoing further study, and endocardial as well as epicardial approaches exist.

There will be many more devices seeking approval from the FDA for clinical use in the years to come. Hopefully, the problems with peri-device leaks and device-related thrombus formation occasionally seen with current devices will be solved with new generations of devices. Further studies will be required to determine the best mechanism of LAA closure and the best treatment strategy for specific patient populations.

References

1. Asmarats L, Rodes-Cabau J. The spectrum of devices for percutaneous left atrial appendage occlusion. Cardiac Interv Today. 2018;12(3):34–9.
2. Saw J, Holmes DR, Cavalcante JL, et al. SCAI/HRS expert consensus statement on transcatheter left atrial appendage closure. Catheter Cardiovasc Interv. 2023;2:100577.
3. Asmarats L, Rodes-Cabau J. Percutaneous left atrial appendage closure: current devices and clinical outcomes. Circ Cardiovasc Interv. 2017;10:e005359.
4. Bavishi C. Transcatheter left atrial appendage closure: devices available, pitfalls, advantages, and future directions. US Cardiol Rev. 2023;17:e05.
5. Chava R, Turagam MK, Lakkireddy D. Left atrial appendage occlusion: what are the options and where is the evidence? J Innov Cardiac Rhythm Manage. 2018;9(4):3095–106.
6. Turagam MK, Neuzil P, Hala P, et al. Intracardiac echocardiography-guided left atrial appendage closure with a novel foam-based conformable device. JACC Clin Electrophysiol. 2022;8(2):197–207.
7. Wong GX, Kar S, Smith TW, et al. Transcatheter left atrial appendage exclusion. JACC Cardiovasc Interv. 2023;16(11):1347–57.
8. Reinthaler M, Grosshauser J, Schmidt T, et al. Preclinical assessment of a modified Occlutech left atrial appendage closure device in a porcine model. Sci Rep. 2021;11:2988.
9. Zhang X, Hou S, Liu W, et al. Percutaneous left atrial appendage closure with a novel LAA Occluder for stroke prevention in atrial fibrillation. JACC Asia. 2022;2(5):547–56.

Chapter 15
Concomitant Left Atrial Appendage Closure and Catheter Ablation for Atrial Fibrillation

Mohammed Wazzan, Ali Azeem, Jawad Almajad, and Mauricio Arruda

Highlights
- Atrial fibrillation (AF) is a highly prevalent arrhythmia accounting for significant morbidity and mortality.
- Rhythm control strategy by catheter ablation for AF reduce symptoms, hospitalization, stroke, and mortality in select populations.
- AF catheter ablation is a Class Ia recommendation in select populations patients in the 2023 ACC/AHA/HRS Atrial Fibrillation guidelines.
- Left atrial appendage occlusion (LAAO) is appropriate for non-valvular AF patients with high thromboembolic risk and contraindication for long-term oral anticoagulation, Class IIa.
- The OPTION trial will assess the safety and efficacy of concomitant AF catheter ablation and LAAO with a randomized controlled trial.

Introduction

Atrial fibrillation (AF) is a very prevalent arrhythmia with a high burden of downstream morbidity and mortality, as outlined in Chap. 1 ("Epidemiology: Atrial fibrillation, anticoagulation, and stroke"). One key domain in the treatment of patients with atrial fibrillation is the choice of rate vs. rhythm control. There is a growing body of evidence [1–4] supporting a rhythm control strategy to reduce hospitalizations, stroke, and mortality in select populations. In particular, there is a growing role of AF catheter ablation to electrically isolate the pulmonary veins and other

M. Wazzan (✉) · A. Azeem · J. Almajad · M. Arruda
Division of Cardiology, Harrington Heart & Vascular Institute, University Hospitals Cleveland Medical Center, Cleveland, OH, USA
e-mail: Mohammed.wazzan@uhhospitals.org

S. J. Filby et al. (eds.), *A Contemporary Manual of Left Atrial Appendage Closure*, https://doi.org/10.1007/978-3-031-68441-8_15

potential triggers of atrial fibrillation as a safe and effective intervention in specific patient populations, with several class 1 recommendations for catheter ablation in the treatment of select patients with atrial fibrillation in the 2023 ACC/AHA/HRS Atrial Fibrillation guidelines [5].

However, one necessary prerequisite for a rhythm control strategy in general and with catheter ablation for atrial fibrillation in particular anticoagulation to reduce the risk of left atrial appendage thrombus and to protect from thromboembolism after restoring sinus rhythm. Several studies as outlined in the 2024 JACC State-of-the-Art Review [6] by Di Biase et al. highlight the central role of anticoagulation pre- and intraprocedurally to reduce the risk of thromboembolism. Current guidelines recommend continuation of anticoagulation to reduce thromboembolism based on risk assessment between thromboembolism and bleeding regardless of catheter ablation outcomes. Real-world registry data suggests that discontinuation of anticoagulation is common (roughly 20%) and that there is likely an increased risk of thromboembolism when anticoagulation is withheld after catheter ablation [7, 8]. The OCEAN trial will prospectively assess the role of anticoagulation 1 year after catheter ablation [9]. This need for continued protection from thromboembolism is of particular importance when electrical isolation of the left atrial appendage in addition to pulmonary vein isolation is pursued in an attempt to maintain sinus rhythm, as this electrical disconnection of the left atrial appendage from the remainder of the left atrial can result in significant disruption of the left atrial appendage mechanical function and provide a substrate to raise the risk of thromboembolism, even if the remainder of the atrium is in sinus rhythm.

This poses a challenging treatment decision for patients who stand to benefit significantly from catheter ablation to help maintain sinus rhythm for atrial fibrillation (i.e., younger patients with heart failure and lower comorbidity burden) but are at significant bleeding risk. Left atrial appendage occlusion (LAAO) is an established intervention to reduce the risk of thromboembolism in select patients (Chap. 2: Current indications and evidence for left atrial appendage closure).

Concomitant catheter ablation for atrial fibrillation with LAAO is an emerging approach under investigation to mitigate the risk of thromboembolism. The implications of combining these two procedures in the same setting include the use of a single transseptal access to perform both procedures as outlined below in "Practical Considerations" and has the potential to be safer and more efficient than performing both procedures in separate settings, but the left atrial dwell time (amount of time catheters and other equipment are inside the left atrium) is higher with concomitant procedure and may increase thromboembolic risk of procedure. Moreover, there may be an interaction between the mechanical effect of the atrial fibrillation ablation and the success of LAAO. To date, there are no randomized trials to date regarding the role of LAAO in and around catheter ablation for atrial fibrillation. In this chapter, we will review the available registry, observational evidence of this practice, and the upcoming OPTION ("Comparison of Anticoagulation with Left Atrial Appendage Closure After AF Ablation") trial [10] in which patients with AF at standard bleeding risk and elevated thromboembolic risk are randomized to anticoagulation vs LAAO with either recent catheter ablation (within 90–180 days) or concurrent LAAO at the time of the catheter ablation and discuss practical considerations of concomitant AF ablation and LAAO.

Registries of Concomitant AF Ablation and LAAO

The largest registry of concurrent AF ablation and LAAO included 349 patients with AF across 5 centers from 2009 to 2015 [11]. In this registry, catheter ablation was first performed with radiofrequency ablation to achieve pulmonary vein isolation with additional ablation targets left to the physician's discretion. All of the included patients had non-valvular AF and were scheduled for combined CA and LAAC procedure per local and international guidelines at the time. The ablation was limited to pulmonary vein isolation in 37% of patients, and the remainder of the patients had other lesions delivered at the discretion of the operator; it is not specified if the left atrial appendage was isolated in these cases. After catheter ablation, the transseptal sheath for ablation was exchanged for the Watchman sheath with the subsequent deployment of the Watchman under TEE guidance. TEE at the time of procedure showed complete closure in 92.6% of patients with minimal residual flow (<5 mm) in 7.4% of patients with a mean total procedural time of 154 +/− 61 min and a mean fluoroscopy time of 28 +/− 12 min. The overall complication-free rate was 92.8% with observed complications including minor groin hematoma (4.4%) and pericardial effusion requiring intervention (1.5%). One patient had a minor stroke (0.3%) several hours after the procedure despite the use of an oral anticoagulant with TEE showing the appropriate position of the Watchman device with no residual flow and no device-related thrombus.

Regarding LAAO outcomes from this registry, imaging follow-up was available in 78% of patients with successful sealing in 99% of patients (70%, complete occlusion of LAA; 29%, residual flow <5 mm). In one patient, the Watchman had dislodged and was eventually found to be in the abdominal aorta and was extracted percutaneously. In three patients (1.1%), there was device-related thrombus leading to a temporary continuation of anticoagulation until resolution, followed by transition to antiplatelet therapy.

Regarding rhythm outcomes of this registry, 42 patients (12%) had implantable loop recorder, and the remainder underwent routine clinical surveillance, typically multiday Holter monitor. After a median follow-up of 34 months, 51% of patients had a documented recurrence of atrial tachyarrhythmias. There were 29 (11%) re-do ablations, 5 (1.4%) required pacemaker and AV nodal ablation, and 5 (1.4%) underwent thoracoscopic or surgical AF ablation.

Regarding bleeding and ischemic outcomes, at 3 months, 11% of patients were on anticoagulation (mostly VKA, only 3% of patients on DOAC), 42% on SAPT, and 44% on DAPT. By the end of follow-up, only 11% of patients were on therapeutic anticoagulation, with 73% of patients on SAPT and 5% of patients on DAPT. A total of 11 patients (3.2%) had major bleeding during the 34.5 months of follow-up. There was one intracranial bleed (0.3%) in the registry, which occurred after thrombolysis for ischemic stroke. The observed annualized bleeding rate was 1.1%, which was lower than the expected 3.7% bleeding rate as expected by HAS-BLED score. There were 2 strokes (0.6%) after full Maze IV with LAA ligation and removal of Watchman. Among patients with an active Watchman, there were 7 (2.0%) ischemic strokes, with a resultant annualized stroke rate of 0.7% which is lower than the projected annualized stroke risk of 3.2% as projected by CHA2DS2-VASc scores. Overall, these results are comparable to similar outcomes of standalone Watchman or catheter ablation procedures for rhythm and ischemic/bleeding outcomes, respectively.

This is the largest registry to date of concomitant AF catheter ablation and LAAO and is promising regarding the efficacy, safety, and efficiency of a combined procedure. These outcomes are in line with other smaller case series and registries of concomitant AF ablation and LAAO as outlined in a recent review article [12]. Though detailed and informative, this registry's ability to inform clinical practice is limited by the realities of real-world registry data with the limitations of unmeasured confounders, potential for incomplete follow-up, and the lack of a true control arm. The upcoming OPTION trial will help answer this question regarding the safety and efficacy of concomitant AF ablation and LAAO with a randomized controlled trial.

The OPTION Trial

The OPTION trial [10, 13] was designed with the goal of answering if LAAO with Watchman FLX is a reasonable alternative to oral anticoagulation following catheter ablation for atrial fibrillation. To answer this, the study is a prospective, multicenter, global trial with 1:1 randomization to DOAC vs. WATCHMAN FLX. The randomization will also be stratified by sequential vs. concomitant planned ablation +/− Watchman implantation, which will also inform the safety and efficacy of concurrent LAAO + catheter ablation of atrial fibrillation. The trial has completed an enrollment of 1600 participants across 130 sites.

The key inclusion criteria are as follows:

- Either underwent a prior catheter ablation 90–180 days prior (sequential arm) or to be performed at time of WATCHMAN (concomitant).
- Is able to undergo TEE.
- Is able to undergo the planned pharmacologic anticoagulant/antiplatelet regimen.
- CHA2DS2-VASc score 2 or more in men or 3 or more in women.

The key exclusion criteria are the following:

- An alternate indication for long-term anticoagulation (i.e., venous thromboembolism).
- Unsuitable for long-term anticoagulant or antiplatelet therapy (i.e., high bleeding risk).

- Recent or planned other major cardiac procedures during the study period (i.e., percutaneous coronary intervention, other ablation, cardiac surgery).
- Stroke or transient ischemic attack within the past 60 days.
- Myocardial infarction within the past 90 days.
- Anatomic contraindication (prior ASD/PFO closure, prior surgical closure of LAA, active infection, cardiac tumor).
- Life-limiting comorbidity with life expectancy <2 years or NYHA Class IV heart failure or LVEF <30%.
- Echo parameters—existing echo-free space >5 mm, high-risk PFO with atrial septal aneurysm >15 mm or length >15 mm, high risk patent foramen ovale with large shunt, or significant mitral stenosis with mitral valve area <1.5 cm^2.

For patients randomized to WATCHMAN, a pre-procedural TEE is used for device sizing and for excluding left atrial appendage thrombus. For patients in the concomitant AF ablation and LAAO group, the WATCHMAN FLX implant and catheter ablation are performed by standard-of-care methods for both procedures by operators who have performed the manufacturers implantation course. Aspirin was started 1 day prior to the procedure, and post-implant were treated with oral anticoagulant (typically DOAC) + aspirin for 90 days followed by aspirin alone for at least 12 months post-implant. Follow-up imaging (TEE or CT) is obtained at 3 and 12 months post-implant. The control arm would be treated oral anticoagulant alone as in line with the current standard of care.

The two pre-specified primary endpoints are the following:

- Stroke, all-cause-mortality, and systemic embolism at 36 months (noninferiority).
- Non-procedural bleeding: ISTH major bleeding and clinically relevant non-major bleeding (superiority, 36 months).

The pre-specified secondary outcome measure is ISTH major bleeding (including procedural bleeding) at 36 months.

The OPTION trial will further inform the risks and benefits of LAAO in standard-risk patients undergoing catheter ablation for atrial fibrillation. If shown to be safe and effective, this has the potential to significantly improve procedural efficiency, safety, and cost-effectiveness by lowering overall exposure of the patient to the sources of risk in the two procedures given the significant overlap of both procedures.

Practical Aspects

Performing both procedures concomitantly using a single transseptal access reduces patient exposure to procedural risk of undergoing two separate transseptal punctures. Most published experiences of combing both procedures describe a workflow of performing catheter ablation first prior to LAAO, as the LAAO device may impair maneuverability of the ablation catheter to the ridge between the LAA and the left pulmonary veins, which would lower long-term success rate if the left-sided pulmonary veins are not isolated. Moreover, if LAAO is performed first, then there is a risk of mapping or ablation catheters dislodging the LAAO device resulting in device embolization, though there are no published cases of this. In one observational study [14], 107 sequential patients were stratified to catheter ablation first then LAAO (n = 61) or LAAO first then catheter ablation (n = 46). TEE did show an increase in left atrial ridge thickness (4.6 + 0 0.4 mm to 6.8 + − 0.6 mm) after catheter ablation likely due to increased edema. The group of patients who had catheter ablation first had a higher rate of peri-device leak on TEE at 45 days (46% vs 4%) and at 12 months (15% vs 2%), which could be a signal to use pre-ablation measurements in sizing the LAAO device given the possibility of transiently changing the dimensions of the LAA orifice due to edema from ablation.

Conclusions

Concomitant atrial fibrillation ablation with LAAO is an emerging treatment strategy to potentially reduce the risk of periprocedural complications and total exposure to anticoagulation. This may be particularly useful for patients at elevated bleeding risk and anticipated to benefit the most from catheter ablation (younger, more-symptomatic patients with heart failure). The OPTION trial will help clarify the risk of procedural-related complications and if there is a significant interaction between the two procedures in the safety or efficacy of either procedure.

References

1. Roy D, Talajic M, Nattel S, Wyse DG, Dorian P, Lee KL, Bourassa MG, Arnold JM, Buxton AE, Camm AJ, Connolly SJ, Dubuc M, Ducharme A, Guerra PG, Hohnloser SH, Lambert J, Le Heuzey JY, O'Hara G, Pedersen OD, Rouleau JL, Singh BN, Stevenson LW, Stevenson WG, Thibault B, Waldo AL. Atrial fibrillation and congestive heart failure Investigators. Rhythm control versus rate control for atrial fibrillation and heart failure. N Engl J Med. 2008;358(25):2667–77. https://doi.org/10.1056/NEJMoa0708789.
2. Sohns C, Fox H, Marrouche NF, Crijns HJGM, Costard-Jaeckle A, Bergau L, Hindricks G, Dagres N, Sossalla S, Schramm R, Fink T, El Hamriti M, Moersdorf M, Sciacca V, Konietschke F, Rudolph V, Gummert J, Tijssen JGP, Sommer P, CASTLE HTx Investigators. Catheter ablation in end-stage heart failure with atrial fibrillation. N Engl J Med. 2023;389(15):1380–9. https://doi.org/10.1056/NEJMoa2306037. Epub 2023 Aug 27.
3. Marrouche NF, Brachmann J, Andresen D, Siebels J, Boersma L, Jordaens L, Merkely B, Pokushalov E, Sanders P, Proff J, Schunkert H, Christ H, Vogt J, Bänsch D, Investigators CASTLE-AF. Catheter ablation for atrial fibrillation with heart failure. N Engl J Med. 2018;378(5):417–27. https://doi.org/10.1056/NEJMoa1707855.
4. Kirchhof P, Camm AJ, Goette A, Brandes A, Eckardt L, Elvan A, Fetsch T, van Gelder IC, Haase D, Haegeli LM, Hamann F, Heidbüchel H, Hindricks G, Kautzner J, Kuck KH, Mont L, Ng GA, Rekosz J, Schoen N, Schotten U, Suling A, Taggeselle J, Themistoclakis S, Vettorazzi E, Vardas P, Wegscheider K, Willems S, HJGM C, Breithardt G, EAST-AFNET 4 Trial

Investigators. Early rhythm-control therapy in patients with atrial fibrillation. N Engl J Med. 2020;383(14):1305–16. https://doi.org/10.1056/NEJMoa2019422. Epub 2020 Aug 29.

5. Joglar JA, Chung MK, Armbruster AL, Benjamin EJ, Chyou JY, Cronin EM, Deswal A, Eckhardt LL, Goldberger ZD, Gopinathannair R, Gorenek B, Hess PL, Hlatky M, Hogan G, Ibeh C, Indik JH, Kido K, Kusumoto F, Link MS, Linta KT, Marcus GM, McCarthy PM, Patel N, Patton KK, Perez MV, Piccini JP, Russo AM, Sanders P, Streur MM, Thomas KL, Times S, Tisdale JE, Valente AM, Van Wagoner DR, Peer Review Committee Members. 2023 ACC/AHA/ACCP/HRS guideline for the diagnosis and Management of Atrial Fibrillation: a report of the American College of Cardiology/American Heart Association joint committee on clinical practice guidelines. Circulation. 2024;149(1):e1–e156. https://doi.org/10.1161/CIR.0000000000001193. Epub 2023 Nov 30. Erratum in: circulation. 2024 Jan 2;149(1):e167. Erratum in: circulation. 2024 Feb 27;149(9):e936.
6. Di Biase L, Lakkireddy DJ, Marazzato J, Velasco A, Diaz JC, Navara R, Chrispin J, Rajagopalan B, Natale A, Mohanty S, Zhang X, Della Rocca D, Dalal A, Park K, Wiley J, Batchelor W, Cheung JW, Dangas G, Mehran R, Romero J, Electrophysiology ACC, Councils I. Antithrombotic therapy for patients undergoing cardiac electrophysiological and interventional procedures: JACC state-of-the-art review. J Am Coll Cardiol. 2024;83(1):82–108. https://doi.org/10.1016/j.jacc.2023.09.831.
7. Noseworthy PA, Yao X, Deshmukh AJ, Van Houten H, Sangaralingham LR, Siontis KC, Piccini JP Sr, Asirvatham SJ, Friedman PA, Packer DL, Gersh BJ, Shah ND. Patterns of anticoagulation use and Cardioembolic risk after catheter ablation for atrial fibrillation. J Am Heart Assoc. 2015;4(11):e002597. https://doi.org/10.1161/JAHA.115.002597. PMID: 26541393; PMCID: PMC4845220
8. Freeman JV, Shrader P, Pieper KS, Allen LA, Chan PS, Fonarow GC, Gersh BJ, Kowey PR, Mahaffey KW, Naccarelli G, Reiffel JA, Singer DE, Go AS, Hylek EM, Steinberg BA, Peterson ED, Piccini JP. Outcomes and anticoagulation use after catheter ablation for atrial fibrillation. Circ Arrhythm Electrophysiol. 2019;12(12):e007612. https://doi.org/10.1161/CIRCEP.119.007612. Epub 2019 Dec 13.
9. Verma A, Ha ACT, Kirchhof P, Hindricks G, Healey JS, Hill MD, Sharma M, Wyse DG, Champagne J, Essebag V, Wells G, Gupta D, Heidbuchel H, Sanders P, Birnie DH. The optimal anti-coagulation for enhanced-risk patients post-catheter ablation for atrial fibrillation (OCEAN) trial. Am Heart J. 2018;197:124–32. https://doi.org/10.1016/j.ahj.2017.12.007. Epub 2017 Dec 8.
10. ClinicalTrials.gov [Internet]. Bethesda (MD): National Library of Medicine (US). 2000 Feb 29 – . Identifier NCT03795298, Comparison of Anticoagulation With Left Atrial Appendage Closure After AF Ablation (OPTION); first posted 2019 Jan 07, last updated 2024 Mar 22 [cited 2024 Mar 24]; [about 8 screens]. Available from: https://clinicaltrials.gov/study/NCT03795298.
11. Wintgens L, Romanov A, Phillips K, Ballesteros G, Swaans M, Folkeringa R, Garcia-Bolao I, Pokushalov E, Boersma L. Combined atrial fibrillation ablation and left atrial appendage closure: long-term follow-up from a large multicentre registry. EP Europace. 2018;20(11):1783–9. https://doi.org/10.1093/europace/euy025.
12. Mills MT, Calvert P, Velavan P, Lip GYH, Gupta D. Concurrent percutaneous left atrial appendage occlusion and catheter ablation for atrial fibrillation: state-of-the-art review. Trends Cardiovasc Med. 2023;S1050-1738(23):00100-7. https://doi.org/10.1016/j.tcm.2023.11.003. Epub ahead of print.
13. Wazni OM, Boersma L, Healey JS, Mansour M, Tondo C, Phillips K, Doshi R, Jaber W, Hynes E, Allocco DJ, Reddy VY. Comparison of anticoagulation with left atrial appendage closure after atrial fibrillation ablation: rationale and design of the OPTION randomized trial. Am Heart J. 2022;251:35–42. https://doi.org/10.1016/j.ahj.2022.05.003. Epub 2022 May 6.
14. Li XX, Tian Y, Shi L, Wang YJ, Zeng LJ, Huang LH, He SN, Li JP, Liu XP. One-stop hybrid procedure combining catheter ablation and left atrial appendage closure increases long-term risk for adverse events in patients with atrial fibrillation. Pacing Clin Electrophysiol. 2020;43(11):1358–65. https://doi.org/10.1111/pace.14084. Epub 2020 Oct 10.

Chapter 16
Femoral Venous Access Technique and Vascular Closure for Left Atrial Appendage Occluder Implantation

C. Barton Gillombardo, Jun Li, and Mehdi Shishehbor

Abbreviations

ACT	Activated clotting time
GSV	Greater saphenous vein
LAAO	Left atrial appendage occlusion
NCDR	National Cardiovascular Data Registry
RCT	Randomized clinical trial
US	Ultrasound
VCD	Vascular closure device

Highlights

- Safe and effective management of vascular access is an essential aspect of the left atrial appendage occlusion (LAAO) procedure.
- Use of a micropuncture technique with ultrasound (US) guidance has been associated with reduced complications and is considered best practice for LAAO.
- Following LAAO, hemostasis may be obtained using a variety of techniques including manual compression, vascular closure devices (VCD), and figure-of-8 skin sutures.

C. B. Gillombardo · J. Li (✉) · M. Shishehbor
University Hospitals Harrington Heart and Vascular Institute, Cleveland, OH, USA

Case Western Reserve University School of Medicine, Cleveland, OH, USA
e-mail: Jun.Li@UHhospitals.org

S. J. Filby et al. (eds.), *A Contemporary Manual of Left Atrial Appendage Closure*, https://doi.org/10.1007/978-3-031-68441-8_16

Introduction

Safe and effective management of vascular access is one hallmark of a high-quality interventional cardiology practice. Recent analysis of the National Cardiovascular Data Registry (NCDR) Left Atrial Appendage Occlusion (LAAO) Registry, which includes data from more than 38,000 patients, found that major bleeding or major vascular complication occurred in approximately 1–2% of cases [1]. This nontrivial event rate is important to recognize, as vascular complications can lead to considerable morbidity and mortality. Strict adherence to best practices and meticulous attention to detail have been shown to reduce both the likelihood of vascular complication as well as procedure times, with positive impact on patient satisfaction, comfort, and safety [2, 3]. In this chapter, we will begin with a comprehensive step-by-step guide to obtaining large bore femoral venous access. We will then review various techniques for achieving safe hemostasis.

Femoral Venous Access

Anatomical assessment of the femoral head is a critical first step in any femoral access procedure, with fluoroscopic guidance to help confirm location. Use of a micropuncture technique with ultrasound (US) guidance has been shown to correlate with higher first-attempt success rates, a decrease in inadvertent femoral artery punctures, and a reduction in the incidence of groin hematomas [3, 4]. Additionally, it ensures optimal entry site and angle for femoral venipuncture, facilitating the delivery of subsequent equipment.

1. Prepare femoral access site in the usual sterile fashion. Preference is given to the right femoral vein for its advantageous alignment during transseptal puncture and sheath navigation [4, 5].
2. Anatomical assessment for the femoral head, with confirmation on fluoroscopy. Proximity of access to the femoral head allows for appropriate manual compression against a bony landmark if bleeding occurs.
    (a) Patients with protuberant abdominal habitus may benefit from pannus retraction to assist in the appropriate location of the access site. Puncture should be below the inguinal ligament.
3. Apply liberal amounts of lidocaine for local anesthesia under US guidance. Adjust the US to an appropriate depth, positioning the probe perpendicularly to the femoral vein's axis. The vein is situated medial to the artery just below the inguinal ligament [6]. For the vast majority of clinical situations, the vascular probe provides adequate depth for visualization of the anatomical structures. If additional depth is needed, the curvilinear probe may be needed.

   (a) Operators should familiarize themselves with the appearance of superficial femoral artery, profunda femoris artery, and greater saphenous vein (GSV) junction with the common femoral vein. Typically, large bore access should be obtained above the GSV junction; augmentative smaller bore access can be obtained inferior to the GSV if needed.

4. Insert the 21-gauge micropuncture needle at roughly a 45° angle to the skin, mindful of the depth of subcutaneous tissue. For patients with larger habitus, the insertion site should be approximately 1–2 cm caudal to the US probe to ensure needle entry into the vessel corresponds with the ultrasound plane. Following skin puncture, apply negative pressure to the syringe as the needle is guided into the femoral vein under ultrasound visualization.

   (a) Venous access typically results in backwall puncture due to pliability of the wall structure. After accessing the vein under US guidance, the US probe should be removed from the site to allow venous flow.

      (i) This is then followed by a methodical negative traction on the syringe along with a slow retraction of the needle while simultaneously decreasing the angulation of the needle toward 15–20°. This allows better alignment with the intravascular component of the vein.
      (ii) In patients who are hypovolemic, methods to improve flow during this maneuver include Valsalva or reverse Trendelenburg positioning. Fluid bolus can also be administered if needed.

5. Upon confirming the intraluminal position with the free flow of blood, disconnect the syringe and advance the micropuncture wire, ensuring its smooth passage without resistance. Verify its placement with fluoroscopy. The use of slip-tip syringes can facilitate this step.
6. Over the wire, exchange the needle for a micropuncture sheath and dilator.
7. Withdraw both the wire and the inner dilator from the sheath.
8. Introduce a 0.035″ guidewire into the right atrium.
9. With the J wire in situ, remove the micropuncture sheath and progressively dilate the tract to accommodate a 15 French delivery sheath.
10. If additional secondary venous access is indicated for intracardiac echocardiogram imaging, the steps can be replicated for the 9 French secondary access in the same vein, positioning the entry point approximately 1.5 cm distal to the primary site.

   (a) Some operators may choose to retain a 0.035″ guidewire or micropuncture sheath in the one access site (without completing the final upsizing) while obtaining the second access site to minimize the intravascular footprint affecting the active phase of access. Others may obtain the smaller bore, distal access first. Any sequence of events is reasonable and should be left to the discretion of the operator and his or her comfort level.

Large Bore Femoral Venous Closure Techniques

Recognizing risk factors for vascular access site complications is vital. This includes female sex, age >70 years old, body mass index <20 kg/m^2, renal dysfunction with creatinine clearance <60 mL/min, and those with ongoing antiplatelet or anticoagulant therapy [7]. The large sheath sizes required for LAAO procedures compound these risks. Given that approximately 70% of LAAO patients have a history of significant bleeding events, the selection of an effective hemostasis technique becomes paramount [1]. Although manual compression, figure-of-8 sutures, and various vascular closure devices (VCD) are commonly employed, the lack of comprehensive randomized controlled trials (RCT) leaves a gap in determining the most effective method. This underscores the need for targeted research to develop an evidence-based standard for post-procedure hemostasis.

The figure-of-8 suture technique is highly regarded for its hemostasis efficacy in LAAO procedures, potentially reducing the need to reverse periprocedural anticoagulation. A small-scale RCT has demonstrated its advantages over manual compression, notably in reducing time to hemostasis and lowering complication rates without affecting vascular integrity [8]. Interestingly, a relatively small RCT involving 40 patients found the figure-of-8 suture to be comparable to the Perclose system in terms of safety and efficacy for large bore venous access [9]. In contrast, the AMBULATE Clinical Trial, which enrolled 1223 patients undergoing a variety of electrophysiology procedures, highlighted the effectiveness of the Vascade MVP Vascular Closure System. This system notably shortened the time to ambulation, enhanced patient satisfaction, and reduced opioid use post-procedure compared to manual pressure. These outcomes highlight the Vascade MVP's role in improving recovery and minimizing complications in patients undergoing cardiovascular interventions [10]. These diverse findings indicate the necessity for more focused research, including cost-benefit analysis, to determine the optimal closure technique.

Significantly, more data is available regarding the relative safety and efficacy of vascular closure techniques following percutaneous femoral arterial access for cardiac or endovascular procedures. A comprehensive meta-analysis of 52 studies, involving over 19,000 participants, compared manual compression and surgical closure with collagen-, metal clip-, and suture-based VCDs. The findings suggest that, in general, VCDs outperform manual compression by enabling quicker hemostasis, earlier patient mobilization, faster discharge, and improved patient satisfaction. Notably, collagen-based VCDs were associated with a lower incidence of groin hematomas in comparison to manual compression (OR 0.46, 95% CI 0.40 to 0.54; 25 studies, 10,247 participants). While these results may hint at potential advantages for managing large-bore femoral venous access, extrapolation requires caution, and further investigation is essential [2].

Manual Compression and Bedrest

Manual compression followed by bedrest has historically been the standard method for achieving hemostasis once vascular access is no longer required. This technique's primary disadvantages are its slower achievement of hemostasis and delayed patient ambulation, often leading to postponed discharge eligibility. It is also labor-intensive for medical staff and may cause patient discomfort due to extended pressure at the access site as well as extended bedrest. Nonetheless, its simplicity and cost-effectiveness remain advantageous. Protocols may vary slightly between institutions, but several key steps are commonly shared, detailed below:

1. Confirm an activated clotting time (ACT) of less than 170 s.
2. Administer IV pain medication judiciously for patient comfort.
3. Aspirate and flush the sheath to minimize the risk of thrombus formation and embolism.
4. Ensure pre-measured doses of atropine and phenylephrine are available bedside to counteract increased vagal tone from femoral vessel compression.
5. Remove the vascular sheath.
6. Permit bleeding from the access site for 1–2 cardiac cycles to dislodge any clot along the venotomy track.
7. Apply pressure 1–2 cm proximal to the sheath's entry point on the skin along with a simultaneous 1–2 cm distal to skin entry point to control venous inflow. Allow visualization of the entry point to observe for active bleeding.
   (a) Given the low-pressure state of the venous system, it is reasonable to remove both the primary and secondary access sites simultaneously and hold pressure.
   (b) Smaller venous access sites will achieve hemostasis within a 10-min period of continuous pressure hold.
   (c) Base the duration of manual compression on the sheath size removed—for most clinical scenarios involving venous access, 1–2 min per French size is typically adequate.
8. Following 4 h of strict bedrest, the patient may be safely mobilized.

It is important to adapt these steps to individualized patient needs and align them with each institution's specific protocols.

Figure-of-8 Suture

Employing a figure-of-8 suture for hemostasis effectively provides manual compression using the patient's soft tissue. It presents a cost-effective and efficient alternative to manual compression and is less labor-intensive for medical staff. This method is versatile, requiring no specialized equipment for implementation. There is a minor learning curve, requiring technical proficiency and experience. Typically, the figure-of-8 stitch can be removed at 4 h post-procedure, which provides time for ACT to return to a normal range. Below is a step-by-step guide to suture placement:

1. Partially retract the large bore access sheath within the vein.
2. Employ a #1 non-absorbable silk suture, or larger, with a curved needle for suturing.
3. Insert a suture loop subcutaneously, approximately 0.5 to 1 cm distal to the puncture site. The needle should penetrate the medial to the access point and emerge lateral to it, capturing a substantial amount of subcutaneous tissue in a "horizontal" fashion. Replicate the loop placement proximal to the sheath insertion, mirroring the initial loop (Fig. 16.1a, b).

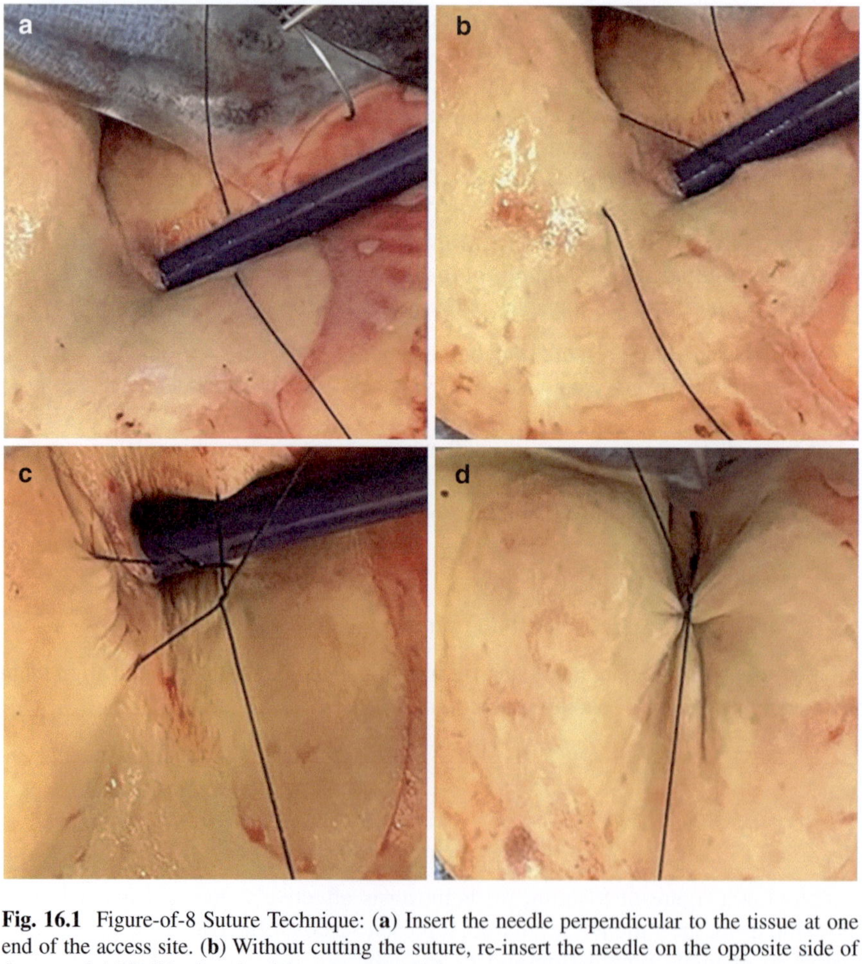

Fig. 16.1 Figure-of-8 Suture Technique: (**a**) Insert the needle perpendicular to the tissue at one end of the access site. (**b**) Without cutting the suture, re-insert the needle on the opposite side of the wound. (**c**) Pull both ends of the suture material to approximate the wound edges. Tie the suture with a surgical knot to secure the loops in place. The figure-of-8 pattern should now be visible, with the suture crossing over the wound in an "X" shape. (**d**) Secure the suture with additional knots as needed to ensure that it stays in place without causing excessive tension or tissue trauma

   (a) Alternatively, some operators use a "vertical" deployment method, by which the first needle drive is on the lateral aspect of the vessel, from caudal toward cranial. The suture is brought across the access site, just medial to the sheath(s), and the loop placement is replicated, from caudal to cranial fashion.
   (b) Both of these methods ultimately formulate an 8 figure on the surface of the skin, which can be cinched to provide pressure from the subcutaneous tissue onto the venous access site(s) (Fig. 16.1c).
   (c) Care should be taken not to inadvertently puncture the femoral vessels in particularly smaller patients.

4. Secure the suture with square knots. Typically, the first knot is thrown and tightened on the site, while the sheath(s) is extracted by an assistant. Using a dilator or Kelley clamp to "hold" the first knot by an assistant, the second knot is formed. Rapid retraction of the dilator or clamp will allow tightening of the second knot atop the first to allow appropriate locking. A third knot can be formed without additional maneuvers as a final securement of the square knots (Fig. 16.1d).

   (a) If there is ongoing bleeding, a second figure-of-8 stitch may be needed. Typically, if the "horizontal" method is used first, the second suture added may be more advantageous using the "vertical" method to allow a perpendicular tissue interaction.
   (b) An alternative to knotting is the use of a 3-way stopcock for suture management. Thread the suture tails through the stopcock, tighten at skin level, and then rotate the valve to lock. This enables easy suture removal and re-tightening if necessary [11, 12].

5. In patients who are exhibiting frequent increases intra-abdominal pressure (e.g., coughing spells), it may be reasonable to add a pressure dressing to prevent oozing from the venous site during the coughing spells.
6. Following a minimum of 4 h of bed rest, the suture may be removed. Following removal of the suture, an additional 2–4 h of bed rest is typically advised prior to patient mobilization.

   (a) These timeframes serve only as guidelines, and operators should utilize an individualized approach to duration of figure-of-8 for hemostasis.

Perclose Device

The Perclose device, receiving FDA clearance in 2013, is a closure system that applies a polyester suture directly to the arteriotomy or venotomy site. Given it is a suture-based system without a large intravascular footprint, vessel re-access can be performed immediately without limitations. The Perclose ProStyle, a 6-French-compatible system, accommodates a broad range of femoral access sizes from 5 French to 21 French and venous access from 5 French to 24 French. For arterial sheaths larger than 8 French, dual Perclose systems may be needed [11]. Pre-close, a method of deploying the polypropylene monofilament sutures before advancement of a larger sheath, with one device is sufficient typically for venous access closure, regardless of French size.

Advantages of Perclose for hemostasis over manual compression include less labor-intensive compression for medical staff, improving patient comfort and satisfaction, and allowing for immediate hemostasis. These benefits contribute to shorter times for ambulation and discharge eligibility. However, Perclose does require a higher level of operator skill, and its success is associated with a learning curve. Both the figure-of-8 stitch and the Perclose device carry the risk of suture-related complications; however, the Perclose suture material remains permanently in place and does not require subsequent removal. The cost of the Perclose device is considerably higher than the direct costs associated with manual compression and the figure-of-8 stitch. Nevertheless, the Perclose device provides a valuable tool for vascular closure in appropriate clinical scenarios, offering a balance between immediate closure and flexibility for future vascular access.

The following is a step-by-step approach to deploying a Pre-close prior to conversion to larger bore venous access:

1. Following routine access as noted above with US guidance, the venous access can be pre-dilated to 6 French.
2. The Perclose device is flushed in the usual fashion, and 6 French dilator is exchanged for the device over a 0.035″ guidewire.
3. Dilation of the tract with a Kelley clamp may be appropriate if scar tissue or thicker skin is encountered.
4. Thread the Perclose device over the guidewire and advance it into the vein until the wire exit port nearly reaches the skin surface.
5. Remove the guidewire.
6. Advance the Perclose device further until dark blood is observed from the marker lumen, confirming correct intravenous placement. If venous blood return is not visible, due to the low pressure within the venous system, apply gentle pressure to the abdomen to facilitate blood return.
7. Confirm the position of the Perclose device by withdrawing it slowly until the bleeding stops and then readvancing until the bleeding resumes.
8. Position the device at approximately 45 degrees to the skin surface and elevate the lever to deploy the footplate (Fig. 16.2).
9. Keep the device steady and pull back until you feel resistance from the vessel wall.
10. Press the plunger to release the suture (Fig. 16.2).
11. Separate the needles and plunger from the device and trim the suture with the integrated cutting instrument (Fig. 16.2).
12. Re-enter back into the lumen of the vein and lower angulation of the device to parallel the thigh prior to returning the footplate lever to its original position (Fig. 16.2).
13. Gently withdraw the Perclose device until the guidewire exit port is visible above the skin, and readvance the 0.035″ guidewire.

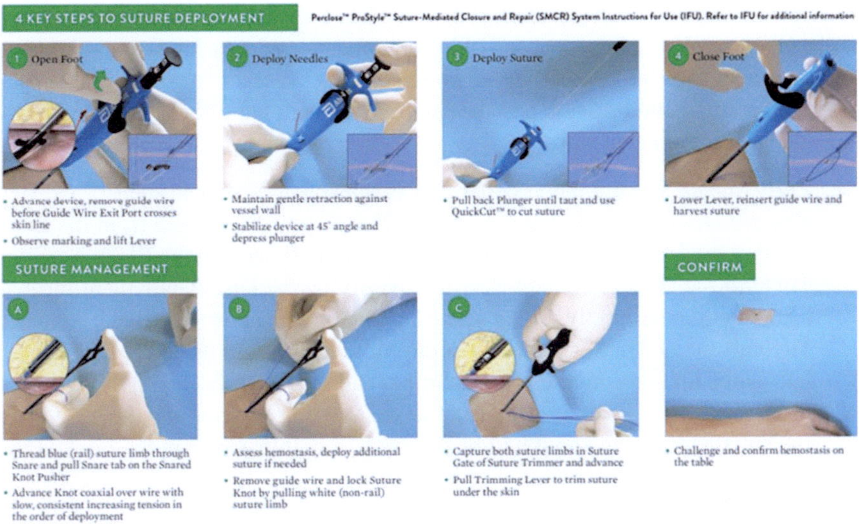

Fig. 16.2 Perclose Closure Device Procedure: Key steps for suture deployment and management. (Courtesy of Abbot Vascular, Redwood City, CA.)

14. The sutures are secured away from the 0.035″ guidewire usually by sterile stickers or Kelley clamp onto the drape, ensuring that neither suture is inadvertently tightened.
15. The Perclose is removed and the larger sheath is advanced (with or without further pre-dilatation, depending on size of sheath).
16. Following conclusion of LAAO, sheath is removed, and 0.035″ guidewire is usually retained during the initial completion stage of the Perclose.
17. Coil the blue limb around your index finger and secure with a knot pusher into the venotomy site, using a gentle forward traction on the pusher (Fig. 16.2).
18. Check for sufficient hemostasis and, if confirmed, remove the 0.035″ guidewire. Further tighten the blue limb, and then simultaneously tug on the white limb to lock the knot (Fig. 16.2).
19. Snip the suture below the level of the skin using the designated suture cutter (Fig. 16.2).

Vascade Closure Device

Vascade is an extravascular and bioabsorbable closure system for femoral access, garnered FDA approval in 2013 [13]. Initially designed for the closure of femoral arterial access sites, it has since been adopted for large bore venous access closures in current medical practices. The advantages of timing to hemostasis, ambulation, and discharge are akin to other closure devices [14]. Compared to Perclose, Vascade provides an extravascular closure and does not leave unabsorbed material intraluminally. However, Vascade's bioabsorbable components do necessitate a period during which re-access of the vessel may be more complex. Vascade may be more expensive than manual compression and the figure-of-8 stitch but offer indirect cost savings due shorter hospital stays.

1. *Flush Sheath*: Ensure the vascular access sheath is properly flushed.
2. *Prepare Device*: Check that the Yellow-Blue Key is disengaged from the Lock and that the Black Sleeve is locked in position. Pull back on the Black Actuator Tip until the Green Segment is visible, verifying the Disc deployment mechanism functions correctly. Collapse the Disc by pressing down the Black Actuator Tip until the Green Segment is hidden. Momentarily dip the VCS Catheter tip into saline up to the White Marker Stripe, and then remove it quickly.
3. *Insert Catheter*: Gently insert the collapsed Vascade catheter into the introducer sheath hub, ensuring about half of the Lock is visible. Confirm the Lock is not fully inserted into the sheath (Fig. 16.3a).
4. *Deploy Disc*: Securely hold the Silver Handle and pull back the Black Actuator until it locks (Fig. 16.3b).
5. *Remove Sheath*: Gently withdraw the sheath without compressing the access site or holding the Catheter. As the sheath slides over the Catheter, grasp the Catheter near the Lock as it exits the sheath. Continue to slide the sheath over the Catheter, and then discard the sheath (Fig. 16.3c).
6. *Achieve Hemostasis*: Apply gentle tension on the Black Actuator until temporary hemostasis is achieved. Check if any part of the White Marker Stripe near the distal aspect of the Black Sleeve is visible above the skin. If visible, the tissue tract might be shorter than 2.5 cm.
7. *Apply Clip*: Once hemostasis is achieved, place the Clip on the Black Sleeve at skin level (Fig. 16.3d).
8. *Expose Collagen Patch*: Unlock the Black Sleeve by sliding the Yellow-Blue Key into the Lock until no blue is visible. While holding the Lock, remove the Clip and slide the Lock back to retract the Black Sleeve. The Sleeve will move freely after initial resistance. A second resistance point may be felt after moving the sleeve about 1.6 cm (0.6 inch) (Fig. 16.3e,f).
9. *Retract Sleeve and Swell Patch*: Fully retract the Black Sleeve toward the Silver Handle to expose the Collagen Patch. Allow the Collagen Patch to swell at the venotomy site for up to 30 s. Reapply the Clip with minimal tension on the Catheter during the swell period.
10. *Remove Catheter*: After the patch swell time ($\leq$30 s), remove the Clip. Rest your palm on the patient, and grasp the green tube with your thumb and index finger. With slack in the catheter, collapse the Disc by pressing the Black Actuator Tip. Ensure the Green Segment is not visible for a 6/7F device, or only a small portion (about 1 mm) for a 5F device. Keeping the green tube stationary, pull back the Catheter proximally. The Catheter Handle will move about 1.5 cm while the green part remains stationary. Let go of the Green Tube and apply gentle manual compression at the venotomy site. Finally, remove the Vascade catheter and assess hemostasis (Fig. 16.3g).

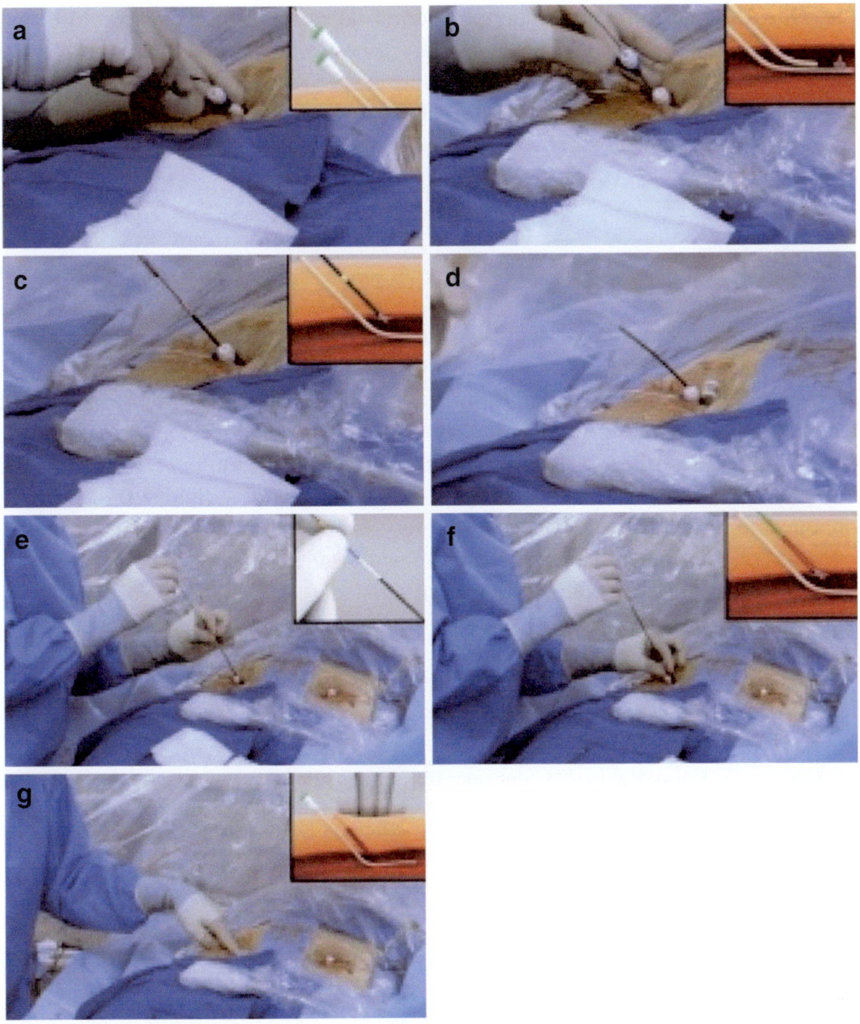

Fig. 16.3 Vascade Closure Device Procedure: (**a**) Insert the collapsed Vascade catheter into the introducer sheath hub. (**b**) Deploy Disc. (**c**) Withdraw the vascular access sheath while maintaining the position of the disc at the venotomy site. (**d**) Place the Clip on the Black Sleeve at skin level. (**e, f**) Expose collagen patch. (**g**) Apply gentle manual compression at the venotomy site. (Courtesy of Haemonetics Corporation, Boston, MA)

Clinical Practice at University Hospitals Harrington Heart and Vascular Institute

At University Hospitals Harrington Heart and Vascular Institute, our primary objective is to minimize bleeding risks and promote rapid patient rehabilitation, ensuring a safe and prompt discharge. Our approach is pragmatic, as we tailor it to meet the specific needs of each patient. In our standard protocol, we administer protamine at the end of the case to reverse periprocedural heparin. We use one Perclose in a Preclose fashion for the 15 French primary access site and one Vascade for the 8 French secondary access. If an overnight stay is necessary, or if we anticipate a need to re-access the vessel in the near future, hemostasis is achieved with manual compression or a figure-of-8 stitch.

Conclusions

Meticulous access technique with US guidance is the most critical aspect of any intravascular procedure to minimize adverse outcomes. Closure techniques are plentiful and vary among different institutions and practitioners. Given a lack of formal data to support one technique over another, a personalized approach to care, with consideration of each patient's unique risk factors and future healthcare needs, remains the best practice. By adhering to this philosophy of individualized care, we not only uphold the highest standards of safety and efficacy but also ensure that each intervention resonates with the patient's lifestyle and preferences, thereby enhancing both institutional outcomes and patient satisfaction.

References

1. Freeman JV, Varosy P, Price MJ, Slotwiner D, Kusumoto FM, Rammohan C, et al. The NCDR left atrial appendage occlusion registry. J Am Coll Cardiol. 2020;75(13):1503.
2. Robertson L, Andras A, Colgan F, Jackson R. Vascular closure devices for femoral arterial puncture site haemostasis. Cochrane Database Syst Rev. 2016;3:CD009541.
3. Brass P, Hellmich M, Kolodziej L, Schick G, Smith AF. Ultrasound guidance versus anatomical landmarks for subclavian or femoral vein catheterization. Cochrane Database Syst Rev. 2015;1:Cd011447.
4. Glikson M, Wolff R, Hindricks G, Mandrola J, Camm AJ, Lip GYH, et al. EHRA/EAPCI expert consensus statement on catheter-based left atrial appendage occlusion - an update. Europace. 2020;22(2):184.
5. Saw J, Holmes DR, Cavalcante JL, Freeman JV, Goldsweig AM, Kavinsky CJ, et al. SCAI/HRS expert consensus statement on Transcatheter left atrial appendage closure. J Soc Cardiovasc Angiogr Interv. 2023;2(3):100577.
6. Tsui JY, Collins AB, White DW, Lai J, Tabas JA. Placement of a femoral venous catheter. N Engl J Med. 2008;358(26):e30.
7. Rashid S, Hughes S. Risk factors for femoral arterial complications and management. Br J Cardiol. 2016;23(4):155.
8. Pracon R, Bangalore S, Henzel J, Cendrowska-Demkow I, Pregowska-Chwala B, Tarnowska A, et al. A randomized comparison of modified subcutaneous "Z"-stitch versus manual compression to achieve hemostasis after large caliber femoral venous sheath removal. Catheter Cardiovasc Interv. 2018;91(1):105.
9. Lodhi H, Shaukat S, Mathews A, Maini B, Khalili H. Comparison of figure-of-eight suture and Perclose ProGlide suture-mediated closure in large bore venous access hemostasis: a randomized controlled trial. Am J Cardiol. 2023;15(209):181–3.

10. Natale A, Mohanty S, Liu PY, Mittal S, Al-Ahmad A, De Lurgio DB, et al. Venous vascular closure system versus manual compression following multiple access electrophysiology procedures: the AMBULATE trial. JACC Clin Electrophysiol. 2020;6(1):111.
11. Pershad A, Gade V, Wiesner P. Vascular access, management, and closure: best practices. 1st ed. Shroff A, Pinto D, vol. 1. Washington, DC: The Society for Cardiovascular Angiography and Interventions (SCAI); 2019. pp. 40–135.
12. Bui QT, Kolansky DM, Bannan A, Herrmann HC. "Double wire" Angio-seal closure technique after balloon aortic valvuloplasty. Catheter Cardiovasc Interv. 2010;75(4):488.
13. Case BC, Kumar S, Medranda GA, Yerasi C, Forrestal BJ, Satler LF, et al. Contemporary post-marketing adverse events and modes of failure related to VASCADE vascular closure system: the utility of the MAUDE database. Catheter Cardiovasc Interv. 2022;99(3):822.
14. Hermiller JB, Leimbach W, Gammon R, Karas SP, Whitbourn RJ, Chiu Wong S, et al. A prospective, randomized, pivotal trial of a novel extravascular collagen-based closure device compared to manual compression in diagnostic and interventional patients. Vol. 27 136-7 25740964, J Invasive Cardiol 2015.

Chapter 17
Surgical Treatment for Left Atrial Appendage Closure

Mustafa M. Houmsse, Pablo Ruda-Vega, and Gregory D. Rushing

Abbreviations

NVAF	Non-valvular atrial fibrillation
LAA	Left atrial appendage
OAC	Oral anticoagulation
NOAC	Non-vitamin K antagonist oral anticoagulants
TEE	Transesophageal echocardiography
TIA	Transient ischemic attack

Highlights

- Surgical left atrial appendage (LAA) occlusion (LAAO) during cardiac surgery is a significantly more effective preventive procedure for ischemic stroke and systemic embolism in patients with non-valvular atrial fibrillation (NVAF) when compared to valvular atrial fibrillation (VAF).
- Surgical LAAO should be considered during cardiac surgery in patients with a diagnosis or history of atrial fibrillation.
- Surgical LAAO during cardiac surgery and oral anticoagulation therapy (OAC) is a significantly more effective preventive therapy for ischemic stroke and systemic embolism when compared to OAC's alone.
- Surgical LAAO should be evaluated intraoperatively via trans-esophageal echocardiogram (TEE) in order to confirm no communication between LAA and Left atrial (LA) with a residual LAA stump <1 cm in depth.

M. M. Houmsse
College of Graduate Studies, Northeast Ohio Medical University, Rootstown, OH, USA

P. Ruda-Vega · G. D. Rushing (✉)
Division of Cardiac Surgery, University Hospitals Harrington Heart and Vascular Institute, Case Western Reserve University College of Medicine, Cleveland, OH, USA
e-mail: Gregory.rushing@uhhospitals.org

S. J. Filby et al. (eds.), *A Contemporary Manual of Left Atrial Appendage Closure*, https://doi.org/10.1007/978-3-031-68441-8_17

- Surgical methods of LAA exclusion via external compression with a clip device result in superior LAAC with increased efficacy and minimal device-related complications.

Introduction

Atrial fibrillation (AF) is a cardiac arrhythmia that is commonly encountered in clinical practice. AF is classified into valvular atrial fibrillation (VAF), including patients with mechanical cardiac valves, rheumatic, non-rheumatic disease, and non-valvular atrial fibrillation (NVAF) [1]. Patients with AF are at risk for ischemic stroke from systemic embolization, driven by atrial remodeling which decreases atrial contractility, blood flow, and velocity. This potentially results in stagnation of blood, thrombus formation within the left atrium and left atrial appendage (LAA), increasing the likelihood of thromboembolic events and ischemic stroke (Fig. 17.1). As such, stasis-related LA thrombi is a strong predictor of TIA and ischemic stroke [2, 3].

Oral anticoagulation (OAC) is the first-line recommended therapy to prevent thrombus formation. However, only 60% of OAC-eligible patients receive this treatment [4]. For those receiving treatment, adherence to OACs remains to be a challenge. A retrospective cohort analysis including 64,661 patients with NVAF found that only 40.2% of patients taking vitamin K antagonist (warfarin) and 47.5% of patients taking non-vitamin K antagonist oral anticoagulants (NOACs) had greater than 80% adherence after 1 year [5].

Mechanical exclusion of the LAA is an effective alternative preventive procedure for thromboembolic formation and ischemic stroke if patients are intolerant to OACs. It is important to note that the exclusion of the LAA is more effective in preventing thromboembolic events and ischemic stroke in patients with NVAF. This is due to different sources of left atrial thrombi among patients with valvular versus

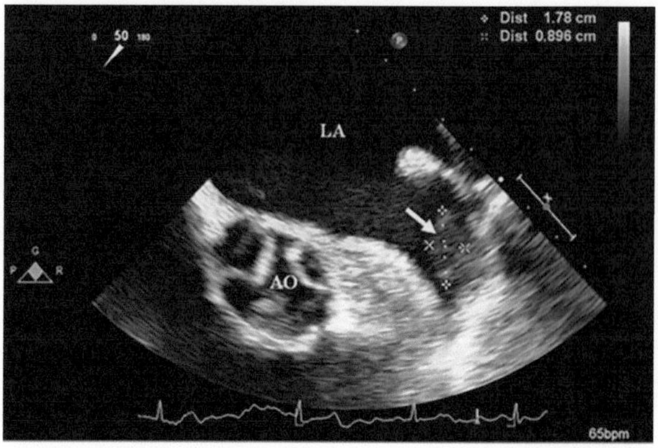

Fig. 17.1 Intraoperative TEE evaluation of thrombus in the left atrial appendage

non-valvular and nonrheumatic AF. A literature review of 23 studies found that for patients with VAF, 254 of 446 (57%) of the total observed left atrial thrombi were located in the left atrium cavity, whereas in patients with NVAF, 201 of 222 (91%) of left atrial thrombi were instead located in the left atrial appendage. This illustrates the value of LAA closure for thromboembolic events and stroke prevention in patients with NVAF [6].

There are multiple approaches to excluding the LAA. By far, the most utilized are percutaneous endocardial devices, as well as surgical exclusion techniques implemented in clinical practice. Surgical LAA exclusion is considered a standalone procedure, or more commonly, during concomitant cardiac surgery and has been shown to reduce the risk of stroke and embolization, after adequate intraoperative transesophageal echocardiography (TEE) evaluation (Fig. 17.1). One study investigating the incidence of both stroke and systemic embolization in AF patients who either did or did not undergo LAA occlusion during cardiac surgery found higher incidences (7% vs 4.8%) of both stroke and systemic embolisms in the non-occlusion group [7]. Regarding current surgical techniques, simple neck ligation, purse string suturing, excision and over-sewing, external clip compression, and surgical stapling can be employed for mechanical LAA exclusion.

Methods of Exclusion

Multiple studies evaluating the impact of surgical LAA exclusion during cardiac surgery demonstrate efficacy in the prevention of ischemic stroke and systemic embolization. Surgical LAA exclusion can be achieved through different techniques including simple neck ligation, purse-string techniques, and surgical stapling to seal off the LAA from circulation. The following is a review of the most pivotal studies in confirming the benefits of surgical exclusion of LAA during cardiac surgery for stroke prevention.

In the EXCLUDE study, 71 patients undergoing elective cardiac surgery with stroke scores greater than 2 were eligible for concomitant AtriClip® (Atricure Inc., Westchester, Ohio) device placement. AtriClip® were placed in patients undergoing sternotomy, on or off cardiopulmonary bypass. One patient had an LAA that was too small to be eligible for clip placement, resulting in 70 patients being included in the analysis. Intraprocedural success of LAA occlusion using the AtriClip® device was confirmed in 67 of 70 patients (95.7%). There were no reported complications that were related to the device. During a 3-month follow-up, successful LAA occlusion was confirmed by computed tomography angiography or TEE in 98.4% of patients. The investigators concluded that the AtriClip® is a safe and efficacious device in achieving LAA occlusion with >95% of successful occlusions 3 months follow-up cardiac imaging [8]. This study led to FDA approval of this device and its widespread use by cardiac surgeons.

Whitlock and associates in the LAAOS (left atrial appendage occlusion study) trial assessed the efficacy and safety of surgical LAA exclusion during coronary artery bypass grafting (CABG) procedures. Seventy-seven patients who were at increased risk of stroke were randomized into LAA occlusion or no LAA occlusion groups. The LAA was occluded via suture or a surgical stapling device. Complete LAA occlusion was confirmed by TEE. There were no significant differences in cardiopulmonary bypass duration, perioperative heart failure, AF, or bleeding between the 2 groups. During surgery, there were 9 appendage tears, all of which were immediately repaired with sutures. Stapling was demonstrably more effective in achieving complete LAA occlusion in 72% (24/33) compared to 45% (5/11) of cases which utilized sutures to occlude the LAA. The learning curve improved the rate of LAA occlusion by individual surgeons from 43% (9/21) to 87% (20/23) after performing 4 cases ($P = 0.0001$). The LAAOS study confirmed that LAAOS during CABG is a safe improvement of LAA occlusion especially when utilizing surgical stapling devices [9].

In a follow-up trial, LAAOS III, Whitlock and colleagues demonstrated that surgical exclusion of the LAA during cardiac surgery for patients with AF prevented ischemic stroke and systemic embolization. LAAOS III included 4811 patients with a history of AF, with increased risk for ischemic stroke and systemic embolism, (CHADS-VASc >2). Patients undergoing cardiac surgery were randomized into 2 groups. The treatment arm included 2400 patients who underwent cardiac surgery and LAA occlusion (LAAO group). The control arm included 2411 patients who underwent cardiac surgery without LAA occlusion (no occlusion group). The patients, research team, and primary care physicians (other than the surgeons) were blind to the study-group assignments. Post-procedure, all patients resumed usual care including oral anticoagulation (OAC) and monitored across 3 years. The adherence to OAC's between both groups was comparable with 75.3% in the LAAO group and 78.2% in the control group. There was a statistically significant reduction of ischemic stroke or non-cerebral systemic embolism in the LAAO group, 4.8% compared to 7.0% in the no occlusion group (hazard ratio, 0.67; 95% confidence interval, 0.53 to 0.85; $P = 0.001$). There was no significant difference in the incidence of perioperative bleeding, heart failure, or death between the study groups [8].

Surgical Techniques for LAA Occlusion

1. *Surgical excision and over-sew*: Surgical removal of the appendage and oversewing of the base of the left atrium is a simple, inexpensive, and effective technique. Surgeons may use Teflon felt strips to buttress the friable thin left atrial wall from tearing, one of the complications from this technique. Care must be taken to watch for the proximity of the left circumflex coronary artery, to avoid injury. This technique does take more time and prolongs cross-clamp time but not by an excessive amount.
2. *Staple and excision*: There are several models of GIA stapling devices that are used to ligate and excise the left atrial appendage. Multiple (usually 3) linear staple rows are fired across the base of the left atrial appendage; care is taken to

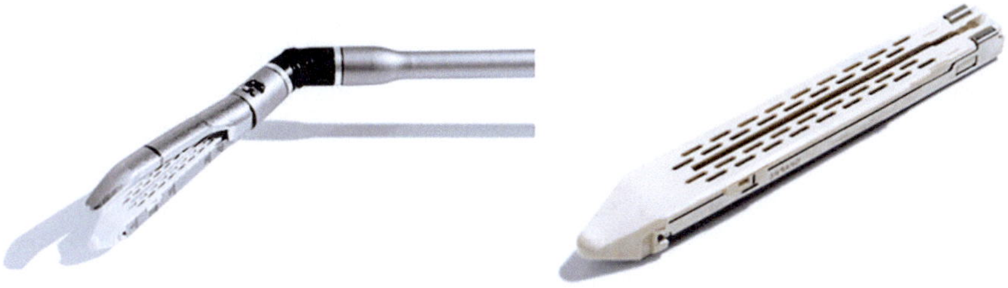

Fig. 17.2 Ethicon Endo-GIA vascular stapling device

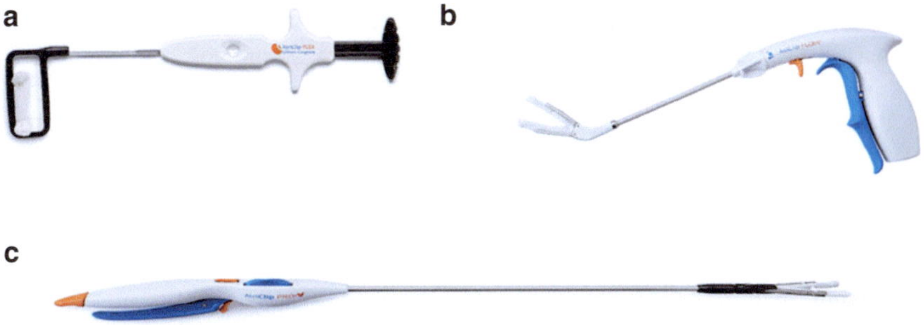

Fig. 17.3 AtriCure AtriClip® (**a**) ACHV, (**b**) Flex V, (**c**) Pro –V

avoid the left circumflex coronary artery. The stapling device also enables concomitant scalpel excision of the left atrium above the staple lines. Buttress material such as bovine pericardial strips are often used in conjunction with these staple loads, given the thin friable nature of the left atrial tissue (Fig. 17.2).

3. *AtriClip®*: The AtriClip® is an epicardial applied exclusion device that prevents blood flow into the LAA once it has been deployed at its base. The clips construction consists of two titanium tubes that utilize nitinol springs housed in a woven polyester sheath. There are a number of iterations of the AtriClip® including the flex, pro, long, V, and standard AtriClip® system devices. All AtriClip® devices come in 35 mm, 40 mm, 45 mm, and 50 mm clip sizes. The most recent Flex-V and Pro-V clips are all titanium construction and can be used in patients with Nickel allergy. The clip can most readily be applied during open cardiac surgery to exclude the LAA through its non-piercing application. Minimally invasive delivery devices are available for stand-alone or video-assisted thoracoscopic surgical (VATS) application (Fig. 17.3).
4. *TigerPaw*: the TigerPaw was an epicardial LAA occlusion system that features a jaw-like implantable fastener to be externally placed at the base of the LAA. The U-shaped fastener has opposing male and female sides that are both housed in silicone, allowing conformation and a custom fit to the morphology of the LAA. The male side of the fastener contains a series of titanium needle barbs

which are conical in shape and contain no sharp edges. The female side holds the connectors directly parallel to the male needle barbs, which allow for the connection of the two opposing sides of the fastener when the fastener is deployed. Similar to the AtriClip system, the TigerPaw fastener could be applied during open cardiac surgery [8]. Concerns for bleeding and failure to close appropriately led to the FDA class I recall of this device from the market in 2015.

5. *Penditure®*: The Penditure® device is the most recent to receive FDA approval for LAA management. It is an epicardial applied exclusion device that prevents blood flow into the LAA once it has been deployed at its base. The clip is made of poly ethyl-ethyl kinase (PEEK) and a nitinol spring. The clip is curvilinear, designed to conform to the shape of the left atrium. There is no Dacron, fabric, or tissue enveloping the clip, possibly making minimally invasive application easier. One unique feature is the ability to fully recapture and re-deploy the clip (Fig. 17.4).

Current Practice/Problems with Existing Techniques

In a study including 137 patients undergoing LAA exclusion followed by TEE to evaluate the success of various surgical techniques for LAA excision and exclusion, patients either underwent LAA excision (surgical excision or amputating stapling device) or exclusion (suture or staple exclusion). Only 55 of 137 (40%) LAA closures were successful, with 73% of those 55 patients having undergone excision compared to the 23% with suture exclusion, with no successful closures resulting from staple exclusion. Residual stumps larger than 1 cm were found in 14 (27%) of patients who underwent LAA excision. Additionally, as confirmed by TEE, it was found that 6 (11%) of patients with successful and 12 (15%) with unsuccessful LAA closure procedures showed evidence of strokes or transient ischemic attack (TIA) [10].

One study evaluating the AtriClip® success of exclusion both intraoperatively and at a 3-month follow-up period by TEE or computed tomography angiography (CTA), in 70 patients. Sixty-seven of 70 (95.7%) patients had successful intraoperative LAA exclusion with no reported incidences of bleeding or damage to the appendage or surrounding arteries. Of the 61 patients who returned for their follow-up meeting and agreed to TEE or CTA imaging, 60 (98.3%) patients had apparent

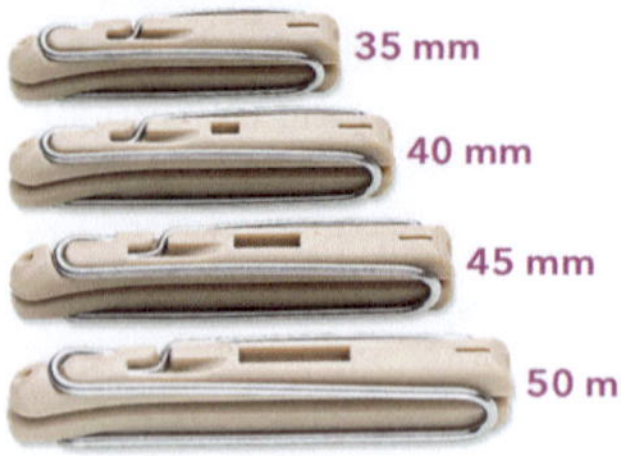

Fig. 17.4 Medtronic Penditure® Devices

complete exclusion of the LAA. This means that only one patient of the initial three who did not undergo initial successful LAA exclusion remained unsuccessful at the time of the 3-month follow-up [11].

Reported malfunctions of the Tigerpaw® device include incomplete closure of the fasteners which, in some cases, resulted in a tear and severe bleeding of the LAA when attempting to remove the device. As a result, a Class I recall was issued by the US Food and Drug Administration, effectively removing the device from the market [12].

Future Direction/Studies

The future of surgical LAA occlusion may lie in preventative procedures to minimize the risk of stroke in individuals who are at risk for but may not necessarily have yet developed AF. Epicardial clip devices have shown promising results, most notably with the AtriClip® system, as it has demonstrated high efficacy with minimal device-related complications. The Left Atrial Appendage Exclusion for Stroke Prevention (LeAAPS™) is a recently announced large-scale randomized clinical trial that will include up to 6500 patients across 250 healthcare centers. This will be the largest randomized clinical trial for surgical LAA exclusion but will also evaluate the efficacy of using the AtriClip® device as a means of reducing stroke risk in individuals without a previous AF diagnosis. This study is using a combination of physiology (CHA2DS2-VASc >2) parameters as well as anatomic (LAA dimension >4.5 cm) to screen patients at increased risk of developing AF or stroke/TIA. Additionally, new epicardial clips for LAA exclusion are in development and may deliver promising results. Medtronic is looking to implement the usage of the Penditure® LAA exclusion system as it has recently added the device to its cardiac surgery portfolio as of November 2023. The device is a single-use, externally deployed clip system that comes in 35 mm, 40 mm, 45 mm, and 50 mm sizes. The clip is curved which may help with providing a secure fit at the base of the LAA, as well as being free of any fabric to reduce any device-related adverse effects like trauma to the appendage or inflammation. Another key feature of its design is the ability for surgeons to fully recapture and redeploy the clip to optimize placement at the LAA base. The post-market study, exClusion of the Left atrIal appendage with PendITure™ (CLIP-IT), was recently launched in 2024. The study will enroll 150 patients in a non-randomized interventional study which will further investigate the safety and efficacy of the Penditure® system in LAA exclusion.

References

1. Joglar JA, et al. 2023 ACC/AHA/ACCP/HRS guideline for the diagnosis and management of atrial fibrillation: a report of the American College of Cardiology/American Heart Association Joint Committee on Clinical Practice Guidelines. Circulation. 2023;148:e00–e00. https://doi.org/10.1161/CIR.0000000000001193.
2. Stoddard MF, Singh P, Dawn B, Longaker RA. Left atrial thrombus predicts transient ischemic attack in patients with atrial fibrillation. Am Heart J. 2003;145(4):676–82. https://doi.org/10.1067/mhj.2003.91.
3. Goldman ME, Pearce LA, Hart RG, et al. Pathophysiologic correlates of thromboembolism in nonvalvular atrial fibrillation: I. Reduced flow velocity in the left atrial appendage (The Stroke Prevention in Atrial Fibrillation [SPAF-III] study). J Am Soc Echocardiogr. 1999;12(12):1080–7.
4. Marzec LN, Wang J, Shah ND, Chan PS, Ting HH, Gosch KL, Hsu JC, Maddox TM. Influence of direct oral anticoagulants on rates of oral anticoagulation for atrial fibrillation. J Am Coll Cardiol. 2017;69(20):2475–84. https://doi.org/10.1016/j.jacc.2017.03.540.
5. Yao X, Abraham NS, Alexander GC, Crown W, Montori VM, Sangaralingham LR, Gersh BJ, Shah ND, Noseworthy PA. Effect of adherence to oral anticoagulants on risk of stroke and major bleeding among patients with atrial fibrillation. J Am Heart Assoc. 2016;5(2):e003074. https://doi.org/10.1161/JAHA.115.003074.
6. Blackshear JL, Odell JA. Appendage obliteration to reduce stroke in cardiac surgical patients with atrial fibrillation. Ann Thorac Surg. 1996;61(2):755–9. https://doi.org/10.1016/0003-4975(95)00887-X. PMID: 8572814.
7. Whitlock RP, Belley-Cote EP, Paparella D, Healey JS, Brady K, Sharma M, Reents W, Budera P, Baddour AJ, Fila P, Devereaux PJ, Bogachev-Prokophiev A, Boening A, Teoh KHT, Tagarakis GI, Slaughter MS, Royse AG, McGuinness S, Alings M, Punjabi PP, Mazer CD, Folkeringa RJ, Colli A, Avezum Á, Nakamya J, Balasubramanian K, Vincent J, Voisine P, Lamy A, Yusuf S, Connolly SJ, LAAOS III Investigators. Left atrial appendage occlusion during cardiac surgery to prevent stroke. N Engl J Med. 2021;384(22):2081–91. https://doi.org/10.1056/NEJMoa2101897. Epub 2021 May 15. PMID: 33999547.
8. Ailawadi G, Gerdisch MW, Harvey RL, Hooker RL, Damiano RJ Jr, Salamon T, Mack MJ. Exclusion of the left atrial appendage with a novel device: early results of a multicenter trial. J Thorac Cardiovasc Surg. 2011;142(5):1002–9. https://doi.org/10.1016/j.jtcvs.2011.07.052. Epub 2011 Sep 8. PMID: 21906756
9. Healey JS, Crystal E, Lamy A, Teoh K, Semelhago L, Hohnloser SH, Cybulsky I, Abouzahr L, Sawchuck C, Carroll S, Morillo C, Kleine P, Chu V, Lonn E, Connolly SJ. Left Atrial Appendage Occlusion Study (LAAOS): results of a randomized controlled pilot study of left atrial appendage occlusion during coronary bypass surgery in patients at risk for stroke. Am Heart J. 2005;150(2):288–93. https://doi.org/10.1016/j.ahj.2004.09.054. PMID: 16086933
10. Kanderian AS, Gillinov AM, Pettersson GB, Blackstone E, Klein AL. Success of surgical left atrial appendage closure: assessment by transesophageal echocardiography. J Am Coll Cardiol. 2008;52(11):924–9. https://doi.org/10.1016/j.jacc.2008.03.067.
11. Slater AD, Tatooles AJ, Coffey A, Pappas PS, Bresticker M, Greason K, Slaughter MS. Prospective clinical study of a novel left atrial appendage occlusion device. Ann Thorac Surg. 2012;93(6):2035–40. https://doi.org/10.1016/j.athoracsur.2011.12.077.
12. Ventosa-Fernandez G, Quintana E, Castellá M, Pereda D. Exclusion of the left atrial appendage with the TigerPaw II system: a word of caution. Interact Cardiovasc Thorac Surg. 2015;21(6):803–4. https://doi.org/10.1093/icvts/ivv256.

Part III
Post-procedural Management

Chapter 18
Complications Following Percutaneous Left Atrial Appendage Occlusion

Rafey Feroze, Nawaf Alhabdan, Puneet Kang, Mohammed A. Alghammass, Luis Augusto Palma Dallan, and Steven J. Filby

Highlights

- Pericardial effusion (PE) with associated tamponade is the most common serious complication following left atrial appendage occlusion (LAAO), but its incidence has reduced with improved technique and newer generation devices.
- Device-related thrombus is an infrequent but significant complication after LAAO and requires continued oral anticoagulation.
- Procedure-associated thromboembolism may occur from clot formation in the heart due to subtherapeutic intraprocedural anticoagulation or air embolism from inadequate deairing of equipment.
- Device embolization is a rare but potentially lethal complication and may require surgical extraction of the device depending on location.
- Peri-device leaks have been associated with an increased risk of thromboembolism and may be treated with endovascular plugs, radiofrequency ablation, or coil embolization depending on size.

R. Feroze · M. A. Alghammass · L. A. P. Dallan (✉) · S. J. Filby
Division of Cardiology, Harrington Heart & Vascular Institute, University Hospitals Cleveland Medical Center, Cleveland, OH, USA
e-mail: luisaugusto.palmadallan@uhhospitals.org

N. Alhabdan · P. Kang
Division of Internal Medicine, University Hospitals Cleveland Medical Center, Cleveland, OH, USA

S. J. Filby et al. (eds.), *A Contemporary Manual of Left Atrial Appendage Closure*, https://doi.org/10.1007/978-3-031-68441-8_18

Introduction

Percutaneous left atrial appendage occlusion (LAAO) has become a viable alternative to oral anticoagulation (OAC) for atrial fibrillation (AFIB) patients. Following FDA approval of the WATCHMAN 2.5 device in 2015 due to noninferiority compared to Coumadin in the pivotal PROTECT-AF and PREVAIL randomized controlled trials, the number of implants in the United States have increased exponentially and are being performed by both electrophysiologist and interventional cardiologists in various hospital settings. While being a relatively safe procedure with adverse events ranging from only 1.8–8.7%, there are several post-procedure complications that require high-fidelity monitoring and specific management. This chapter enumerates the common complications following LAAO and expounds on their respective mechanisms, reported incidences, timing following procedure, prognosis, and various management strategies.

Pericardial Effusion

Mechanism

Pericardial effusion (PE) is the most common adverse event and reported cause of death following LAAO. The left atrium (LA) and left atrial appendage (LAA) are both low-pressure and thin-walled structures. In fact, the LAA has been described as the "most lethal human attachment" due to fragile tissue between pectinate muscles. As such, equipment used for transeptal puncture or manipulation of large bore sheaths and occlusion devices during implantation can cause trauma and macroperforation of the right atrium, LA, LAA, or left superior pulmonary artery resulting in hemorrhagic PE. This risk is increased with device recapture, repositioning, or replacement and mitigated by the use of atraumatic wires and pigtail catheters. Figure 18.1 illustrates the presence of a hemorrhagic PE suggested by the high attenuation of pericardial fluid on CT following AMULET implantation (PE indicated by white arrows). Additionally, both the WATCHMAN FLX and AMULET Occluders (LAAO devices that are most frequently utilized in the United States) have fixation anchors that predispose to some degree of microperforation which may lead to PE. Patients undergoing LAAO are given intraprocedural heparin and antiplatelet/anticoagulation following implantation which albeit necessary enhances the risk of hemorrhagic PE and development of cardiac tamponade.

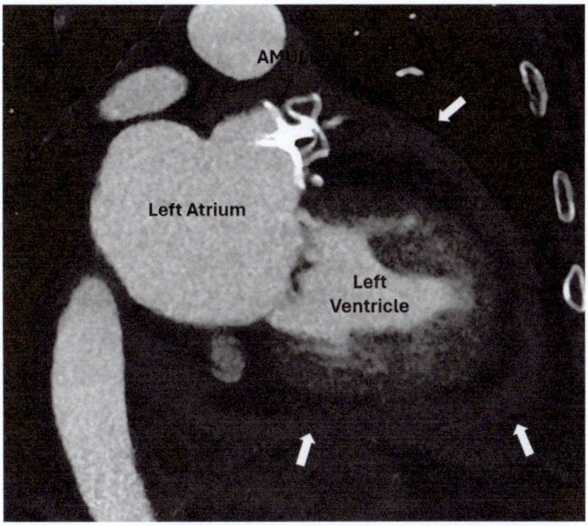

Fig. 18.1 Cardiac computed tomography image of circumferential pericardial effusion in a patient following left atrial appendage occlusion (LAAO) with the AMULET device

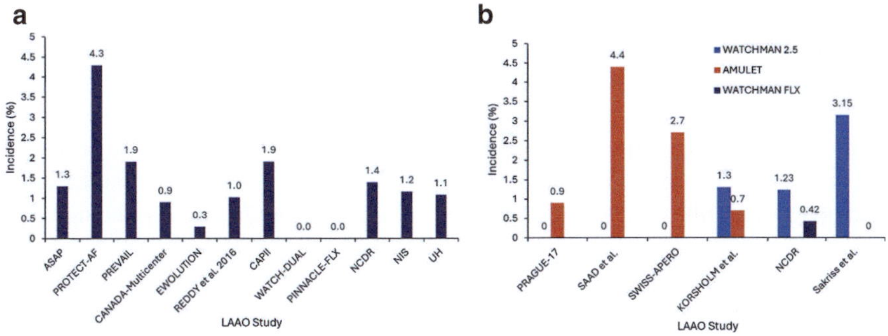

Fig. 18.2 (**a**) Incidence of pericardial effusion (PE) requiring drainage in major left atrial appendage occlusion (LAAO) studies in chronological order from left to right. (**b**) Incidence of PE requiring drainage across LAAO studies each comparing 2 devices

Incidence

The initial PROTECT-AF trial demonstrated an incidence of PE requiring intervention at 4.8%. However, newer generation devices and improved operator technique and experience decreased the incidence to 1.9% in the subsequent PREVAIL trial, and European/US studies have demonstrated PE rates of 1.24–1.50%. PE incidence in our own LAAO experience was 1.35%. Figure 18.2a illustrates the incidence of PE requiring drainage reported in major LAAO randomized controlled trials (RCTs) and observational studies.

Risk Factors

Clinical factors pre-disposing to post-LAAO PEs include female sex, obesity, older age, decreased albumin, elevated CHADS2VASC score, prior bleeding events, and pre-procedural antiplatelet therapy. Interestingly, sinus rhythm and paroxysmal atrial fibrillation have also been independently associated with PE. Mechanistically, LAA contraction during sinus rhythm may accentuate mechanical interaction between the LAA and device anchors leading to microperforation and hemopericardium. Whether a greater prevalence of LAAO PE is associated with the presence of atrial flutter as opposed to AFIB is yet to be determined.

Timing

The vast majority of post LAAO PEs manifest within hours to days following LAAO and are attributed to intraprocedural macroperforation. In fact, all PEs reported in the PROTECT-AF trial occurred within 7 days following LAAO. As such, a post-procedural transthoracic echocardiogram (TTE) has become a routine part of post-LAAO surveillance at large centers. Relatively little has been reported on delayed PEs presenting more than a month following LAAO. In the absence of clear LAA/coronary artery macroperforation, very delayed PEs are expected to occur due to pericardial microperforations in the LAA leading to hemopericardium and pericardial inflammation and have been observed more frequently among those on anticoagulation compared to patients on antiplatelet therapy alone or no antithrombotic medication. Delayed PEs are expected to accumulate slowly, but further investigation is required to determine if they are less likely to progress to tamponade.

Association of Device Design and PE

Certain device characteristics may also play a role in PE development. The Boston Scientific registry featuring the earlier generation WATCHMAN 2.5 device revealed a PE rate of 1.02%. Similarly, a 1% incidence of PEs was reported with newer generation WATCHMAN FLX device in the PINNACLE FLX study at 12-month follow-up, though notably all of these occurred >7 days post LAAO with half occurring at >1 month post-LAAO. Our experience reproduced these findings with more PEs seen past 7 days with the WATCHMAN FLX compared to the WATCHMAN 2.5. However, head-to-head comparisons have revealed an overall lower rate of PE with the FLX compared to the older generation WATCHMAN. A possible explanation for these findings may be a more traumatic distal end of the WATCHMAN FLX due to folded back tines reducing the risk of macroperforation, but the presence of 8 more lateral fixation anchors may cause an increased risk of microperforation.

Head-to-head comparisons of the AMULET and WATCHMAN devices have reported a higher incidence of PEs in the former (2.4–4.4% vs. 0.0–1.2%), as shown in Fig. 18.2b, with a significantly greater proportion of post-AMULET PEs occurring >2 day post-procedure. This may partially be due to the AMULET having 2.2 times longer fixation anchors creating a lower threshold for microperforation leading to PE. Regardless, the higher rate of PE with AMULET was largely driven by subclinical Pes, and AMULET was not associated with increased risk of cardiac tamponade or death; however, these studies were not powered to detect such differences.

Clinical Impact and Management

Periprocedural PEs have been associated with prolonged length of stay, lower likelihood of discharge on antiplatelet therapy predisposing to device thrombus and stroke, tamponade requiring percutaneous/surgical intervention, and rarely death. Examination of LAAO outcomes from the MAUDE procedural complications database revealed 71% of post-LAAO PEs to require pericardiocentesis with 26% requiring surgical drainage and 5.7% resulting in death. As such, clinical vigilance and careful surveillance is required in high-risk patients. A large perforation might necessitate emergent surgical consultation and reversal of heparin. Smaller macroperforations will usually require a pericardiocentesis with drain placement and continued drainage for 48–72 h. Colchicine may be used for its anti-inflammatory effects and to mitigate associated chest discomfort. Delayed PEs presenting weeks to months following LAAO may or may not require drainage depending on presence of hemodynamic impact of PE. Delayed effusions may be managed conservatively with an anti-inflammatory regimen of colchicine and corticosteroids to curb the development of effusive-constrictive pericarditis, but a high index of suspicion is required to make this diagnosis following PE resolution.

Device-Related Thrombus

Mechanism

While LAAO has emerged as a pivotal intervention for AF patients, device-related thrombus (DRT) poses a unique challenge wherein the device meant to obviate the need for OAC directly compels continued OAC in a population that is unsuitable for such treatment. This is naturally demoralizing for both patients and providers. The formation of DRT involves a complex interplay of factors related to LAAO device, patient physiology, and the post-procedural environment. DRT primarily form due to inadequate endothelialization of the LA side of the LAAO device creating a surface prone for thrombus formation. Additionally, turbulence and stasis of flow in the LAA following LAAO along with blood pooling in fibrillating LA also contribute to clot formation on the device. However, why some patients developed DRT while others don't is incompletely understood.

DRTs have typically been detected via surveillance TEEs as an echo-dense mass that is adherent to the LA side of the LAAO device as illustrated in Fig. 18.3. However, cardiac CT has been demonstrated to have increased sensitivity in DRT detection and with its growing use various morphologies have been detected and characterized on the device face. Following LAAO, the majority of patients will have hypoattenuated thickening (HAT) on device face, which may not be readily evident on TEE. HAT encompasses a spectrum of changes occurring at the device surface where low-grade HAT (flat, sessile, and <3 mm of thickness from the face of the device) may represent benign device healing with temporary platelet aggregation and fibrin deposition (early subclinical thrombus) followed by time-dependent neoendothelialization over 2–3 months. Low-grade HATs are not associated with greater risk of ischemic stroke/thromboembolism and appear to resolve by 12 months without OAC. They have been visualized more frequently at 8 weeks following LAAO in WATCHMAH FLX cases vs. AMULET implants (40% vs. 6%) likely due to a polyethylene terephthalate membrane on the former which promotes neoendothelialization. High-grade HAT (pedunculated, asymmetric, with an irregular surface, >3 mm in thickness, and without continuity with the LA wall) is deemed to be more consistent with DRT. Design differences between AMULET and WATCHMAN along with the absence of standardized imaging protocols and HAT

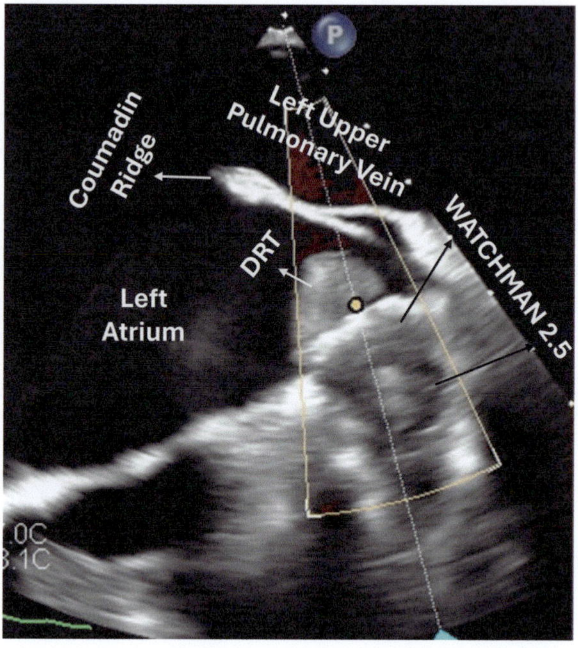

Fig. 18.3 Transesophageal echocardiogram illustrating device-related thrombus (DRT) on the atrial side of WATCHMAN 2.5 device discovered over a year following implantation

measurements have made routine characterization challenging and largely preclinical at this point.

Incidence and Risk Factors

Fortunately, DRTs are rare with an incidence of 3.74% in the landmark PROTECT-AF, PREVAIL trials, and their continued registries featuring the WATCHMAN 2.5 device. Of note, this was on a regimen of ASA + warfarin for 6 weeks followed by ASA + clopidogrel until the 6-month time-point followed by ASA monotherapy. Figure 18.4a illustrates the incidence of DRTs in major LAAO studies. Risk factors associated with DRT are summarized in Table 18.1 and include hypercoagulable disorder, renal insufficiency, high CHADS2VASC score, prior history of stroke/thromboembolic disease, greater frequency of AF (portending greater atrial size and myopathy), low LVEF (leading to depressed LA emptying), larger device size (requiring greater coverage by a neoendothelium), and larger LAA diameter. Deep implantation (defined by at least 10 mm distance of uncovered pulmonary vein ridge) of LAAO devices may leave trabeculated portions of the residual, proximal LAA in contact with static blood precipitating thrombus formation on the device face and has been associated with DRT. In fact, pulmonary ridge coverage with AMULET resulted in reduced rates of DRT (1% vs. 27%) with an associated reduction in stroke (1.3% vs. 6.5%). Thereby, depth of implantation may be the major modifiable procedural factor to reduce DRT. LAAO-associated PEs have been predictive of early DRT, likely due to interruption of periprocedural antithrombotic agents. More frequent, larger peri-device leak (PDL) and higher number of PDLs/patient have been identified among DRT patients, with PDL found to be an independent predictor of DRT at >180 days but not early DRT. A mechanistic connection between PDLs and DRTs has been hypothesized due to the extension of the thrombus from behind the device, but mixed data have made this association inconclusive.

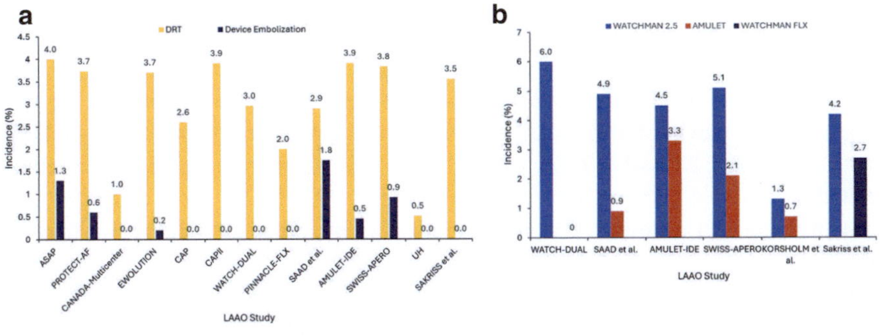

Fig. 18.4 (**a**) Incidence of device-related thrombus (DRT) and device embolization in major left atrial appendage occlusion (LAAO) studies in chronological order from left to right. (**b**) Incidence of DRT across LAAO studies each comparing 2 devices

Table 18.1 Clinical and procedural risk factors associated with device related thrombus (DRT)

DRT risk factors
Hypercoagulable disorder
LAAO associated pericardial effusion
Greater atrial fibrillation burden
Depth of implantation >1 cm from the pulmonary vein ridge
Renal insufficiency
Prior history of stroke
Peri-device leak
Higher CHADS2VASC score
Depressed LVEF
Larger LAAO device size
Larger LAA diameter

From a subset of the aforementioned risk factors, a DRT risk score consisting of 5 factors (weighted loosely based on respective ORs from multivariate models testing association to DRT) has been proposed by Simard et al. with the following breakdown:

1. Hypercoagulability disorder: 4 points
2. Pericardial effusion: 4 points
3. Renal insufficiency: 1 point
4. LAAO depth of implantation >10 mm from pulmonary vein limb: 1 point
5. Non-paroxysmal AFIB: 1 point

A total score of ≥2 suggested a 2.1-fold greater risk for DRT development. No association between LAA morphologies or dual antiplatelet duration and DRT has been found.

Association of Device Design with DRTs

DRTs have been most frequently found on the device cap facing the LA (55.3%) followed by the metal screw (12.7%). Head-to-head comparisons between the two major LAAO device types have consistently revealed a lower incidence of DRT with the AMULET (AMULET: 0.8–3.3% vs. WATCHMAN: 1.3–5.5%) as illustrated in Fig. 18.4b. This is surprising given that the AMULET is not equipped with a membrane that promotes endothelialization. A hypothetical mechanism may be that the outer disc of the AMULET covers the entire LAA ostium leaving no room for a pulmonary ridge as may be seen with deep implantation with the plug type WATCHMAN design. This would theoretically lead to reduced risk of a residual proximal pocket of the LAA, which could serve as a nidus for thrombus formation. The newer WATCHMAN FLX has demonstrated reduced incidence of DRT

(0–2.7%) compared to the earlier generation WATCHMAN 2.5. This is expected given that the FLX has a less exposed metal screw on the face of the device and folded back distal nitinol tines resulting in a reduced metal footprint and decreased thrombogenicity. Additionally, the FLX allowed for more proximal implantation (without a higher rate of device embolization), thereby promoting less residual patent LAA neck (measured from the pulmonary vein ridge to the device face) further contributing to reduced DRT risk. Future device iterations made with antithrombotic coatings on the atrial surface may eliminate DRTs altogether.

DRT Timing

Discerning the precise timing of DRT formation has been challenging as they are usually detected on surveillance imaging or during work-up of a thromboembolic event. Most studies feature initial surveillance imaging at 45 days and serial repeat imaging at an interval of a few months at a time to assess for DRT resolution. However, DRTs are most commonly detected within 180 days following LAAO (63.7%) with some delayed DRTs presenting more than 1 year following LAAO (20.3%). With more frequent imaging, the detection of DRTs and their perceived prevalence would be higher.

Clinical Impact

The association of DRT with thromboembolic events has been challenging to establish due to the low frequency of DRTs and even lower incidence of thromboembolic events after LAAO. An international multicenter study examining 237 DRTs at 37 centers demonstrated an almost fivefold higher rate of ischemic stroke without an increase in all-cause mortality. Similarly, a post-hoc pooled analysis of the PROTECT-AF/PREVAIL trails and their associated multicenter registries of the WATCHMAN 2.5 device revealed an almost threefold higher risk of ischemic stroke/thromboembolism with DRT without differences in cardiovascular or all-cause mortality. Despite this, it is important to note that the majority of patients with DRT (73.8%) did not sustain a stroke/systemic embolism, and, conversely, the majority of strokes/embolic events (~90%) took place in patients without any detected DRT. Furthermore, patients with DRT still had a 28% relative risk reduction in ischemic stroke compared to their expected rate (based on average CHADS2VASC score) in the absence of OAC. DRTs were also associated with a higher rate of major bleeding and hemorrhagic strokes, likely potentiated by the use of OAC for stroke prevention.

Management

Given the persistent signal that DRT is associated with an increased risk of stroke, OAC remains the cornerstone of management and should ideally be continued after detection (with concomitant de-escalation of DAPT to SAPT) and until thrombus resolution on follow-up imaging. While most DRTs are largely immobile and adherent to the LA side of the LAAO device, rarely large/hypermobile DRTs may require surgical excision due to high risk of significant thromboembolism. A short course of OAC following LAAO has been shown to reduce DRT development. DRTs usually resolve with OAC, but continued DRT has been observed in 20–25% of patients on OAC. Persistent large DRT may require surgical excision of LAAO device. Recurrent DRT has been reported in 35% of cases (though none associated with thromboembolism) and in 75% of patients who were on no antithrombotic medication, 38% who were on single/double antiplatelet therapy, and 0% on OAC following resolution of initial DRT. Due to the incidence of DRT recurrence, it is prudent to repeat device imaging at 12 months post-implant with either TEE or CTA. Taken together, these results suggest that the absence of all antithrombotic therapy creates significant DRT risk, while OAC can both prevent and treat DRT to great effect, but its use must be balanced with bleeding risk which is particularly high in the LAAO patient population.

Procedural Thromboembolism

Embolic strokes are an ever-present risk in all left-sided percutaneous cardiac procedures and are often avoidable for LAAO cases if adequate care is taken. Prior to LAAO procedures, TEE or cardiac CT imaging is necessary to rule out LA/LAA thrombus which otherwise may embolize from wire/sheath manipulation during LAAO. Intraprocedurally, an activated clotting time of ≥250 s should be achieved and maintained using unfractionated heparin (or bivalirudin with a concomitant diagnosis of heparin induced thrombocytopenia) to prevent de novo thrombus formation on procedural equipment. During equipment preparation, sheaths and the LAAO delivery system must be adequately flushed and de-aired to prevent the development of air embolism. The delivery system should be inspected thoroughly to ensure no air is visible prior to insertion.

A thorough intraprocedural neurologic assessment is virtually impossible for patients under the influence of general anesthesia and challenging in the case of moderate sedation. As such, ST segment changes on telemetry can hint at an intraprocedural coronary event. If intracardiac thrombus is visualized intraprocedurally, prior to the LAAO device being placed in the LAA, the procedure should be aborted. If the device has already been positioned in the LAA, then deployment should be completed rapidly followed by removal of equipment. Consideration should be given to aspiration thrombectomy using a large sheath, if possible, while conservative management would require intensive anticoagulation and thorough surveillance imaging. The MAUDE procedural complications database reported a 0.1% incidence of intracardiac thrombus (extrapolated across 43,802 procedures) most frequently in the LA followed by the LAA and RA (1.7% of WATCHMAH associated deaths from pulmonary embolism) with 16% of cardiac thrombi undergoing aspiration thrombectomy. A post-procedural neurologic assessment should be undertaken routinely on every patient with consideration for thrombolysis if deficits are uncovered.

Despite a significant number of procedural steps that can introduce air or thrombus, procedure-associated embolic events are low. The initial PROTECT-AF and PREVAIL trials reported 0.70–1.90% incidence of procedure related stroke. However, with increased procedural experience and refined device preparation, the more contemporary US NCDR-LAAO and European EWOLUTION registries have reported a much lower incidence at 0.09% and 0.10%, respectively. Incidence of air embolism has been reported at 0.1–0.2% in earlier LAAO studies. Air embolization may involve any arterial system but is most concerning when involving the coronary arteries or the cerebral circulation. MAUDE database reports described air emboli to be most commonly observed in the left ventricle, followed by the LAA and LA, but also in the coronary arteries (especially the right coronary artery), brain, aorta, and pericardium. Fifty-five percent of air emboli were associated with coronary ischemia with 28% aspirated intraprocedurally and 5.6% implicated in procedural mortality.

Device Embolization

Mechanism and Incidence

Device embolization remains a rare but dramatic complication following LAAO. While many embolizations are clinically silent, some may present with fulminant hemodynamic collapse and require urgent intervention. Embolization is expected to occur in the setting of device implantation that may be too proximal, use of an undersized device, off-axis device orientation, or presence of significant torsion during device placement.

Similar to PEs, the incidence of device embolization has decreased over time. With the initial WATCHMAN 2.5 device, device embolization was observed in 0.25–0.60% of implants. However, with greater operator experience and newer generator devices, there were no device embolizations noted with the WATCHMAN FLX. Figure 18.4a illustrates the incidence of device embolization in major LAAO studies. The aggregate of three head-to-head comparisons between AMULET and WATCHMAN devices have revealed a numerically higher rate of device embolization with the former (AMULET: 8.7% vs. WATCHMAN: 2.5%), but these differences did not reach significance. As such, the embolization potential, risk of myocardial/vascular damage, and ease of extraction between the two device types are not clear.

Clinical Presentation and Impact

Due to the rarity of device embolizations, it has been challenging to do large-scale analyses regarding this complication. However, a systemic review featuring the WATCHMAN 2.5 and AMULET devices described 31 device embolizations with 65% of cases presenting within 4 days of LAAO and 30% of cases occurring at 4 weeks or greater following LAAO. The majority of these patients were largely asymptomatic with embolization detected due to palpitations, new LBBB, or on routine TEE. One patient was presented with cardiogenic shock. Similarly, in 143 device embolizations examined from the MAUDE database, only 5 resulted in cardiac arrest (4 deaths). Given the large number of device embolizations that were discovered routinely, imaging surveillance in the form of transesophageal echocardiography or computed tomography should be conducted to evaluate for this uncommon but significant complication. Combining these aforementioned studies, embolization to the aorta and distal vessels occurred in 51.3% of cases, with 24.7% of implants embolizing to the left ventricle, and 19.5% becoming dislodged and remaining in the LA and/or interacting with the mitral valve. Despite incomplete information regarding many of these cases, it appears that larger devices embolized much less frequently past the aortic valve.

Management

Across a post-FDA approval experience with the WATCHMAN 2.5 provided by the PROTECT -AF investigators, the aforementioned systematic review and MAUDE analysis, and a multicenter experience across 8 US hospitals, we were able to compile treatment approaches for 155 embolizations with 60% undergoing percutaneous device removal and 40% managed via surgical extraction. Percutaneous retrieval is the preferred method of device removal whenever possible, particularly when the dislodged device is in the LA. Pigtail catheter placement across the mitral inflow can prevent further embolization into the LV. Reports have described the use of 10 mm to 30 mm snares (or biopsy bioptomes/vascular retrieval forceps in some cases) for device grabbing and stabilization followed by retraction into transeptal sheaths that are larger (2–4 Fr larger) than the one used for device delivery. The Raptor™ grasping device (Diagmed Healthcare) may be well suited for retrieval, but large devices (e.g., WATCHMAN 35 mm FLX) are unlikely to be removed percutaneously. Snares have been successfully used for embolized devices in the aorta. However, when the dislodged device becomes entangled with the mitral apparatus, urgent surgical consultation should be considered as acute valvopathy can trigger cardiogenic shock, and percutaneous retrieval is accompanied by a high risk of valvular damage. Device migration to the LV has frequently required surgical extraction in comparison to embolization to the LA or aorta which have proven to be more amenable to percutaneous removal.

Device Leaks

Endothelialization and Leak

While LAAO has proven to be an effective strategy in stroke prevention for AFIB patients in the absence of anticoagulation, the concern for LAA patency due to device leak remains a specter for embolus formation and potential stroke. During implantation, the goal is to seal the entire LAA orifice and ideally not allow blood to flow around the perimeter of the device. Additionally, the face of the device is expected to endothelialize over time closing off the LAA from the LA cavity. However, communication between the LA lumen and LAA cavity (patent LAA) can happen either from flow through the device, peri-device leak (PDL), or the simultaneous presence of both. Flow through the device is not considered a device leak and results from incomplete endothelialization of the face of the LAA Occluder, leading to the passage of blood and contrast during CT evaluation *but not thrombus* from the LA cavity into the LAA lumen across the permeable device cap. PDLs occur due to a gap between the LAA Occluder edge and the adjacent LAA tissue, resulting in a conduit between the LAA cavity and LAA lumen. PDLs are often identified using contrast CT imaging or doppler flow on TEE. On the other hand, flow through the device is not as well detected by TEE as with CT and is often seen when CT imaging is acquired within 3 months of implantation, as device endothelialization is expected to require 3 months for completion.

Characterization and Surveillance

Examination of leaks following LAAO has been challenging as varying definitions and size criteria across several studies have precluded direct comparisons. Most studies define large/severe PDLs to be >5 mm in diameter with a subset using >3 mm as a threshold. However, PDLs of <3 mm have universally been accepted to be small leaks, though these cutoffs are largely arbitrary and not grounded upon patient outcomes. Understanding leaks has been further hindered by the absence of a standardized method and timepoint for leak evaluation. However, the majority of studies feature the use of CT and/or TEE at 45 days following implantation.

Incidence

In the initial PROTECT-AF trial featuring the WATCHMAN 2.5 device, a high PDL rate of 40.9% was observed with 7.7% of leaks being <1 mm, 59.9% being between 1 and 3 mm and 32.4% measured >3 mm by TEE. The NCDR LAAO registry (51,333 patients) with the WATCHMAN 2.5 device identified 25.8% of patients with PDLs of <5 mm and 0.7% having PDLs of >5 mm. In contrast, the newer WATCHMAN FLX was associated with much lower PDL rates with 17.2% of patients having PDLs of <5 mm and no patients with a PDL of >5 mm. Figure 18.5a demonstrates the incidence of PDL observed across various major LAAO studies. Of note, head-to-head comparisons between the WATCHMAN 2.5/FLX and AMULET devices have consistently shown AMULET to be associated with fewer PDLs as shown in Fig. 18.5b. However, AMULET was found to have more patent LAAs when compared to WATCHMAN FLX.

Risk Factors

LAA anatomy, procedural aspects, and device design are all expected to play crucial roles in leak development and are enumerated in Table 18.2. The presence of PDL has been associated with permanent AFIB, elevated CHADS2VASC score, larger landing zone, lower device compression ratio, and off-axis device position. Since the LAA ostium is often an eccentric and elliptical structure, while the WATCHMAN and AMULET have circular faces, some degree of geometric mismatch is unavoidable leading to PDLs. Furthermore, shallower device implantation in tapering proximal LAAs, while reducing a residual neck and decreasing the risk of DRT, may functionally create a larger landing zone predisposing to PDL development. Although LAA orifice eccentricity/irregularity has been associated with

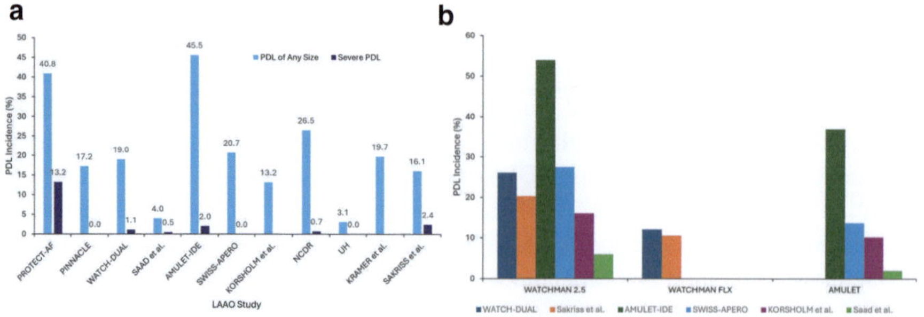

Fig. 18.5 (**a**) Incidence of peri-device leak (PDL) in major left atrial appendage occlusion (LAAO) studies in chronological order from left to right with severe PDL being >3 mm or 5 mm as defined by the study. (**b**) Incidence of PDL with respect to device type across LAAO studies

Table 18.2 Clinical and procedural risk factors associated with peri-device leak (PDL)

PDL risk factors
Permanent atrial fibrillation
Elevated CHADS2VASC score
Eccentric LAA orifice
Larger LAA orifice and device landing zone
Low device compression ratio
Off-axis device implantation

post-closure PDL, the anatomy of the rest of the LAA has not been found to be implicated in leak following LAAO.

Association of PDL/IDL and Device Design

The disparate leak rates between WATCHMAN 2.5 and AMULET are explained by their different designs. The WATCHMAN device employs a single plug mechanism which is implanted within the ostium and anchored at the neck of the LAA. The LA side of the device is covered with a polyethylene terephthalate (PET) membrane which continues to the side of the device for a few millimeters and is expected to promote endothelialization. A PDL will arise if there is an incomplete apposition of the device with the LAA ostium, which may occur in irregularly shaped or multi-lobed ostia. A PDL that is large/deep enough to allow passage of blood/contrast past the side portion of the membrane will result in a patent and thereby inadequately occluded LAA. In fact, while device under-sizing is intuitively expected to predispose to PDLs, oversizing has been associated with fewer PDLs of >5 mm. In contrast, the AMULET features a dual sealing mechanism with a proximal disc which covers the LAA orifice and an anchoring lobe that sits within the neck of the LAA. With the proximal disc sealing the entirety of the LAA ostium, appendage closure is theoretically less dependent on the shape of the ostium, and even if there is a PDL at the level of the disc, the more distal lobe serves to reinforce anatomic closure. This single vs. dual occlusive mechanism may explain the higher rates of PDL observed with WATCHMAN 2.5. Despite adhering to a single plug mechanism, the newer generation WATCHMAN FLX has yielded a lower PDL rate in 3 head-to-head comparisons with the earlier WATCHMAN 2.5. This may partially be due to a wider size range (to accommodate larger LAA landing zones), longer fabric membrane around the side of the device (reducing side leaks), greater number of struts (18 vs. 10), and most importantly greater delayed radial device expansion at 3-month follow-up effectively increasing closure of the LAA ostium. A lower rate of flow through the device was also observed with WATCHMAN FLX (21.3% vs. 40%) along with thicker HATs likely due to a thicker PET membrane on the FLX promoting faster endothelialization and lower device permeability.

Leak Timing and Evolution

Given that device endothelialization, LAA ostium remodeling following LAAO (particularly in the setting of enlarging LA from AF and/or mitral regurgitation), and device expansion are dynamic processes occurring over the course of months following LAAO, leaks are expected to change with time. Flow through the device may resolve over time with endothelialization, but the rate of resolution is unknown and likely device-dependent. Temporal evaluation revealed new PDL development in 8.3% of WATCHMAN patients and 4.2% of AMULET patients at 12 months. Twenty-two percent of PDLs of ≤3 mm and 6% of PDLs that were >3 mm underwent complete resolution at 1 year in WATCHMAN patients. Additionally, 31–41% of PDLs in WATCHMAN patients and 52% of AMULET PDLs were >3 mm regressed to <3 mm at 1 year follow-up. Afzal et al. showed that for WATCHMAN patients, 69% of such PDLs actually increased in size with 29% developing PDLs of >5 mm. Conversely, only 8.3–14% of WATCHMAN PDLs and 4.1% of AMULET PDLs were <3 mm evolved to >3 mm, while the remaining majority regressed (mean size decrease from 2.2 mm to 1.6 mm in WATCHMAN patients) or remained stable. Collectively, these results demonstrate that PDLs of >3 mm are unlikely to close, while PDLs of <3 mm have a good chance of regressing at 12 months following LAAO. These changes are likely due to LA remodeling, device expansion, or neoendothelization between the device edge and LAA ostial wall and should be taken into consideration when developing patient-specific leak management strategies.

Clinical Impact

While leak detection and characterization is one part of the puzzle, data examining the association of leaks with subsequent thromboembolic events has been inconsistent. Leaks >5 mm are deemed to be theoretically significant requiring medical or mechanical management. However, the significance of smaller leaks has been a source of active investigation. In the original PROTECT-AF trial, PDL was not associated with a higher incidence of thromboembolic events; however, this study was underpowered to identify such an association. Combined long-term follow-up from PROTECT-AF, PREVAIL, and CAPII registry identified an almost twofold increased risk of stroke/systemic embolism (9.9% vs. 5.1%, largely driven by non-disabling stroke) over 5-year follow-up in patients who had a PDL <5 mm at 1 year following WATCHMAN 2.5 implantation. Similarly, Afzal et al. reported a higher incidence of TIA/stroke in patients with PDL (8.3 vs. 2.7%) and those with PDL of <5 mm (7.4 vs. 2.7%). While significant, this risk is still much smaller than the risk of stroke predicted for AFIB patients by the CHADS2VASC score. Similarly, the large-scale NCDR-LAAO registry with WATCHMAN 2.5 found PDLs of <5 mm to be associated with a slightly increased (10–15%) risk of systemic embolism at

1 year. Conversely, no such association was identified for PDLs >5 mm, likely because there were very few such cases, and they were all placed on long-term OACs due to the high perceived risk of thromboembolism. The AMULET-IDE trial revealed a numerically higher (yet insignificant) incidence of stroke/systemic thromboembolism with the presence of PDL and PDLs >3/5 mm (with the effect more pronounced with WATCHMAN vs. AMULET), but the clinical implications remain unclear. Collectively, the aggregate data does support the signal of even small PDLs (<5 mm) conferring an increased risk of stroke/systemic thromboembolism over time. However, whether this risk is truly different for patients with PDLs of <5 mm vs. >5 mm or the efficacy of OAC to mitigate this risk remains to be established.

Management

The critical leak size that warrants closure has not been determined, with no leak being preferable to small or large leaks. Furthermore, the timing for leak imaging is not standardized, and this adds another layer of complexity as leaks change over time. However, most institutions obtain initial surveillance TEE or CT imaging at approximately 45 days following LAAO. At present, it is widely accepted to prescribe OAC while considering secondary closure for PDLs ≥5 mm. The decision to pursue closure for smaller leaks is predicated on patient-specific thromboembolism risk and operator discretion, though the aforementioned findings suggest that this may also be required for smaller leaks that fail to regress with time. The decision to continue OAC is dependent on whether there is continued leak on serial imaging.

Various devices have been employed for leak closure largely featuring endovascular plugs radiofrequency ablation (RFA) and coil embolization. Similar to LAAO procedures, catheters for these approaches are inserted using femoral vein access followed by advancement into the right atrium with subsequent transeptal puncture to gain entry to the LA and access the LAA.

Endovascular plugs such as the Amplatzer™ Vascular Plug and Amplatzer™ Vascular Plug II (Abbott) are Occluders typically made from a nitinol mesh and occlusive fabric. They come in a variety of sizes (smaller than WATCHMAN and AMULET) with the appropriate device size chosen based on imaging-based leak assessment to allow for 50% device compression. They are advanced in a sheath to the area of the leak and deployed at the neck of the leak with an atrial side and LAA side. Steerable systems such as the Agilis NxT introducer (Abbott) are often useful in reaching these leaks, and TEE imaging is helpful for intraprocedural guidance. A "tug test" is used to ensure device stability. The decision for leak closure should be undertaken cautiously as these devices have the potential for device embolization and DRT. Nonetheless, endovascular plugs have demonstrated a 100% efficacy without any residual leak at follow-up and without adverse events (DRT, device embolization, stroke, major bleeding, death) in multiple studies.

RFA is performed with an ablation catheter advanced at the site of the leak, and radiofrequency energy is delivered for 30–45 s at each segment of the leak with a reported average RFA time of 249 s/case. This approach may be most applicable to eccentric leaks where plug positioning is challenging and perhaps not ideal for large leaks which will require greater amounts of RFA potentially increasing complication risk or the chance of residual leak following resolution of acute edema. All RFA cases achieved complete immediate closure in the LAA leak study. However, closure rates reduced to 83.3–85.9% at follow-up imaging with a 0.9% PE rate without other significant adverse events. The delayed resurgence of leak was likely the result of tissue contraction from scarring after the healing of initial tissue injury.

Lastly, coil embolization involves advancing a catheter to the leak site and deploying coils to fill the gap. These coils are thrombogenic by design leading to the formation of a coil-thrombus mass which serves as a mechanical plug preventing flow from the LA to the LAA. All coil cases achieved complete post-procedural closure in the LAA leak study. However, closure rates reduced to 83.3% at follow-up imaging with a 3.1–6.1% risk of PE but without other adverse events.

Contrast angiography and TEE can be used to ensure leak closure intraprocedurally with follow-up TEE or CT to assess for residual leak. All three of the aforementioned approaches have proven quite effective in leak closure, but imaging-based pre-procedural planning and surveillance are key to an ideal result. Figure 18.6 provides a framework for leak assessment and management predicated on existing literature. With future iterations of LAAO having lower incidence of leaks, it may be challenging for operators to learn these highly specialized techniques requiring unique education opportunities to ensure proficiency.

Vascular Complications

Access for LAAO is most frequently obtained in the femoral vein with access site complication prevention centered around achieving hemostasis. This is commonly done using manual compression, percutaneous vascular closure devices, or figure-of-8 sutures placed at the end of the procedure and removed within 24 h. Additionally, the use of ultrasound guidance to obtain vascular access has been associated with lower rates of post-procedural bleeding and pain.

Hematomas are a potential complication following LAAO and usually happen following sheath removal with inadequate hemostasis. Symptoms include groin pain or swelling with a potential drop in hemoglobin levels. Hematomas account for 40% of access site complications following LAAO. Generally, access site groin hematomas are self-limited and resolved with the application of manual pressure. Rarely, hematomas might lead to nerve compression requiring surgical evacuation.

Pseudoaneurysms can occur with inadvertent arterial puncture. A growing or pulsatile swelling is concerning for a pseudoaneurysm. Duplex ultrasound is used to confirm the diagnosis, with color flow Doppler for confirmation of “To and Fro” flow pattern typical of pseudoaneurysms. Pseudoaneurysms account for 8.6% of

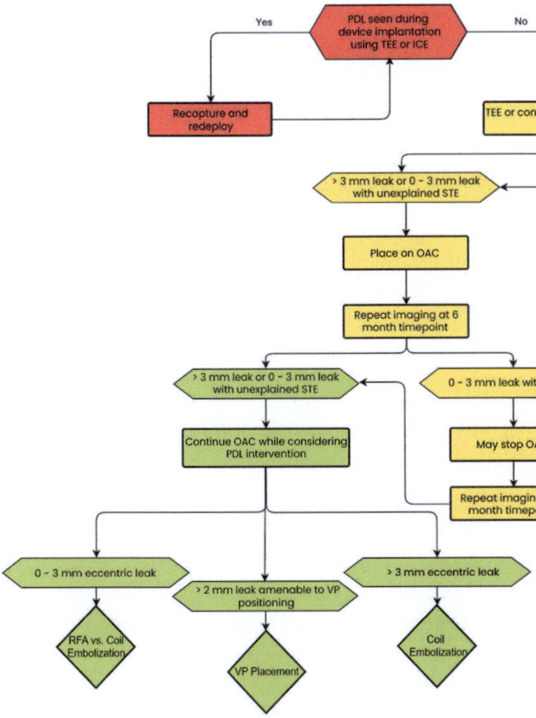

Fig. 18.6 Proposed algorithm for assessment and management of peri-device leaks (PDL)

post-LAAO vascular access complications. Management includes observation for asymptomatic patients with small pseudoaneurysms, ultrasound-guided thrombin injection (UGTI) for uncomplicated cases >3 cm, and endovascular repair with covered stents for cases that do not resolve with observation or UGTI. More complex pseudoaneurysms including those with hemodynamic instability, neurovascular deficits, and expanding hematomas often require open surgical repair. While no studies have compared those approaches in the LAAO patient population, only 22% of pseudoaneurysms were found to resolve with compression following AFIB ablation, while a small randomized controlled trial reported a 100% rate of successful thrombosis achieved with UGTI compared to 13% in patients with ultrasound-guided compression.

Arteriovenous fistulae may form due to inadvertent arterial puncture, present with abnormal vibratory sensation in the groin, and may lead to distal ischemic symptoms. Diagnosis is made via duplex ultrasound, with Doppler waveform showing high resistance and low velocity flow. Management for arteriovenous fistula follows a similar trend to that of pseudoaneurysm, with observation or ultrasound-guided compression for uncomplicated patients. Patients with persistent symptoms warrant open surgical repair or endovascular repair with covered stents among those who are not surgical candidates.

The incidence of major vascular complications with LAAO is low and was reported to be around 0.15% in the National Cardiovascular Data Registry (NCDR) registry. While there is not a large body of literature specific to LAAO vascular access complications, venous access for LAAO is similar to that seen in mitral transcatheter edge-to-edge repair or atrial arrythmia ablations, and lessons regarding complication prevention and management can be extrapolated to the LAAO population.

Conclusions

Numerous randomized controlled trials and multicenter registries over the past decade have provided a wealth of information regarding complications following LAAO. Increased operator experience and widespread adoption of LAAO implantation techniques have led to a substantial decrease in acute and severe complications such as device embolization and major thromboembolism. However, it is important to note that the vast majority of data available is with the earlier generation WATCHMAN 2.5 device in patients with fewer comorbidities than the contemporary population undergoing LAAO. Pericardial effusion with associated cardiac tamponade remains the most feared complication following LAAO, albeit with a substantially reduced incidence with the incorporation of the WATCHMAN FLX. Long-term assessment of LAAO patients will continue to feature surveillance and management of DRT and device leak, which may become less prevalent with newer LAAO devices with faster endothelialization, reduced thrombogenicity, and the ability to conform to a wide range of LAA orifice morphologies.

References and Suggested Readings

1. Afzal MR, Gabriels JK, Jackson GG, et al. Temporal changes and clinical implications of delayed Peridevice leak following left atrial appendage closure. JACC Clin Electrophysiol. 2022;8:15–25.
2. Alkhouli M, Du C, Killu A, et al. Clinical impact of residual leaks following left atrial appendage occlusion: insights from the NCDR LAAO registry. JACC Clin electrophysiol. 2022;8:766–78.
3. Boersma LV, Ince H, Kische S, et al. Efficacy and safety of left atrial appendage closure with WATCHMAN in patients with or without contraindication to oral anticoagulation: 1-year follow-up outcome data of the EWOLUTION trial. Heart Rhythm. 2017;14:1302–8.
4. Charate R, Ahmed A, Della Rocca DG, et al. Evaluation of multimodality LAA leak closure methods following incomplete occlusion: the LAA leak study. JACC Cardiovasc Interv. 2022;15:2158–70.
5. Dukkipati SR, Kar S, Holmes DR, et al. Device-related thrombus after left atrial appendage closure: incidence, predictors, and outcomes. Circulation. 2018;138:874–85.
6. Freixa X, Cepas-Guillen P, Flores-Umanzor E, et al. Pulmonary ridge coverage and device-related thrombosis after left atrial appendage occlusion. EuroIntervention. 2021;16:e1288–94.

7. Galea R, De Marco F. Amulet or Watchman device for percutaneous left atrial appendage closure: primary results of the SWISS-APERO randomized clinical trial. Circulation. 2022;145:724–38.
8. Galea R, Mahmoudi K, Gräni C. Watchman FLX vs. Watchman 25 in a dual-center left atrial appendage closure cohort: the WATCH-DUAL study. Europace. 2022;24:1441–50.
9. Holmes DR Jr, Kar S, Price MJ, et al. Prospective randomized evaluation of the Watchman left atrial appendage closure device in patients with atrial fibrillation versus long-term warfarin therapy: the PREVAIL trial. J Am Coll Cardiol. 2014;64:1–12.
10. Kar S, Doshi SK, Sadhu A, et al. Primary outcome evaluation of a next-generation left atrial appendage closure device: results from the PINNACLE FLX trial. Circulation. 2021;143:1754–62.
11. Korsholm K, Kramer A, Andersen A, et al. Left atrial appendage sealing performance of the Amplatzer Amulet and Watchman FLX device. J Interv Card Electrophysiol. 2023;66:391–401.
12. Lakkireddy D, Thaler D, Ellis CR, et al. Amplatzer Amulet left atrial appendage Occluder versus Watchman device for stroke prophylaxis (Amulet IDE): a randomized. Control Trial. 2021;144:1543–52.
13. Ledesma PA, Uzomah UA, Yu X, et al. MAUDE database analysis of post-approval outcomes following left atrial appendage closure with the Watchman device. Am J Cardiol. 2021;152:78–87.
14. Reddy VY, Sievert H, Halperin J, et al. Percutaneous left atrial appendage closure vs warfarin for atrial fibrillation: a randomized clinical trial. JAMA. 2014;312:1988–98.
15. Simard T, Jung RG, Lehenbauer K, et al. Predictors of device-related thrombus following percutaneous left atrial appendage occlusion. J Am Coll Cardiol. 2021;78:297–313.

Chapter 19
Post-procedural Antiplatelet and Anticoagulant Strategies

Nawaf Alhabdan, Mohammed Alghammass, Rafey Feroze, and Anselma Intini

Highlights

- Left atrial appendage closure (LAAC) devices are thrombogenic and require post-procedural anti-thrombotic therapy.
- The majority of patients undergoing LAAC have some degree of contraindication to anticoagulation, complicating the decision to choose a specific regimen for post-LAAC anti-thrombotic therapy.
- Initial regimens based on vitamin K antagonists (VKA) have been falling out of practice.
- Newer regimens including direct oral anticoagulants (DOACs) are becoming more popular.
- Multiple ongoing randomized trials will guide future recommendations.

Introduction

The need for antithrombotic therapy following LAAC stems from the putative thrombogenicity of the initially exposed implants. In LAAC, devices take between 1 and 3 months to endothelialize [14]. During this time period, the bare implant material is exposed to blood elements that can trigger the coagulation cascade.

N. Alhabdan · M. Alghammass · R. Feroze
Division of Cardiology, Harrington Heart & Vascular Institute, University Hospitals Cleveland Medical Center, Cleveland, OH, USA
e-mail: Nawaf.alhabdan@uhhospitals.org

A. Intini (✉)
Louis Stokes Cleveland Veterans Affairs Medical Center, Division of Cardiology, Department of Medicine, Cleveland, OH, USA

S. J. Filby et al. (eds.), *A Contemporary Manual of Left Atrial Appendage Closure*, https://doi.org/10.1007/978-3-031-68441-8_19

There are in general three healing phases after device implantation. The first phase is the acute prothrombotic state triggered by the direct exposure of the device to circulating blood [21]. In patients undergoing LAAC, a comparison of pre- and post-procedural hemostatic markers showed marked activation of the coagulation cascade noted by increased prothrombin fragment 1 + 2 and thrombin-antithrombin III levels, which peaked at 7 days with partial return to baseline at 30 days. Of note, platelet activation was not significantly increased, and the role of platelet function has to be elucidated [21]. The second phase is characterized with neo-endothelialization. In dogs, this phase is completed between 28 and 45 days [14, 23]. Endocardial ingrowth of smooth muscle cells in a proteoglycan-collagenous matrix continues to replace the fibrin deposits and seals the device. The third phase is less active and mainly consists of thrombus evolution and tissue growth in the occluded appendage. However, reports of late device-related thrombus (DRTs) suggest that the new tissue can be damaged or the device might sometimes be incompletely covered by neo-endocardium, reinstating the devices' pro-thrombotic properties [17]. Based on the putative mechanisms of acute and chronic DRT on one side and the patient population inherent risk for bleeding on the other side, several anticoagulation protocols have been designed which will be discussed in this chapter.

Warfarin-Based Regimen: Initial Approval

The FDA approved the WATCHMAN device based on the PROTECT AF and PREVAIL trials, in which warfarin and aspirin were administered for 45 days, and if no device-related thrombosis or peri device leakage of >5 mm was observed on TEE, patients were transitioned to DAPT with aspirin and clopidogrel until 6 months after implant and to aspirin alone afterward [12, 20]. However, following FDA approval, the NCDR LAAO Registry of 31,994 successfully implanted patients showed utilization of varied antithrombotic regimens after LAAC in the United States [11]. The most common discharge medical therapies were warfarin and ASA (36.9%), a DOAC and ASA (20.8%), warfarin alone (13.5%), DOAC alone (12.3%), and DAPT-P2Y12 plus ASA (5.0%). In this registry, discharge after LAAC with WATCHMAN device on DOAC and aspirin was associated with similar outcomes compared with warfarin and aspirin at 45 days and 6 months. Furthermore, discharge on either warfarin or DOAC alone without aspirin was associated with a lower risk of adverse events, largely due to lower rates of bleeding. In the pooled analysis of these two trials and their prospective registries, there was an association between increased risk of adverse event, particularly bleeding, when ASA is added to anticoagulation post-procedure. This finding has been documented in other patient groups (transcatheter aortic valve replacement). Figure 19.1 shows the variation of post-LAAC regimens between different regions (note that the data in the USA and Europe are 2 years older than those in China).

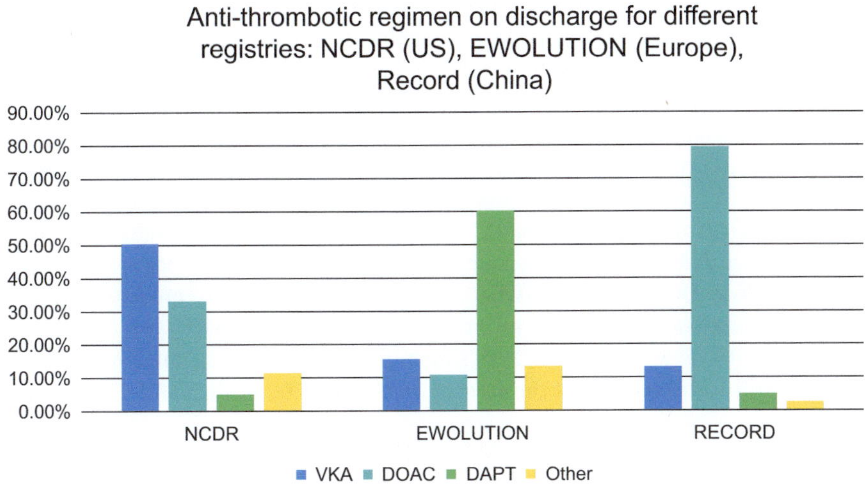

Fig. 19.1 Anti-thrombotic regimen at the time of discharge for different registries: NCDR (United States), EWOLUTION (Europe), Record (China)

Direct Oral Anticoagulants (DOACs)

DOACs have emerged as an alternative to warfarin due to their lower bleeding risk and better efficacy than warfarin [2]. In the PINNACLE FLX study, instead of warfarin, patients received a DOAC (77% apixaban, 20% rivaroxaban) and low-dose aspirin for 45 days and then transitioned to DAPT [15]; there are similar or favorable outcomes in other studies compared with the older pivotal trials. Reduced doses of DOACs have also been compared as a potential anti-thrombotic regimen post - LAAC. Multiple studies have compared the role of reduced dose DOACs as a potential post-LAAC antithrombotic regimen. In the recently presented ADALA trial, patients with atrial fibrillation underwent successful LAAC and then were randomized to a low dose of apixaban (2.5 mg twice daily) or DAPT for 3 months. The mean patient age was 76.6, and two-thirds of participants were men. Almost all (95.6%) had a prior bleeding event, mostly gastrointestinal. Mean CHA2DS2-VASc score was 4.0, and mean HAS-BLED score was 3.5. For the procedure, (67.5%) were treated with an Amplatzer Amulet device, with another 23.3% treated with the Watchman and 8.9% the LAmbre (Lifetech). The trial was stopped early due to an advantage for low-dose DOAC after 90 of a planned 160 patients were randomized [10].

Similarly, a nonrandomized study compared long-term low-dose DOAC vs. the PINNACLE FLX regimen (apixaban 2.5 mg twice a day or rivaroxaban 10 mg once a day +aspirin for 45 days, followed by DAPT for 4.5 months and then aspirin). At 1 year follow-up, the composite endpoint of DRT, thromboembolic events, and major bleeding was significantly lower in the long-term low-dose DOAC (1% vs 9.5%, $p = 0.002$) [6, 7]. In the ADRIFT pilot study, 105 patients were randomized to DAPT with aspirin 81 mg and clopidogrel 75 mg, rivaroxaban 10 mg, and rivaroxaban 15 mg. The primary endpoint was thrombin generation (prothrombin fragments

1 + 2) measured 2 to 4 h after drug intake, and 10 days after treatment initiation. The primary endpoint was lower in patients treated with reduced rivaroxaban doses compared to DAPT. Although the study was not powered for clinical outcomes, no DRT occurred in either of the rivaroxaban groups, and 2 occurred in the DAPT group [9].

There are ongoing studies that will further clarify the use of DOAC vs. DAPT. The FADE-DRT is comparing the standard anticoagulation therapy (DOAC 6 weeks + DAPT until 6 months + aspirin afterward) vs. genetically guided antithrombotic strategy (DOAC for 6 weeks + DAPT (clopidogrel responders) or aspirin plus half-dose OAC (clopidogrel non-responders until 6 months + aspirin afterwards) vs. long term low-dose DOAC. The ANDES study with an estimated enrollment of 350 patients is randomizing patients to one of four DOACs or DAPT with aspirin and clopidogrel for 8 weeks. Table 19.1 summarizes the important ongoing trials. It remains still to be seen what the role of DOAC will be in the future, but, at the

Table 19.1 Current randomized trials comparing antithrombotic therapies following LAAC

Study name	Comparison	Primary outcomes	n	NCT number
Short-Term Anticoagulation Versus Antiplatelet Therapy for Preventing Device Thrombosis Following Left Atrial Appendage Closure (ANDES)	DAPT for 8 weeks vs. DOAC for 8 weeks following LAAC	Device-related thrombosis as evaluated by TEE at 8 weeks	350	NCT03568890
Aspirin Discontinuation After LAAO in Atrial Fibrillation (ASPIRIN-LAAO)	Continuing vs. discontinuing aspirin at 6 months following LAAC	Stroke, systemic embolism, cardiovascular/ unexplained death, major bleeding, acute coronary syndrome, and coronary or periphery artery disease requiring revascularization at 24 months	1120	NCT03821883
Efficacy of Different Anti-Thrombotic Strategies on Device-Related Thrombosis Prevention After Percutaneous Left Atrial Appendage Occlusion (FADE-DRT)	Group1: OAC for 6 weeks followed by DAPT until 6 month-follow-up, then aspirin alone Group2: OAC for 6 weeks followed by DAPT (clopidogrel responders) or aspirin plus half-dose OAC (clopidogrel non-responders) until 6 month-follow-up, and then aspirin alone Group 3: Half-dose DOAC	Composite of stroke, systemic embolism, and device-related thrombosis at 1 year Incidence of major bleeding events at 1 year	360	NCT04502017

present time, it is safe to assume that they can replace warfarin successfully even so with the reduced dose.

Dual Antiplatelet Therapy

In Europe and other parts of the world, the use of post-procedural DAPT (without OAC) after LAAC is common practice. In the Amulet IDE study, 75.7% of patients were discharged on DAPT after Amulet implantation, and the rate of DRT was not different from the WATCHMAN arm, in which 95.8% were on OAC at discharge [16]. The EWOLUTION registry, which followed more than 1000 patients who underwent watchman LAAC in Europe, reported variable antithrombotic regimens following the procedure. Only 16% of patients were discharged on the then FDA-approved regimen of warfarin, with 11% discharged on a DOAC, 60% on DAPT, and 7% on SAPT. This tendency to discharge patients on DAPT is partially explained by the high-risk population in this registry. The mean CHADsVasc score was 4.5, and the mean HASBLED score was 3.2. More than 70% of the patients were ineligible for anticoagulation. Interestingly, at 1 year follow-up, there was no significant difference in the incidence of DRT, stroke, or ischemic events between the different antithrombotic regimens [1]. ASAP was a nonrandomized clinical trial that included patients with absolute contraindication to anticoagulation, who were discharged on 6 months of DAPT followed by SAPT. The results showed comparable rate of stroke reduction to those reported in PREVAIL/PROTECT and a 4% incidence of DRT (vs. 3.8% in PREVAIL/PROTECT) [19]. A propensity-matched comparison, using patients from PREVAIL/PROTECT and their corresponding registries, EWOLUTION and ASAP, compared DAPT to warfarin therapy. The propensity-matched analysis showed a significantly higher incidence of DRT for those on DAPT compared to OAC. This increase in DRT, however, was not associated with any difference in strokes/systemic embolism or major bleeding at 6 months follow-up [25]. The NCDR LAAO Registry showed that discharge on DAPT after WATCHMAN implant was relatively uncommon (5% of implants) but was associated with a similar risk of adverse events compared with warfarin and aspirin at 45 days and 6 months [11]. A large meta-analysis of 83 studies including 12,326 LAAC patients (7900 on antiplatelet and 4151 on OAC) showed no difference in stroke, DRT, bleeding, or overall mortality with antiplatelet versus OAC after LAAC [18]. These results from nonrandomized studies suggest safety and potential equal efficacy for DAPT to anticoagulation. However, and given the lack of randomized clinical studies in this field, DAPT should not always be assumed to be safer than anticoagulation. The ACTIVE-W trial assessed DAPT as a potential alternative to warfarin for stroke prevention in patients with AFIB. Not only was DAPT inferior to warfarin in stroke prevention, but it was also associated with an increased risk of bleeding [4]. The higher incidence of DRT in patients discharged on DAPT could be attributed to clopidogrel resistance. A prospective study aimed to offer a genotypically guided post-LAAC antithrombotic regimen based on clopidogrel resistance pattern. Initially in the study, patients found to be resistant to clopidogrel were placed on aspirin+prasugrel instead of aspirin+clopidogrel. This strategy was abandoned early in the study as high rates of bleeding (10%) were reported in the aspirin+prasugrel group. The authors shifted their strategy to prescribing aspirin+low dose DOAC to clopidogrel non-responders. Results showed that genotypically guided antithrombotic therapy was superior to traditional DAPT regimens in lowering DRT and DRT/thromboembolism rates [6, 7]. These results appear to indicate that DAPT with aspirin and clopidogrel is an excellent option for clopidogrel non-resistant patients.

Device-Related Thrombosis (DRT)

DRT has been reported after 3–5% of LAAC procedures in large clinical trial and registry experiences. DRT has been shown to be more likely in patients with prior stroke, large LAA dimensions, those with permanent AF, and those with previous LA thrombus [8, 24]. The relationship between DRT and long-term adverse cardiovascular events is unclear, but registry-based analyses have found an association between DRT and stroke/transient ischemic attack (TIA) during short-term follow-up. However, most strokes after LAAC occur in patients without DRT; thus, the clinical importance of DRT is not well understood. If DRT is diagnosed on post-LAAC imaging, anticoagulation should be continued. The guidelines recommend that for patients on dual antiplatelet therapy (DAPT), OAC should be started, and DAPT should be discontinued. Repeated imaging at 45- to 90-day intervals can be performed to assess for resolution with eventual cessation of anticoagulation.

Conservative Strategies: No Antithrombotic or Single Antiplatelet Therapy (SAPT)

Patients undergoing LAAC tend to have a high bleeding risk. For a significant number of patients, anticoagulation is absolutely contraindicated. A review of NCDR, EWOLUTION, and Amulet registries showed that between 1.8% and 6.5% of patients were discharged with no antithrombotic therapy following LAAC, and 7–23% were discharged on single antiplatelet therapy [1, 11, 16]. This leads to the question: "Is it feasible to perform LAAO if neither DAPT or anticoagulation can be used afterwards?" The incidence of DRT in patients from the previous registries was not statistically different from other anticoagulation regimens. Multiple smaller studies assessed the feasibility of SAPT or no antithrombotic therapy following LAAC. The results indicate a significant reduction in thromboembolic risk compared to that expected based on the CHADsVASc score [5, 13, 22]. A network meta-analysis of mostly observational studies showed that patients who received no antithrombotic therapy were significantly more likely to develop DRT when compared to those who received DAPT, DOAC, or warfarin [3]. Based on the available evidence, it appears that LAAC in patients with a prohibitive risk of anticoagulation or DAPT is safe and effective in reducing thromboembolic events, even if that risk reduction could be lower than those who can tolerate anticoagulation or DAPT.

Summary and Future Directions

In summary, the studies to date are insufficient to define an optimal postprocedural antithrombotic regimen following LAAC. Discharge on anticoagulation with anticoagulant plus aspirin is well established for WATCHMAN based on the PROTECT AF, PREVAIL, and PINNACLE FLX studies. VKA treatment option is declining in current practice in favor of DOAC.

Discharge on DAPT appears well established for the Amulet device based on the Amulet IDE study and real-world registries. There is also an increasing body of registry evidence supporting DAPT with WATCHMAN. At this juncture, the choice and duration of antithrombotic regimen after LAAC should be made according to the studied regimen for each specific device, potentially individualized based on the patient's bleeding/thrombotic risk and potentially modified if peri-device leak or DRT is seen on post-LAAC imaging surveillance. Patients with low risk of bleeding can receive DOAC for a short duration; intermediate risk patients can receive either a reduced dose of DOAC or DAPT, and a very high bleeding-risk patient can receive SAPT. Newer generation of devices seem to be associated with lower incidence of DRT. The expectation is that future designs will further reduce the incidence of DRT and reduce the need for intense anticoagulation therapy. Figure 19.2 demonstrates a simplified algorithm for post-LAAC antithrombotic regimen.

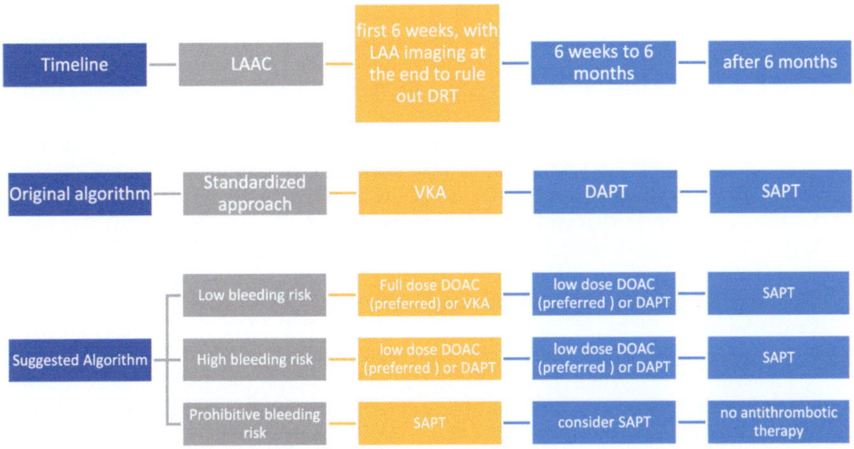

Fig. 19.2 Traditional algorithm for post-LAAC antithrombotic regimen vs. suggested algorithm

References

1. Boersma LV, Ince H, Kische S, Pokushalov E, Schmitz T, Schmidt B, Gori T, Meincke F, Protopopov AV, Betts T, Foley D, Sievert H, Mazzone P, De Potter T, Vireca E, Stein K, Bergmann MW. Efficacy and safety of left atrial appendage closure with WATCHMAN in patients with or without contraindication to oral anticoagulation: 1-year follow-up outcome data of the EWOLUTION trial. Heart Rhythm. 2017;14(9):1302–8. https://doi.org/10.1016/J.HRTHM.2017.05.038.
2. Carnicelli AP, Hong H, Connolly SJ, Eikelboom J, Giugliano RP, Morrow DA, Patel MR, Wallentin L, Alexander JH, Cecilia Bahit M, Benz AP, Bohula EA, Chao TF, Dyal L, Ezekowitz M, Fox KAA, Gencer B, Halperin JL, Hijazi Z, et al. Direct oral anticoagulants versus warfarin in patients with atrial fibrillation: patient-level network meta-analyses of randomized clinical trials with interaction testing by age and sex. Circulation. 2022;145(4):242–55. https://doi.org/10.1161/CIRCULATIONAHA.121.056355.
3. Carvalho PEP, Gewehr DM, Miyawaki IA, Nogueira A, Félix N, Garot P, Darmon A, Mazzone P, Preda A, Nascimento BR, Kubrusly LF, Cardoso R. Network meta-analysis of initial antithrombotic regimens after left atrial appendage occlusion. J Am Coll Cardiol. 2023;82(18):1765–73. https://doi.org/10.1016/J.JACC.2023.08.010.
4. Connolly S, Pogue J, Hart R, Pfeffer M, Hohnloser S, Chrolavicius S, Yusuf S. Clopidogrel plus aspirin versus oral anticoagulation for atrial fibrillation in the atrial fibrillation Clopidogrel trial with Irbesartan for prevention of vascular events (ACTIVE W): a randomised controlled trial. Lancet (London, England). 2006;367(9526):1903–12. https://doi.org/10.1016/S0140-6736(06)68845-4.
5. Darmon A, Couture EL, Stein G, Cormier B, Chevalier B, Lefèvre T, Neylon A, Sanguineti F, Horvilleur J, Garot P. Left atrial appendage closure in patients with atrial fibrillation at very high bleeding risk without Postimplantation antithrombotic therapy. J Invasive Cardiol. 2020;32(10):385–91. https://europepmc.org/article/med/32999093
6. Della Rocca DG, Horton RP, Di Biase L, Gianni C, Trivedi C, Mohanty S, Anannab A, Magnocavallo M, Chen Q, Tarantino N, Bassiouny M, Lavalle C, Natale VN, Forleo GB, Del Prete A, Van Niekerk CJ, Al-Ahmad A, Burkhardt JD, Gallinghouse GJ, et al. Incidence of device-related thrombosis in watchman patients undergoing a genotype-guided antithrombotic strategy. JACC Clin Electrophysiol. 2021a;7(12):1533–43. https://doi.org/10.1016/J.JACEP.2021.04.012.
7. Della Rocca DG, Magnocavallo M, Di Biase L, Mohanty S, Trivedi C, Tarantino N, Gianni C, Lavalle C, Van Niekerk CJ, Romero J, Briceño DF, Bassiouny M, Al-Ahmad A, Burkhardt JD, Natale VN, Gallinghouse GJ, Del Prete A, Forleo GB, Sanchez J, et al. Half-dose direct oral anticoagulation versus standard antithrombotic therapy after left atrial appendage occlusion. J Am Coll Cardiol Intv. 2021b;14(21):2353–64. https://doi.org/10.1016/J.JCIN.2021.07.031/SUPPL_FILE/MMC1.DOCX.
8. Dukkipati SR, Kar S, Holmes DR, Doshi SK, Swarup V, Gibson DN, Maini B, Gordon NT, Main ML, Reddy VY. Device-related thrombus after left atrial appendage closure. Circulation. 2018;138(9):874–85. https://doi.org/10.1161/CIRCULATIONAHA.118.035090.
9. Duthoit G, Silvain J, Marijon E, Ducrocq G, Lepillier A, Frere C, Dimby SF, Popovic B, Lellouche N, Martin-Toutain I, Spaulding C, Brochet E, Attias D, Mansourati J, Lorgis L, Klug D, Zannad N, Hauguel-Moreau M, Braik N, et al. Reduced rivaroxaban dose versus dual antiplatelet therapy after left atrial appendage closure: ADRIFT a randomized pilot study. Circ Cardiovasc Interv. 2020;13(7) https://doi.org/10.1161/CIRCINTERVENTIONS.119.008481.
10. Flores-Umanzor EJ, Cepas-Guillen PL, Arzamendi D, Cruz-González I, Regueiro A, Freixa X. Rationale and design of a randomized clinical trial to compare two antithrombotic strategies after left atrial appendage occlusion: double antiplatelet therapy vs. apixaban (ADALA study). J Interv Card Electrophysiol. 2020;59(2):471–7. https://doi.org/10.1007/S10840-020-00884-X.

11. Freeman JV, Higgins AY, Wang Y, Du C, Friedman DJ, Daimee UA, Minges KE, Pereira L, Goldsweig AM, Price MJ, Reddy VY, Gibson D, Doshi SK, Varosy PD, Masoudi FA, Curtis JP. Antithrombotic therapy after left atrial appendage occlusion in patients with atrial fibrillation. J Am Coll Cardiol. 2022;79(18):1785–98. https://doi.org/10.1016/J.JACC.2022.02.047.
12. Holmes DR, Kar S, Price MJ, Whisenant B, Sievert H, Doshi SK, Huber K, Reddy VY. Prospective randomized evaluation of the watchman left atrial appendage closure device in patients with atrial fibrillation versus long-term warfarin therapy: the PREVAIL trial. J Am Coll Cardiol. 2014;64(1):1–12. https://doi.org/10.1016/J.JACC.2014.04.029.
13. Jalal Z, Dinet ML, Combes N, Pillois X, Renou P, Sibon I, Iriart X, Thambo JB. Percutaneous left atrial appendage closure followed by single antiplatelet therapy: short- and mid-term outcomes. Arch Cardiovasc Dis. 2017;110(4):242–9. https://doi.org/10.1016/J.ACVD.2016.09.006.
14. Kar S, Hou D, Jones R, Werner D, Swanson L, Tischler B, Stein K, Huibregtse B, Ladich E, Kutys R, Virmani R. Impact of Watchman and Amplatzer devices on left atrial appendage adjacent structures and healing response in a canine model. J Am Coll Cardiol Intv. 2014;7(7):801–9. https://doi.org/10.1016/J.JCIN.2014.03.003.
15. Kar S, Doshi SK, Sadhu A, Horton R, Osorio J, Ellis C, Stone J, Shah M, Dukkipati SR, Adler S, Nair DG, Kim J, Wazni O, Price MJ, Asch FM, Holmes DR, Shipley RD, Gordon NT, Allocco DJ, Reddy VY. Primary outcome evaluation of a next-generation left atrial appendage closure device: results from the PINNACLE FLX trial. Circulation. 2021;143(18):1754–62. https://doi.org/10.1161/CIRCULATIONAHA.120.050117.
16. Lakkireddy D, Thaler D, Ellis CR, Swarup V, Sondergaard L, Carroll J, Gold MR, Hermiller J, Diener HC, Schmidt B, MacDonald L, Mansour M, Maini B, O'Brien L, Windecker S. Amplatzer amulet left atrial appendage Occluder versus watchman device for stroke prophylaxis (Amulet IDE): a randomized, controlled trial. Circulation. 2021;144(19):1543. https://doi.org/10.1161/CIRCULATIONAHA.121.057063.
17. Nasser R, Meyten N, Vermeersch P, Prihadi EA. When the solution becomes the problem: left atrial appendage occlusion device-related thrombus after 5 years. Eur Heart J. 2022;43(10):1015. https://doi.org/10.1093/EURHEARTJ/EHAB719.
18. Osman M, Busu T, Osman K, Khan SU, Daniels M, Holmes DR, Alkhouli M. Short-term antiplatelet versus anticoagulant therapy after left atrial appendage occlusion: a systematic review and meta-analysis. JACC Clin Electrophysiol. 2020;6(5):494–506. https://doi.org/10.1016/J.JACEP.2019.11.009.
19. Reddy VY, Möbius-Winkler S, Miller MA, Neuzil P, Schuler G, Wiebe J, Sick P, Sievert H. Left atrial appendage closure with the watchman device in patients with a contraindication for oral anticoagulation: the ASAP study (ASA Plavix feasibility study with watchman left atrial appendage closure technology). J Am Coll Cardiol. 2013;61(25):2551–6. https://doi.org/10.1016/J.JACC.2013.03.035.
20. Reddy VY, Sievert H, Halperin J, Doshi SK, Buchbinder M, Neuzil P, Huber K, Whisenant B, Kar S, Swarup V, Gordon N, Holmes DR, Chinitz L, Douglas P, Gurley J, Sick P, Turi ZG, Hustead ST, Asinger RW, et al. Percutaneous left atrial appendage closure vs warfarin for atrial fibrillation: a randomized clinical trial. JAMA. 2014;312(19):1988–98. https://doi.org/10.1001/JAMA.2014.15192.
21. Rodés-Cabau J, O'Hara G, Paradis JM, Bernier M, Rodriguez-Gabella T, Regueiro A, O'Connor K, Beaudoin J, Puri R, Côté M, Champagne J. Changes in coagulation and platelet activation markers following transcatheter left atrial appendage closure. Am J Cardiol. 2017;120(1):87–91. https://doi.org/10.1016/J.AMJCARD.2017.03.253.
22. Rodriguez-Gabella T, Nombela-Franco L, Regueiro A, Jiménez-Quevedo P, Champagne J, O'Hara G, Bernier M, Macaya C, Rodés-Cabau J. Single antiplatelet therapy following left atrial appendage closure in patients with contraindication to anticoagulation. J Am Coll Cardiol. 2016;68(17):1920–1. https://doi.org/10.1016/J.JACC.2016.08.016.
23. Schwartz RS, Holmes DR, Van Tassel RA, Hauser R, Henry TD, Mooney M, Matthews R, Doshi S, Jones RM, Virmani R. Left atrial appendage obliteration: mechanisms of healing and

intracardiac integration. JACC Cardiovasc Interv. 2010;3(8):870–7. https://doi.org/10.1016/J.JCIN.2010.04.017.

24. Simard T, Jung RG, Lehenbauer K, Piayda K, Pracoń R, Jackson GG, Flores-Umanzor E, Faroux L, Korsholm K, Chun JKR, Chen S, Maarse M, Montrella K, Chaker Z, Spoon JN, Pastormerlo LE, Meincke F, Sawant AC, Moldovan CM, et al. Predictors of device-related thrombus following percutaneous left atrial appendage occlusion. J Am Coll Cardiol. 2021;78(4):297–313. https://doi.org/10.1016/J.JACC.2021.04.098.
25. Søndergaard L, Wong YH, Reddy VY, Boersma LVA, Bergmann MW, Doshi S, Kar S, Sievert H, Wehrenberg S, Stein K, Holmes DR. Propensity-matched comparison of oral anticoagulation versus antiplatelet therapy after left atrial appendage closure with WATCHMAN. J Am Coll Cardiol Intv. 2019;12(11):1055–63. https://doi.org/10.1016/J.JCIN.2019.04.004.

Chapter 20
Post-procedural Imaging and Device-Related Features Management

Sung-Han Yoon, Sara Hazaveh, and Jeremiah P. Depta

Abbreviations

2D	Two-dimensional
3D	Three-dimensional
ASD	Atrial septal defect
CTA	Computed tomography angiography
DAPT	Dual antiplatelet therapy
DRT	Device-related thrombus
LAA	Left atrial appendage
LAAC	Left atrial appendage closure
OAC	Oral anticoagulation
PDL	Peri-device leak (PDL)
TEE	Transesophageal echocardiography

Highlights

- Post-procedural surveillance imaging with transesophageal echocardiography (TEE) or computed tomography angiography (CTA) is recommended at 45–90 days following left atrial appendage closure (LAAC).

Supplementary Information The online version contains supplementary material available at https://doi.org/10.1007/978-3-031-68441-8_20.

S.-H. Yoon (✉) · S. Hazaveh
Department of Cardiology, Hackensack Meridian Health School of Medicine, Hackensack, NJ, USA

J. P. Depta
Sands Constellation Heart Institute, Rochester Regional Health, Rochester, NY, USA

S. J. Filby et al. (eds.), *A Contemporary Manual of Left Atrial Appendage Closure*, https://doi.org/10.1007/978-3-031-68441-8_20

- The primary focus of post-procedural imaging is to assess for peri-device leak (PDL) and device-related thrombus (DRT), which is important for decisions regarding anti-thrombotic management.
- CTA may provide some advantages over TEE in assessing PDL and DRT.

Introduction

After successful LAAC (left atrial appendage closure), post-procedure follow-up imaging is necessary for device surveillance and managing antithrombotic therapy [1, 2]. Device endothelialization of WATCHMAN™ and Amulet™ devices takes approximately 45 days. During this period, patients will be treated with oral anticoagulation (OAC) or dual antiplatelet therapy (DAPT). Transesophageal echocardiography (TEE) or cardiac computed tomography angiography (CTA) is recommended at 45–90 days following device implantation [1, 2]. At this interval, the primary reason for imaging is to assess device endothelialization (i.e., healing) by assessing peri-device leak (PDL) and device-related thrombus (DRT) and determine if OAC or DAPT can be discontinued. Surveillance imaging at 12 months following LAAC can be considered if PDL was present on prior imaging or if there is a clinical concern for DRT [1, 2]. The choice between TEE or CTA should be driven by the center's expertise. CTA has some notable advantages (Chap. 5, Table 5.4), including a higher sensitivity for detecting the presence and potential mechanisms of PDL and DRT [2–4].

Transesophageal Echocardiography (TEE)

Post-procedural TEE should be performed using a transducer with at least a 5 Mhz multiplane transducer. Image optimization is essential to assess the implanted device. The gain and compression should be optimized (fundamental frequency and harmonics) to adequately assess the device, endocardial borders, and Doppler flow. The frame rate of the Doppler signal should be 20 Hz, and spectral Doppler (continuous and pulse wave) interrogation should be parallel to the blood flow with a sweep speed ≥100 mm/s.

Post-device TEE imaging should assess:

- Position (including "shoulder" protrusion of the device) and dimensions of the LAAC device in the LAA including the shape of the device.
- Device seal including the presence and size of PDL and potential mechanism of the defect.
- Presence, size, and mobility of DRT or left atrial thrombus.
- Presence and size of pericardial effusion.
- Presence, size, and direction of flow of the iatrogenic atrial septal defect (ASD).

Post-procedural WATCHMAN™ Images

The post-procedural images for WATCHMAN™ are essential to confirm a successful LAAC procedure and endothelialization of the WATCHMAN™. A suggested post-procedural TEE protocol is detailed in Table 20.1. Reviewing the intra-procedural echocardiographic images is essential to determine if any substantial changes have occurred during the post-procedural period. TEE should be used to assess the WATCHMAN™ device in the LAA. The key points included the device position in comparison to LAA ostium including any protrusion (i.e., shoulders) or shifting, device shape, and compression (as detailed in Chap. 9) in 2D and 3D using the mid-esophageal views (0°, 45°, 90°, 135°) (Fig. 20.1, Video 20.1). Color flow Doppler using a Nyquist settings (20–40 cm/s) should be performed at each of the aforementioned angles to assess for PDL (Video 20.2). If PDL is seen, then it is important to extensively assess the PDL using multiple angles, views, and X-plane imaging in both 2D and 3D images and color Doppler (Fig. 20.2a, Video 20.3; Fig. 20.2b, Video 20.4). Interrogation of the PDL with pulse wave Doppler should be performed to establish if the flow extends into the distal LAA (Fig. 20.2c). The size of the PDL (Fig. 20.2a, b) should be measured as this is often used to determine a patient's antithrombotic regimen (Chap. 20).

Table 20.1 Example of post-procedural TEE protocol

TEE view
<u>LAA device:</u> Mid-esophageal view (0°, 45°, 90°, 135°)
2D and color Doppler
Low-velocity color (i.e., Nyquist) settings (20–40 cm/s).
For PDL:
Measure the vena contracta (i.e., the narrowest cross-sectional plane where the device is closest to the LAA wall).
Doppler box should cover the entire device.
Assess all angulations to measure the size.
Avoid foreshortened views.
Track color flow to the distal edge of the appendage.
Spectral pulsed-wave Doppler to confirm communication between the LA and LAA.
Differentiate color flow from PDL mimics (e.g., left pulmonary vein, left circumflex artery, transverse sinus).
For DRT:
Assess for the presence, size, and mobility of DRT on the atrial-facing side of the device.
<u>Interatrial septum:</u> Mid-esophageal four-chamber (0°–30°), right ventricular inflow-outflow (45°–60°), and bicaval (90°–120°) views
2D and color Doppler assessment of the intertrial septum to assess for the presence and direction of the iatrogenic ASD
Low-velocity color scale settings of 25–40 cm/s.
<u>Other cardiac structures:</u> Mid-esophageal four- (0°), two- (80°–100°), and three- (120°–140°) chamber and transgastric short-axis (0°–20°: Basal, mid-papillary, apical) views
Assess for the presence and size of any pericardial effusion.
Assess for the presence and size of any intracardiac thrombus.
Left ventricular ejection fraction assessment.

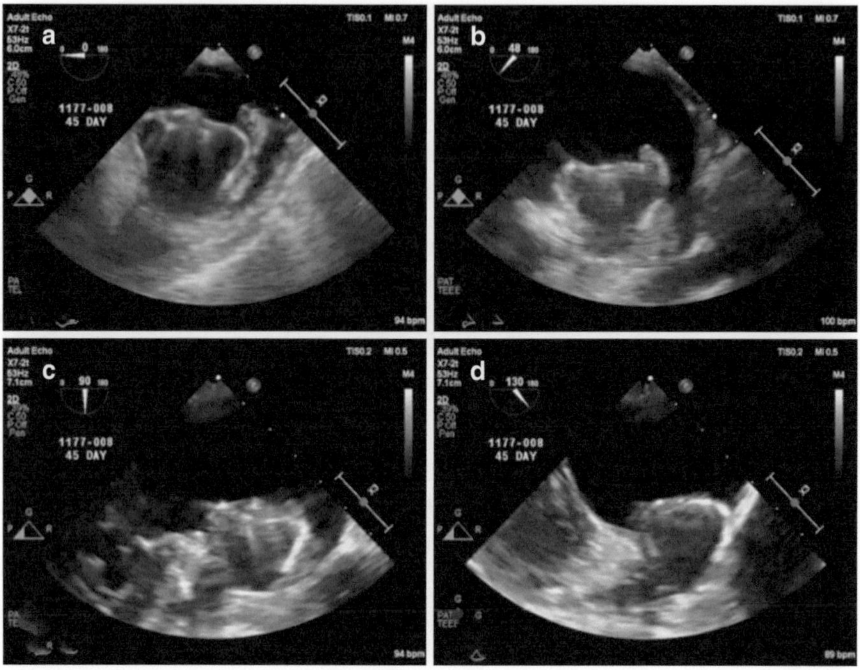

Fig. 20.1 Example of 2D post-procedural TEE images of the WATCHMAN™ device in the LAA. **Panel A,** 0° view; **Panel B,** 45° view; **Panel C,** 90° view; **Panel D,** 135° view. Corresponding videos for 2D and color Doppler are available (Videos 20.1 and 20.2)

Measurements should be taken at vena contracta of the PDL to minimize the risk of overestimating the PDL size. 3D TEE with color can also be performed to determine the circumference of the PDL. A large peri-device leak is often observed in an uncovered lobe which should be assessed carefully with multiplanar reconstruction (Fig. 20.3). DRT should be excluded on the atrial-facing side of the device (Fig. 20.4, Videos 20.7, 20.8, 20.9 and 20.10). Thrombus can form with delayed endothelialization of the device. Some potential causes for delayed endothelialization and DRT formation include the threaded insert on the WATCHMAN™ device, prominent shoulder, and any uncovered LAA lobes or proximal trabeculations. The interatrial septum should be assessed in multiple 2D views and 3D to determine if an iatrogenic ASD is present, its size, and direction of flow. Percutaneous closure of iatrogenic ASD >10 mm may be considered. A complete TEE study should be performed to determine if any substantial changes have occurred in other cardiac and non-cardiac structures since the procedure including a thorough assessment for late pericardial effusion, LA thrombus (Fig. 20.5, Videos 20.11 and 20.12), device erosion, and infection.

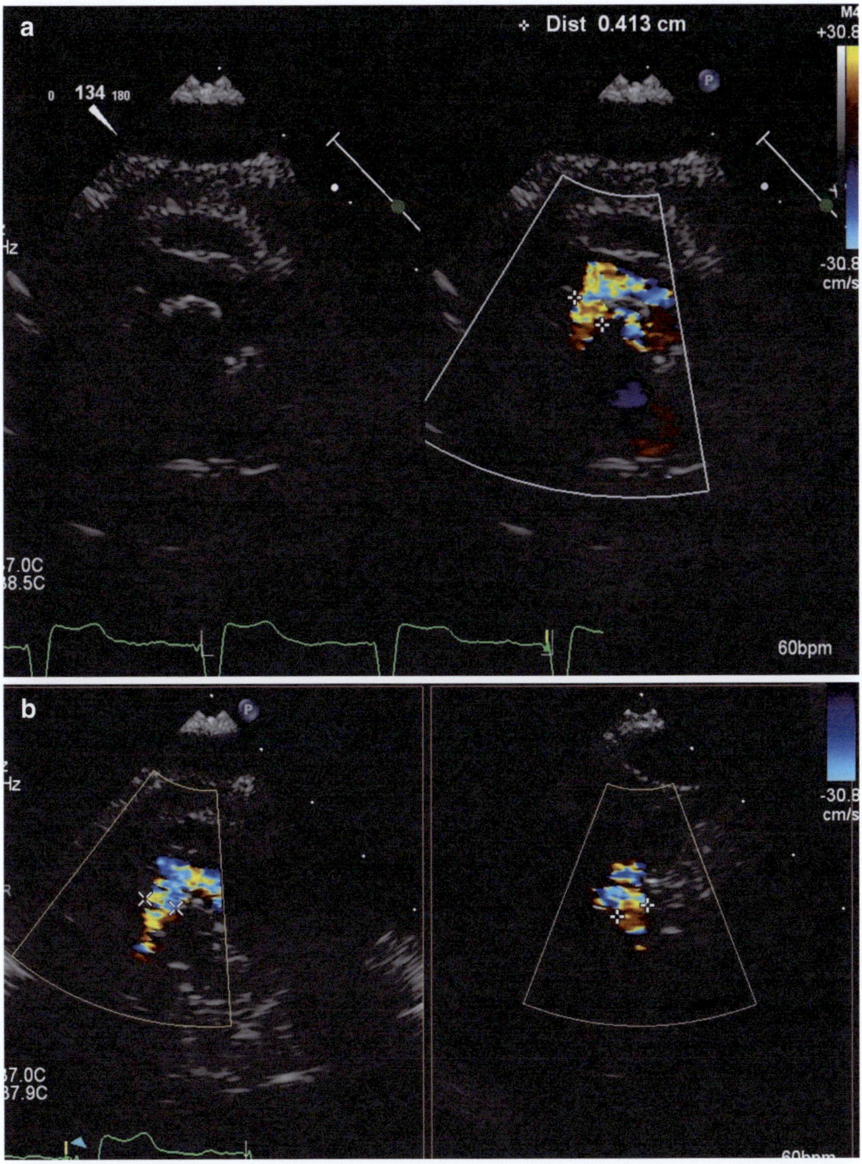

Fig. 20.2 Example of peri-device leak of a WATCHMAN™ device. **Panel A**, Video 20.3, 2D and color Doppler images including measurement of the vena contracta of the leak; **Panel B**, Video 20.4, X-plane imaging of the leak to measure the size of the leak; **Panel C,** pulsed-wave Doppler of the leak to confirm that the leak communicates with the distal appendage. Corresponding videos for 2D and color Doppler are available (Videos 20.3 and 20.4)

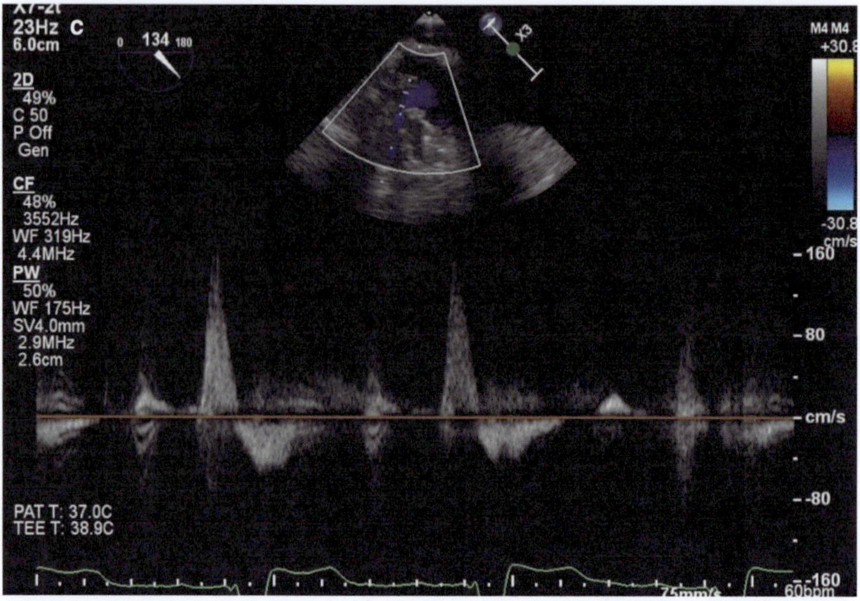

Fig. 20.2 (continued)

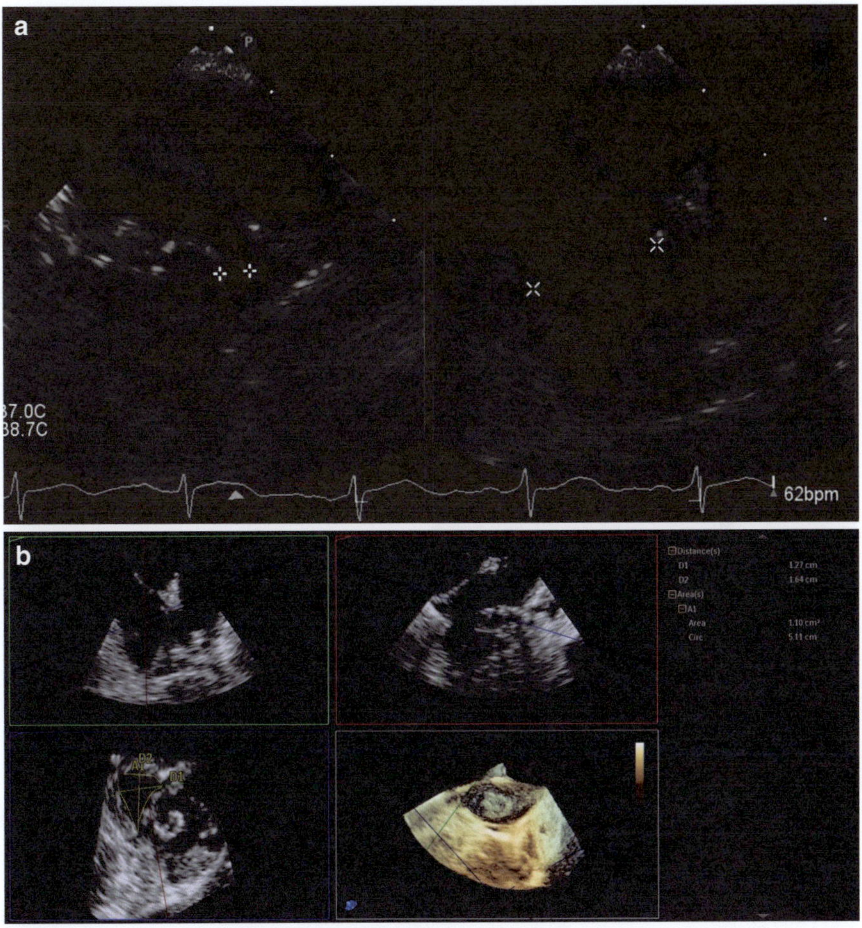

Fig. 20.3 Example of a larger peri-device leak of a WATCHMAN™ device due to an uncovered anterior lobe. **Panel A:** X-plane measurement of leak after color suppression. **Panel B:** 3D multiplanar reconstruction used to further assess the size of the leak and uncovered lobe in cross-section. Corresponding videos for 2D and color Doppler are available (Videos 20.5 and 20.6)

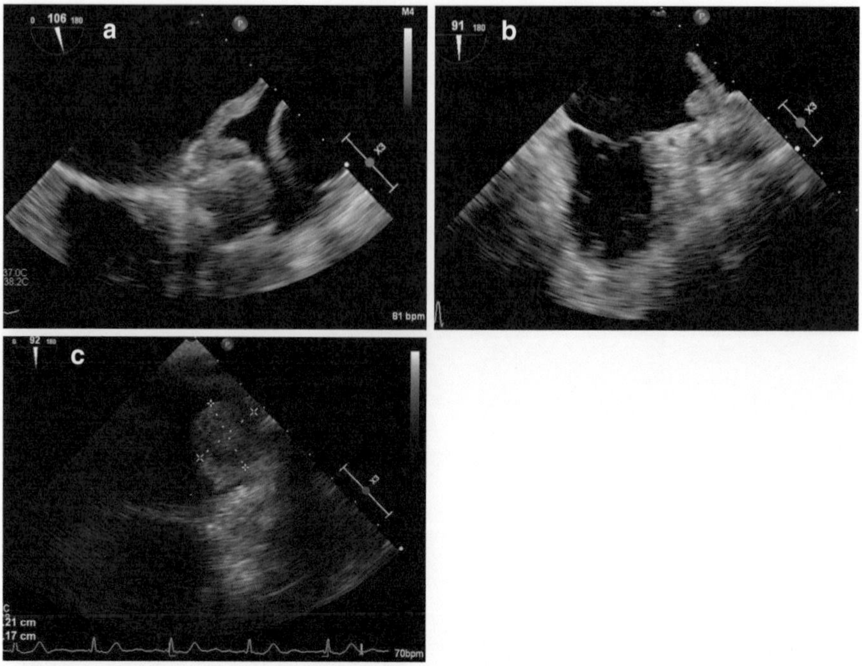

Fig. 20.4 Examples of device-related thrombus on the atrial-facing side of the device in **Panel A** (Video 20.7), **B** (Videos 20.8 and 20.9), and **C** (Video 20.10)

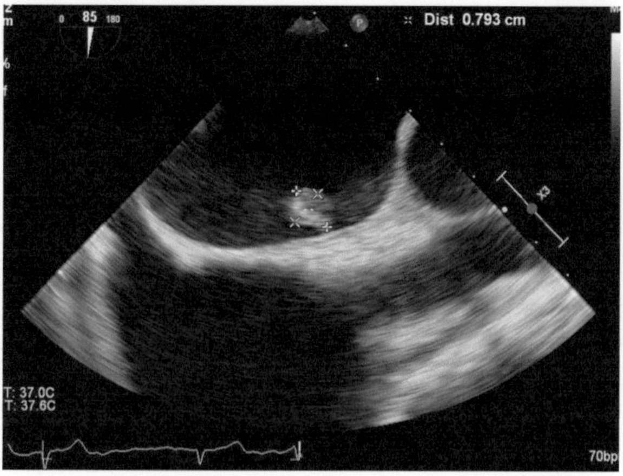

Fig. 20.5 Examples of a left atrial thrombus in 2D and 3D attached to the interatrial septum Videos 20.11 and 20.12)

Post-procedural Amulet™ Images

The post-procedural imaging protocol and assessment of Amulet™ is the same as WATCHMAN™. With Amulet™, the shape of the lobe and disc should be noted and compared with the intraprocedural echocardiographic images. The shape and position of the device lobe and disk, including concavity, should also be noted.

Computed Tomography Angiography (CTA)

CTA has been increasingly used for pre-procedural planning of transcatheter LAAC due to the high spatial and temporal resolution and multiplanar reconstruction capabilities. Considering these advantages, CTA is now used more frequently for post-procedural LAAC surveillance. One of the biggest advantages of post-procedural CTA over TEE is the ability to directly assess LAA patency following LAAC. TEE assesses PDL by detecting flow acceleration of the gap between the device and LAA, whereas CTA can assess PDL and quantify LAA patency and defined as LAA density measured distal to the device $\geq$100 (Hounsfield units [HU]) or $\geq$25% of that of the density measured in the LA [5–7]. Two mechanisms exist for LAA patency on surveillance imaging: PDL and intra-device leak (IDL). The former is defined by the passage of contrast between the device and the adjacent LAA, while the latter occurs when contrast passes through the device into the LAA from incomplete endothelization (Figs. 20.6 and 20.7). TEE can only detect PDL, whereas CTA can detect both PDL and IDL. The sensitivity of CTA for PDL is higher compared with TEE, as evidenced by the higher rates of PDL detected by CTA compared with TEE [3, 6, 7]. In these studies, poor agreement was observed in PDL quantification (e.g., width measurement) between TEE and CTA, where TEE (particularly 2D-TEE) underestimates the measured width of a crescent-shaped PDL compared with CTA.

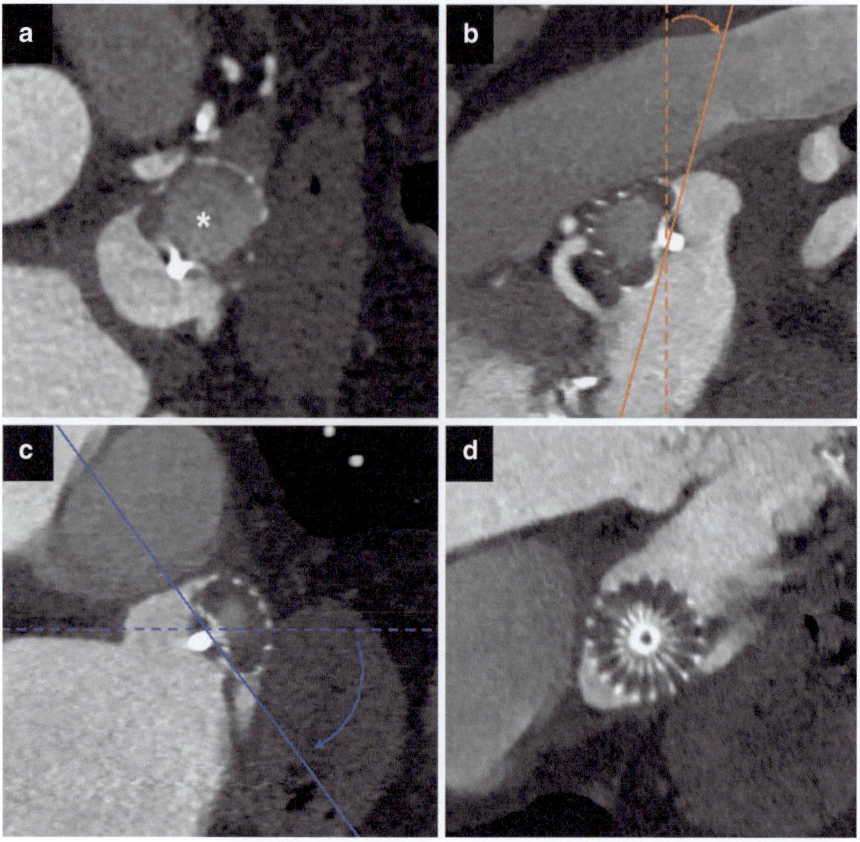

Fig. 20.6 Example of a post-procedural LAAC CTA analysis. **Panels A–C**: WATCHMAN™ FLX in the LAA in the axial, coronal, and sagittal CT images, respectively. The LAA density inside the device (asterisk) was 252 HU. **Panel D:** Multiplanar reconstruction is performed by centering the crosshairs on the central device screw and aligning the orthogonal planes perpendicularly to provide an en-face view of the device. **Panels D–F:** Cross-sectional imaging through the WATCHMAN™ FLX to assess for peri-device leak and a small proximal lobe (arrowhead) is noted in Panel D. **Panels G–L:** Multiple cross-sectional images reveal the continuation of contrast to distal LAA via a peri-device leak (arrows)

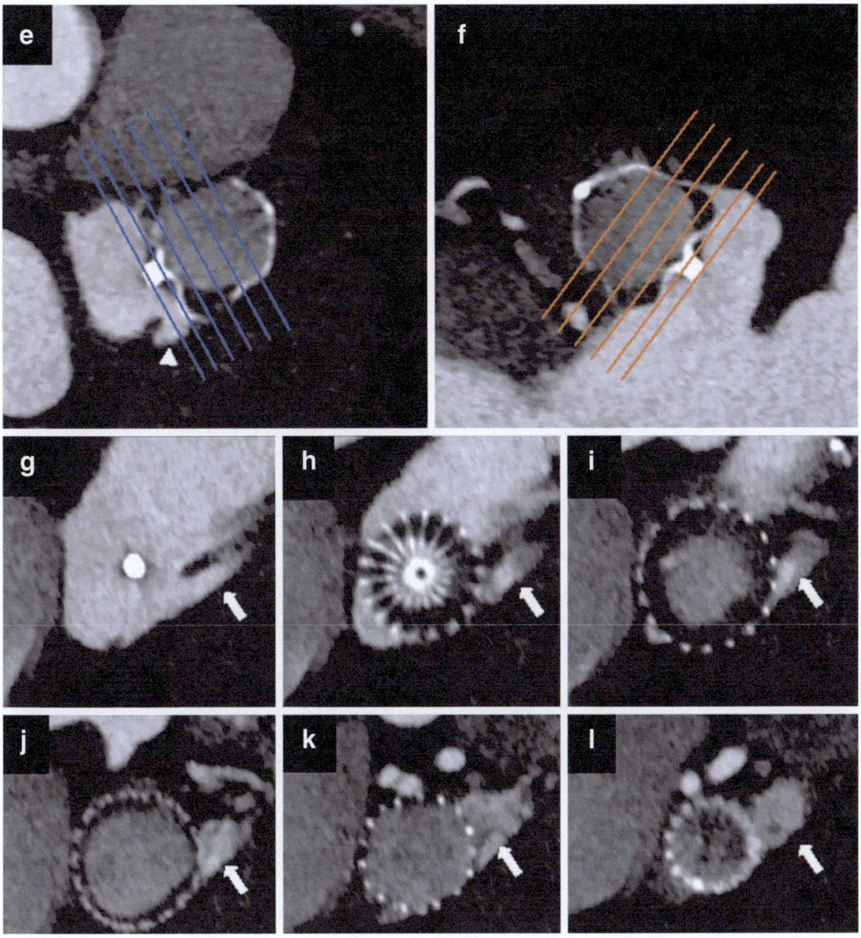

Fig. 20.6 (continued)

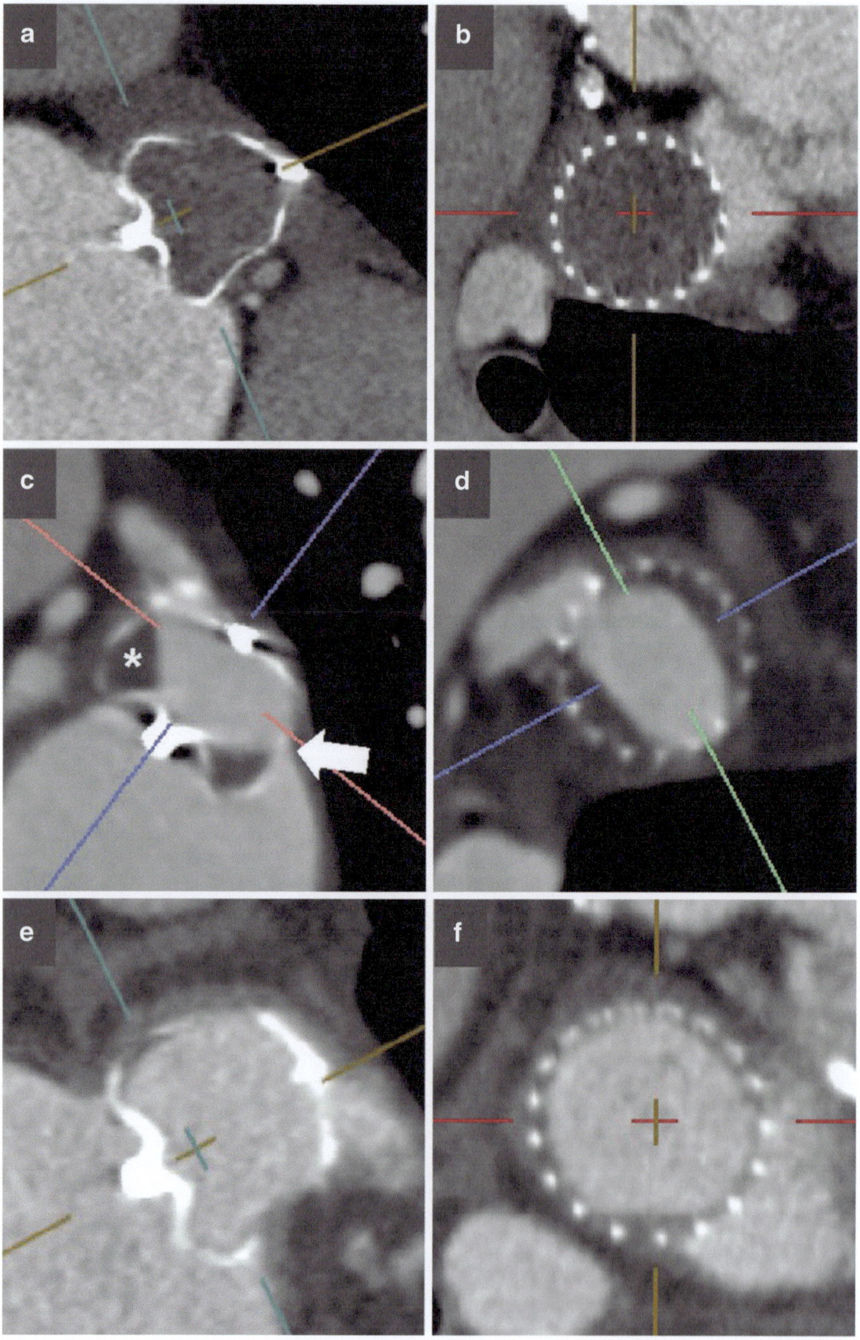

Fig. 20.7 Example CTA Images of a Sealed and Patent LAA. **Panels A and B** reveal a completely sealed LAA by a WATCHMAN™ device. **Panels C–F** demonstrate a WATCHMAN™ device in place with a patent LAA. **Panels C and D** show contrast passage (i.e., direct connection) from the LA to LAA (arrow) behind the fabric of the WATCHMAN™ device and partial endothelialization of the membrane (asterisk). **Panels E and F** demonstrate the absence of endothelialization despite a well-apposed WATCHMAN™ device

Clinical Impact of PDL and LAA Patency

The impact of PDL was not recognized in earlier trials (PROTECT AF trial and the Amulet Observational Study) as these studies were underpowered. However, the National Cardiovascular Data LAAO Registry revealed that small PDLs (<5 mm) were associated with a slightly higher risk of thromboembolic and bleeding events at 1-year follow-up (adjusted hazard ratio [HR]: 1.152; 95% confidence interval [CI]: 1.025–1.294) [8]. Similarly, Dukkipati et al. combined data from 2 FDA randomized clinical trials (PROTECT-AF and PREVAIL) and 1 FDA prospective registry (CAP2) to assess the impact of PDL (<5 mm) by TEE. PDL detected at 1 year, but not at 45 days, was associated with a higher risk of ischemic stroke or systemic embolism at 5 years (adjusted HR: 1.94; 95% CI: 1.15–3.29; $p = 0.014$) [9]. A recent meta-analysis of 48 studies on the prognostic implications of PDL after LAAC revealed that TEE-identified PDL was associated with a higher risk of thromboembolism (pooled odds ratio 2.04, 95% CI: 1.52–2.74) compared with no PDL [10]. Importantly, a positive correlation was noted between PDL size and the risk of thromboembolism (i.e., larger PDL was associated with a higher risk of ischemic stroke).

Despite the increased use of CTSA for post-procedural LAAC imaging, limited data regarding the clinical implications of CTA-based PDL or LAA patency is available. One of the largest studies by Korsholm et al. did not demonstrate a significant association between CTA-based PDL following LAAC with Amulet™ device and adverse events [6]. The SWISS APERO trial (Comparison of Amulet™ Versus Watchman™ FLX Device in Patients Undergoing Left Atrial Appendage Closure) is the first multicenter randomized controlled study comparing LAA patency with Amulet™ versus Watchman™ FLX and comparing TEE and CTA surveillance. At 45 days, LAA patency was surprisingly high with both devices (Amulet™ 67.6% vs. Watchman™ FLX 70%; $p = 0.713$), while TEE-based PDL was modest (Amulet™ 13.7% vs. Watchman™ FLX 27.5%; $p = 0.02$). Follow-up CTA at ~13 months demonstrated persistent high rates of LAA patency (Amulet™ 53.6% vs. Watchman™ FLX 48.4%; $p = 0.537$). A recent meta-analysis also evaluated the impact of CTA-based PDL or LAA patency on clinical outcomes. There was no significant association between thromboembolic risk and LAA patency or PDL (pooled OR 1.45 and 1.04, 95% CI: 0.84–2.50 and 0.52–2.07, respectively). The results of these studies should be interpreted cautiously due to their smaller sample sizes. Future studies with larger sample sizes, longer follow-ups, and systematic methodology for post-procedural LAAO CTA surveillance are warranted.

Device-Related Thrombosis

The incidence of DRT varies (1.7–3.9%) between studies, primarily due to a lack of standard criteria used to define DRT [11–14]. The echocardiographic diagnostic criteria used for DRT include a density on the LA aspect of the device that is (1) not explained by imaging artifact, (2) inconsistent with normal healing/device incorporation, (3) visible in multiple TEE planes, (4) in contact with the LAAC device, and (5) exhibiting independent motion. CTA with multiplanar reconstruction capability provides the ability to assess for DRT and additional findings such as hypoattenuating thickening (HAT). Kramer et al. analyzed 244 patients who underwent LAAC with Watchman™ FLX and surveillance CTA imaging at 8 weeks [15]. Overall, HAT was observed in 64% of patients and classified as subfabric hypoattenuation ($n = 59$), flat sessile HAT ($n = 78$), protruding sessile HAT ($n = 16$), or pedunculated HAT ($n = 7$). A preclinical study of Watchman™ FLX implantation in canine models demonstrated that subfabric hypoattenuation and flat sessile HAT correlated with device healing and endothelialization in histological analyses of explanted devices, suggesting that low-grade HAT may represent a benign process, and protruding or pedunculated HAT may be a precursor for DRT (i.e., high-grade HAT). Several studies have demonstrated that low-grade HAT was not associated with a higher risk of thromboembolic events, whereas high-grade HAT was associated with a higher risk of stroke [4, 15, 16]. Some potential predictors of DRT include prior stroke/TIA, larger LAA orifice, permanent AF, lower ejection fraction/low flow state, and implantation depth [11, 12, 17]. Ongoing clinical studies with novel HAT and DRT CTA classifications will further clarify its prognostic impact. Furthermore, the novel Watchman™ FLX PRO device features a fluoropolymer coating added to the fabric membrane of the device, which facilitates endothelium growth and may inhibit DRT.

Comparison Between CTA and TEE

The latest US and European guidelines recommend either TEE or CT for surveillance imaging following LAAC [1, 2]. The potential advantages of CTA are discussed in Chap. 5 (Table 5.4). The sensitivity of CTA for detecting PDL and DRT (including HAT) is greater than TEE [3, 4]. Additionally, CTA may provide additional information regarding the mechanism of PDL and DRT that may not be readily visible on TEE due to shadowing from the implanted device.

Conclusions

Post-procedural imaging surveillance at 45–90 days ±12 months following LAAC is important to managing LAAC. It provides a complete assessment of the implanted device, including any change that occurred from the intra-procedural imaging. The presence of PDL and DRT need to be assessed and used to determine the choice of antithrombotic therapy. TEE or CTA are both acceptable imaging modalities. CTA may provide some advantages over TEE in assessing PDL and DRT.

References

1. Glikson M, Wolff R, Hindricks G, et al. EHRA/EAPCI expert consensus statement on catheter-based left atrial appendage occlusion—an update. EP Europace. 2019;22:184.
2. Saw J, Holmes DR, Cavalcante JL, et al. SCAI/HRS expert consensus statement on transcatheter left atrial appendage closure. JACC Cardiovasc Interv. 2023;16:1384–400.
3. Qamar SR, Jalal S, Nicolaou S, Tsang M, Gilhofer T, Saw J. Comparison of cardiac computed tomography angiography and transoesophageal echocardiography for device surveillance after left atrial appendage closure. EuroIntervention. 2019;15:663–70.
4. Korsholm K, Jensen JM, Nørgaard BL, Nielsen-Kudsk JE. Detection of device-related thrombosis following left atrial appendage occlusion. Circ Cardiovasc Interv. 2019;12:e008112.
5. Saw J, Fahmy P, DeJong P, et al. Cardiac CT angiography for device surveillance after endovascular left atrial appendage closure. Eur Heart J Cardiovasc Imaging. 2015;16:1198–206.
6. Korsholm K, Jensen JM, Norgaard BL, et al. Peridevice leak following Amplatzer left atrial appendage occlusion: cardiac computed tomography classification and clinical outcomes. JACC Cardiovasc Interv. 2021;14:83–93.
7. Galea R, De Marco F, Meneveau N, et al. Amulet or Watchman device for percutaneous left atrial appendage closure: primary results of the SWISS-APERO randomized clinical trial. Circulation. 2022;145:724–38.
8. Alkhouli M, Du C, Killu A, et al. Clinical impact of residual leaks following left atrial appendage occlusion: insights from the NCDR LAAO registry. JACC Clin Electrophysiol. 2022;8:766–78.
9. Dukkipati SR, Holmes DR Jr, Doshi SK, et al. Impact of peridevice leak on 5-year outcomes after left atrial appendage closure. J Am Coll Cardiol. 2022;80:469–83.
10. Samaras A, Papazoglou AS, Balomenakis C, et al. Residual leaks following percutaneous left atrial appendage occlusion and outcomes: a meta-analysis. Eur Heart J. 2023;45:214–29.
11. Dukkipati SR, Kar S, Holmes DR, et al. Device-related thrombus after left atrial appendage closure: incidence, predictors, and outcomes. Circulation. 2018;138:874–85.
12. Schmidt B, Nielsen-Kudsk JE, Ellis CR, et al. Incidence, predictors, and clinical outcomes of device-related thrombus in the amulet IDE trial. JACC Clin Electrophysiol. 2023;9:96–107.
13. Kar S, Doshi SK, Sadhu A, et al. Primary outcome evaluation of a next-generation left atrial appendage closure device: results from the PINNACLE FLX trial. Circulation. 2021;143:1754–62.
14. Alkhouli M, Busu T, Shah K, Osman M, Alqahtani F, Raybuck B. Incidence and clinical impact of device-related thrombus following percutaneous left atrial appendage occlusion. JACC Clin Electrophysiol. 2018;4:1629–37.
15. Kramer AD, Korsholm K, Jensen JM, et al. Cardiac computed tomography following Watchman FLX implantation: device-related thrombus or device healing? Eur Heart J Cardiovasc Imaging. 2022;24:250–9.
16. Iriart X, Blanc G, Bouteiller XP, et al. Clinical implications of CT-detected hypoattenuation thickening on left atrial appendage occlusion devices. Radiology. 2023;308:e230462.
17. Cepas-Guillén P, Flores-Umanzor E, Leduc N, et al. Impact of device implant depth after left atrial appendage occlusion. JACC Cardiovasc Interv. 2023;16:2139–49.

Chapter 21
Shared Decision-Making and Comprehensive Atrial Fibrillation Management

Ibrahim Alshagjdali and Antonio Sotolongo-Fernandez

Abbreviations

AF	Atrial fibrillation
OAC	Oral anticoagulants
NOAC	Non-vitamin K oral anticoagulants
LAAC	Left atrial appendage closure
PVI	Pulmonary veins isolation
TEE	Transesophageal echocardiogram

Highlights

- Comprehensive atrial fibrillation (AF) treatment should aim to relieve symptoms, improve quality of life, and reduce cardiovascular morbidity and mortality.
- There are four main areas that need to be addressed in the treatment of AF: prevention of systemic thromboembolism, ventricular rate control, sinus rhythm restoration and maintenance, and risk factors modification.
- With the increasing evidence supporting several treatment strategies in atrial fibrillation management, clinicians must consider individualized treatment recommendations and shared decision-making with each patient.

I. Alshagjdali
Division of Cardiology, Harrington Heart & Vascular Institute, University Hospitals Cleveland Medical Center, Cleveland, OH, USA

Devision of Cardiology, Department of Internal Medicine, University of Arkansas for Medical Sciences College of Medicine, Little Rock, AR, USA

A. Sotolongo-Fernandez (✉)
Division of Cardiology, Harrington Heart & Vascular Institute, University Hospitals Cleveland Medical Center, Cleveland, OH, USA
e-mail: Antonio.sotolongo-fernandez@uhhospitals.org

S. J. Filby et al. (eds.), *A Contemporary Manual of Left Atrial Appendage Closure*, https://doi.org/10.1007/978-3-031-68441-8_21

Table 21.1 Main areas to be addressed in the treatment of AF

1. Prevention of systemic thromboembolism
2. Ventricular rate control
3. Sinus rhythm restoration and maintenance
4. Risk factors modification

- AF management after LAAC remains largely the same but with some important considerations in regard to catheter ablation.

Introduction

In general, management of atrial fibrillation (AF) should be focused on identifying and treating underlying causes, symptom reduction, quality of life improvement, and reducing cardiovascular morbidity and mortality associated with AF. There are four main aspects that need to be addressed in the treatment of AF, as seen in Table 21.1: prevention of systemic thromboembolism, ventricular rate control, sinus rhythm restoration and maintenance, and risk factors modification. Therapy is usually influenced by several factors including patient's preference, patient's comorbidities including the presence of heart failure or structural heart disease, presence of symptoms and severity, and lastly the type of AF (i.e., paroxysmal, persistent, etc.).

Shared Decision-Making

Since AF is strongly associated with increased cardiovascular mortality and morbidity, patient involvement should start with proper education about the disease's natural history and progression. Moreover, there are several evidence-based treatment strategies in atrial fibrillation management; therefore, clinicians must consider individualized treatment recommendations and aim for shared decision-making with each patient.

Atrial Fibrillation Management

Oral Anticoagulation (OAC)

Oral anticoagulation (OAC) has served as a mainstay treatment for thromboembolic risk reduction because of its well-documented efficacy but also comes with the cost of increased risk of bleeding. Warfarin is the drug of choice for valvular atrial fibrillation whereas non-warfarin oral anticoagulants (NOAC) are preferred over warfarin for patients with non-valvular AF with elevated CHA_2DS_2-VASc score (2 or more for males or 3 or more for females). However, there have been substantial numbers of patients facing problems with OAC including inadequate therapeutic anticoagulation, non-adherence, and bleeding of different magnitudes from mild to life threatening. As a result, it is estimated that up to 50% of patients with atrial fibrillation are not on anticoagulation. In patients who are poor candidates for long-term oral anticoagulation with an increased risk of stroke, percutaneous LAAC should be considered (2023 AHA/ACC/HRS guidelines Class IIa). The importance of shared decision-making when it comes to LAAC implantation was emphasized by the Centers for Medicare & Medicaid Services (CMS) which requires a formal shared decision-making interaction with an independent non-interventional physician using an evidence-based decision tool on oral anticoagulation prior to LAAC.

Percutaneous Left Atrial Appendage Closure (LAAC)

For patients who are candidates for percutaneous LAAC, management of their atrial fibrillation remains largely the same but with some important considerations. Post-procedural antiplatelet and anticoagulant strategies are discussed separately in Chap. 20. Similar to other patients with AF, management should include rate control, rhythm control if applicable, and addressing risk factors contributing to AF.

Rhythm Control

In regard to rhythm control, electrical cardioversions are a common treatment. Routinely, despite having a LAAC, patients will need to be started on anticoagulation 3 weeks prior to procedure or have transesophageal echocardiogram (TEE) pre-procedurally prior to undergoing cardioversion. Patients will also be kept anticoagulated after the cardioversion for a short period of time. That being said, studies have begun looking into performing cardioversions on patients with LAAC without anticoagulation provided that pre-procedure TEE shows good device position, absence of device-related thrombus, and peri-device leaks smaller than 5 mm. Although results from this study were encouraging, larger studies are warranted to establish safety.

Catheter Ablation

Catheter ablation with pulmonary vein isolation (PVI) is usually recommended for symptomatic patients with paroxysmal or persistent AF who are refractory or intolerant to anti-arrhythmic drugs. The procedure might also be considered as a first-line approach as well as in selected asymptomatic patients. There is a possibility that catheter ablation after LAAC may result in damage to the device, device dislodgement, or catheter entrapment. It is therefore important to have a discussion about future plans for rhythm control if possible prior to LAAC. Percutaneous LAAC and AF ablation can also be combined successfully and safely in a single procedure. Although not ideal, ablation after LAAC has been successfully performed in some high-volume centers with good results. There may also be a role for LAAC in the setting of left atrial appendage electrical isolation. The left atrial appendage has been established as a potential trigger for AF. However, left atrial appendage isolation has led to increase in LAA thrombus formation and thromboembolic risk post-procedure despite anticoagulation. The EHRA/EAPCI expert consensus statement on catheter-based left atrial appendage occlusion stated that, due to increased clinical experience, percutaneous LAAC may be reasonable for those with LAA isolation whose anticoagulation is imperfect. However, data are lacking, and there are no randomized studies comparing oral anticoagulation against LAAC in those patients.

Conclusions

Comprehensive AF treatment should aim to relieve symptoms, improve quality of life, and reduce cardiovascular morbidity and mortality. With the increasing evidence supporting several treatment strategies in atrial fibrillation management, clinicians must consider individualized treatment recommendations and shared decision-making with each patient.

References and Suggested Readings

1. Di Biase L, Burkhardt JD, Mohanty P, Mohanty S, Sanchez JE, Trivedi C, Güneş M, Gökoğlan Y, Gianni C, Horton RP, Themistoclakis S, Gallinghouse GJ, Bailey S, Zagrodzky JD, Hongo RH, Beheiry S, Santangeli P, Casella M, Dello Russo A, Al-Ahmad A, Hranitzky P, Lakkireddy D, Tondo C, Natale A. Left atrial appendage isolation in patients with longstanding persistent AF undergoing catheter ablation: BELIEF trial. J Am Coll Cardiol. 2016;68:1929–40.
2. Du X, Chu H, Ye P, He B, Xu H, Jiang S, Lin M, Lin R, Liu J, Wang B, Feng M, Yu Y, Chen X. Combination of left atrial appendage closure and catheter ablation in a single procedure for patients with atrial fibrillation: multicenter experience. J Formos Med Assoc. 2019;118(5):891–7. https://doi.org/10.1016/j.jfma.2018.10.006. Epub 2018 Oct 25.
3. Elwyn G, Coulter A, Laitner S, Walker E, Watson P, Thomson R. Implementing shared decision making in the NHS. BMJ. 2010;341:c5146.
4. Glikson M, Wolff R, Hindricks G, Mandrola J, Camm AJ, Lip GYH, Fauchier L, Betts TR, Lewalter T, Saw J, Tzikas A, Sternik L, Nietlispach F, Berti S, Sievert H, Bertog S, Meier B. EHRA/EAPCI expert consensus statement on catheter-based left atrial appendage occlusion – an update. EuroIntervention. 2020;15(13):1133–80. https://doi.org/10.4244/EIJY19M08_01.

5. He B, Jiang L-S, Hao Z-Y, Wang H, Miao Y-T. Combination of ablation and left atrial appendage closure as "one-stop" procedure in the treatment of atrial fibrillation: current status and future perspective. Pacing Clin Electrophysiol. 2021;44:1259–66. https://doi.org/10.1111/pace.14201.
6. Holmes DR, Alkhouli M, Reddy V. Left atrial appendage occlusion for the unmet clinical needs of stroke prevention in nonvalvular atrial fibrillation. Mayo Clin Proc. 2019;94:864–74. https://doi.org/10.1016/j.mayocp.2018.09.025.
7. January CT, Wann LS, Calkins H, Chen LY, Cigarroa JE, Cleveland JC Jr, Ellinor PT, Ezekowitz MD, Field ME, Furie KL, Heidenreich PA, Murray KT, Shea JB, Tracy CM, Yancy CW. 2019 AHA/ACC/HRS focused update of the 2014 AHA/ACC/HRS guideline for the management of patients with atrial fibrillation: a report of the American College of Cardiology/American Heart Association Task Force on Clinical Practice Guidelines and the Heart Rhythm Society. Circulation. 2019;140:e125–51. https://doi.org/10.1161/CIR.0000000000000665.
8. Joglar JA, Chung MK, Armbruster AL, Benjamin EJ, Chyou JY, Cronin EM, Deswal A, Eckhardt L, Goldberger ZD, Gopinathannair R, Gorenek B, Hess PL, Hlatky M, Hogan G, Ibeh C, Indik JH, Kido K, Kusumoto F, Link MS, Linta KT, Marcus GM, McCarthy PM, Patel N, Patton KK, Perez MV, Piccini JP, Russo AM, Sanders P, Streur MM, Thomas KL, Times S, Tisdale JE, Valente AM, Van Wagoner DR. 2023 ACC/AHA/ACCP/HRS guideline for the diagnosis and management of atrial fibrillation: a report of the American College of Cardiology/American Heart Association Joint Committee on Clinical Practice Guidelines. Circulation. 2024;149:e1–e156. https://doi.org/10.1161/CIR.0000000000001193.
9. Kim YG, Shim J, Oh S-K, Lee K-N, Choi J-I, Kim Y-H. Electrical isolation of the left atrial appendage increases the risk of ischemic stroke and transient ischemic attack regardless of post isolation flow velocity. Heart Rhythm. 2018;15(12):1746–53. https://doi.org/10.1016/j.hrthm.2018.09.012. ISSN 1547–5271.
10. Rillig A, Tilz RR, Lin T, Fink T, Heeger CH, Arya A, Metzner A, Mathew S, Wissner E, Makimoto H, Wohlmuth P, Kuck KH, Ouyang F. Unexpectedly high incidence of stroke and left atrial appendage thrombus formation after electrical isolation of the left atrial appendage for the treatment of atrial tachyarrhythmias. Circ Arrhythm Electrophysiol. 2016;9:e003461.
11. Sharma SP, Turagam MK, Gopinathannair R, Reddy V, Kar S, Mohanty S, Cheng J, Holmes DR Jr, Sondergaard L, Natale A, Lakkireddy D. Direct current cardioversion of atrial fibrillation in patients with left atrial appendage occlusion devices. J Am Coll Cardiol. 2019;74(18):2267–74. https://doi.org/10.1016/j.jacc.2019.08.1045.
12. Swaans MJ, Post MC, Rensing BJ, Boersma LV. Ablation for atrial fibrillation in combination with left atrial appendage closure: first results of a feasibility study. J Am Heart Assoc. 2012;1(5):e002212. https://doi.org/10.1161/JAHA.112.002212. Epub 2012 Oct 25. PMID: 23316289; PMCID: PMC3541623.
13. Verma N, Knight BP. Left atrial appendage isolation at the time of atrial fibrillation ablation. Heart Rhythm. 2018;15(12):1754–5, ISSN 1547-5271. https://doi.org/10.1016/j.hrthm.2018.09.013.
14. Wintgens LIS, Klaver MN, Swaans MJ, Alipour A, Balt JC, van Dijk VF, Rensing BJWM, Wijffels MCEF, Boersma LVA. Left atrial catheter ablation in patients with previously implanted left atrial appendage closure devices. EP Europace. 2019;21(3):428–33. https://doi.org/10.1093/europace/euy237.

Chapter 22
Future Perspectives for Left Atrial Appendage Closure: CHAMPION-AF and CATALYST Clinical Trials

Ali Azeem and Mauricio Arruda

Highlights

- Atrial fibrillation (AF) increases the risk of stroke and peripheral embolism-related deaths.
- LAAO is a IIa recommendation for non-valvular AF patients with high thrombo-embolic risk and contraindication for oral anticoagulation.
- The role of LAAO in stroke prevention and bleeding risk as compared to DOAC.
- CHAMPION-AF and CATALYST are two upcoming randomized trials that will be comparing DOAC to LAAO with the WATCHMAN FLX and Amulet, respectively, in patients at standard bleeding risk with nonvalvular AF and without contraindication for oral anticoagulation.

Introduction

Oral anticoagulation therapy with warfarin, a vitamin-K antagonist, was the initial therapy shown to reduce the risk of thromboembolism and improve mortality in atrial fibrillation (AF), at the cost of increased bleeding events [1] [2]. Subsequent studies of the direct oral anticoagulants (DOACs) were subsequently shown to be safe and effective when compared to warfarin, though there was still a residual increased bleeding risk. Percutaneous left atrial appendage occlusion (LAAO) currently has a IIa recommendation in the most recent ESC and ACC/AHA/ACCP/HRS guidelines on this matter as an alternative for patients who are at increased risk of stroke but have contraindications to long-term anticoagulation [3, 4]. This

A. Azeem (✉) · M. Arruda
Division of Cardiology, Harrington Heart & Vascular Institute, University Hospitals Cleveland Medical Center, Cleveland, OH, USA
e-mail: ali.azeem@uhhospitals.org

S. J. Filby et al. (eds.), *A Contemporary Manual of Left Atrial Appendage Closure*, https://doi.org/10.1007/978-3-031-68441-8_22

recommendation is primarily on the basis of PROTECT AF and the follow-up PREVAIL which when analyzed in a patient-level meta-analysis showed that patients receiving the device had significantly fewer hemorrhagic strokes than those receiving warfarin, but with an increase of ischemic strokes [5–7]. Given the transition to DOAC's as first-line therapy for anticoagulation in atrial fibrillation and improvements in procedural techniques, two new trials are underway to evaluate the role of LAAO in patients with atrial fibrillation and elevated thromboembolic risk with standard bleeding risk: CATALYST (Abbott Amulet vs. DOAC) and CHAMPION-AF (Boston Scientific WATCHMAN FLX vs. DOAC). These studies are designed to compare LAAO to DOAC therapy in patients with standard bleeding risk that would typically be treated with anticoagulation for the prevention of stroke in AF. There are many ongoing trials addressing the question of whether the indications for LAAO should be expanded, as seen in the timeline of the major clinical trials in Fig. 22.1.

CATALYST

The CATALYST trial is a prospective, randomized, international multicenter trial sponsored by Abbott to evaluate the safety and efficacy of the Amulet LAA Occluder compared to DOAC therapy in patients with non-valvular AF at elevated risk for ischemic stroke and for whom anticoagulation with a DOAC is currently

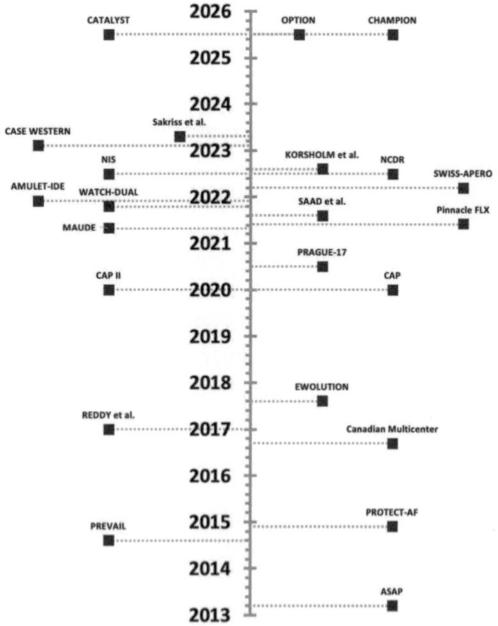

Fig. 22.1 Timeline of the major clinical trials

recommended. CATALYST has started enrolling patients in 7/2020, is projected to enroll 2650 participants, and is projected to be completed in 4/2029.

The exact inclusion and exclusion criteria for CATALYST are enumerated in Table 22.1. In summary, this study is designed to investigate patients who:

- Are adults 18 years of age or greater with AF who are at elevated risk of thromboembolism as a cause of stroke (CHA2DS2-VASc score of ≥3, AF felt not to be due to a reversible cause such as major surgery or hyperthyroidism).
- Are not at elevated risk of stroke from other causes (i.e., cerebrovascular atherosclerosis or risk of left ventricular thrombus).
- Would typically be treated with DOAC in the current treatment paradigm and are expected to be able to adhere to long-term DOAC therapy (in control arm) or antiplatelet regimen (in intervention arm).
- Do not have another indication for long-term anticoagulation or P2Y12 inhibitor.
- Have technically feasible anatomy for the procedure (no ASD or PFO repair or closure, no IVC filter, no contraindication to transesophageal echocardiogram, no hypersensitivity to components of the LAA occlude device, i.e., nickel allergy, LAA is obliterated or surgically ligated).
- Do not have a competing life-limiting comorbidity that would significantly change the risk/benefit ratio of the procedure.
- Do not have rheumatic or congenital mitral valve disease.
- Are not at high bleeding risk with thrombocytopenia (<50,000 platelets per microliter) or anemia (hemoglobin <10 g/dL) requiring transfusion.

This study will randomize patients that meet these criteria in a 1:1 fashion to either the experimental arm of left atrial appendage occlusion with the Amplatzer Amulet LAA Occluder or the control arm of the current standard of care medical anticoagulant therapy with a DOAC.

The anticoagulation/antiplatelet approach in the control arm is to use a DOAC, in keeping with standard practice. The post-implant anticoagulant/antiplatelet strategy in the intervention arm will involve dual-antiplatelet therapy (DAPT) with 75–100 mg aspirin +75 mg clopidogrel if, at the end of the procedure color, Doppler shows no peri-device leak or peri-device leak <5 mm; a patient undergoing LAAO would be continued on DOAC after a successful implant if peri-device leak was >5 mm. DAPT would be continued for 6–12 weeks and then clopidogrel discontinued with continuation of aspirin. Imaging is obtained to evaluate for device-related thrombus and device embolization at 3 months with TEE and at 12 months with TEE or CT. At 1-year post-implant, the decision to continue vs. stop aspirin (i.e., no anticoagulation/antiplatelet) would be left to the discretion of the treating physician [9].

The pre-specified primary outcomes of this trial are a non-inferiority outcome of a composite of ischemic stroke, systemic embolism, or cardiovascular mortality at 2 years, a superiority endpoint of major bleeding or clinically relevant non-major bleeding events (excluding procedure-related events) at 2 years, and a non-inferiority endpoint of composite ischemic stroke or systemic embolism. The pre-specified secondary outcome measures are non-inferiority and superiority of major bleeding

Table 22.1 Inclusion and exclusion criteria for CATALYST [8]

Inclusion criteria
Documented paroxysmal, persistent, or permanent non-valvular AF (documentation must include an electrocardiogram, Holter, or event recorder).
At high risk of stroke or systemic embolism, defined as a CHA2DS2-VASc score of ≥3.
Eligible for long-term NOAC therapy.
Able to comply with the required NOAC medication regimen if randomized to the control group.
Able to comply with the required medication regimen post-device implant if the subject is randomized to the device group or the subject is a roll-in.
Able to understand, and is willing to provide, written informed consent to participate in the trial, prior to any clinical investigation-related procedure or assessment.
18 years of age or older, or the age of legal consent
Able and willing to return for required follow-up visits and assessments.
Exclusion criteria
Requires long-term OAC therapy for a condition other than AF.
Planned cardiac intervention or surgery, which is invasive or requires sedation or anesthesia, within 3 months following randomization, other than study-related procedures such as LAAO and cardiac imaging (if applicable).
Known contraindication to, or allergic to, aspirin, clopidogrel, or OAC medication use.
Indicated for P2Y12 platelet inhibitor for >1 year post-randomization.
In the opinion of the investigator, is considered at high risk for general anesthesia, and general anesthesia is planned for the study procedure.
Has undergone atrial septal defect (ASD) repair or has an ASD closure device present.
Has undergone patent foramen ovale (PFO) repair or has a PFO closure device implanted.
Is implanted with a mechanical valve prosthesis.
Is implanted with an inferior vena cava filter.
History of rheumatic or congenital mitral valve heart disease.
Has any of the customary contraindications for a percutaneous catheterization procedure (e.g., subject is too small to accommodate the ICE probe (if planned) or required catheters, or subject has active infection or bleeding disorder).
Customary contraindications for TEE/TOE (e.g., presence of esophageal varices, esophageal stricture, or history of esophageal cancer).
Experienced stroke or transient ischemic attack (TIA) within 90 days prior to randomization or implant procedure (as applicable).
Underwent any cardiac or non-cardiac intervention or surgery within 30 days prior to randomization.
Underwent catheter ablation for AF or atrial flutter within 60 days prior to randomization.
Experienced myocardial infarction within 90 days prior to randomization.
New York Heart Association Class IV Congestive Heart Failure.
Left ventricular ejection fraction ≤30% (per most recent assessment).
Symptomatic carotid disease (defined as >50% lumen diameter narrowing on CTA, MRA, or TCD with symptoms of ipsilateral transient or visual TIA evidenced by amaurosis fugax, ipsilateral hemispheric TIAs, or ipsilateral stroke); if the subject has a history of carotid stent or endarterectomy, the subject is eligible if there is <50% lumen diameter narrowing.

(continued)

Table 22.1 (continued)

Has known intracranial atherosclerosis and/or intracranial small vessel disease (defined as 6 points on the Fazekas Scale).
Reversible cause of AF (i.e., secondary to thyroid disorders, acute alcohol intoxication, trauma, recent major surgical procedures).
History of idiopathic or recurrent venous thromboembolism.
LAA is obliterated or surgically ligated.
Thrombocytopenia (defined as <50,000 platelets per microliter (<50 × 10^9/L) or anemia (defined as hemoglobin <10 g/dL) requiring transfusions.
Hypersensitivity to any portion of the device material or individual components of the Amulet LAA Occluder device (e.g., nickel allergy).
Actively enrolled in, or plans to enroll in, a concurrent clinical study in which the active treatment arm may confound the results of this trial.
Is pregnant or breastfeeding or pregnancy is planned during the course of the investigation.
Active endocarditis or other infection producing bacteremia.
Transient case of AF (i.e., never previously detected, provoked/induced by surgical or catheter manipulations, etc.).
Severe renal failure (estimated glomerular filtration rate <30 ml/min/1.73 m^2), but not on dialysis.
Life expectancy is less than 2 years in the opinion of the investigator.
Presence of other anatomic or comorbid conditions or other medical, social, or psychological conditions that, in the investigator's opinion, could limit the subject's ability to participate in the clinical investigation or to comply with follow-up requirements or impact the scientific soundness of the clinical investigation results.

or clinically relevant non-major bleeding at 2 years and superiority of disabling or fatal strokes at 2 years.

CHAMPION-AF

The CHAMPION-AF trial is a prospective, randomized, multicenter international trial sponsored by Boston Scientific to evaluate the safety and efficacy of the WATCHMAN FLX device as an alternative for DOAC therapy in patients with non-valvular AF. CHAMPION-AF enrolled 3000 patients at 142 sites from 10/2020 to 11/2022 and is projected to be complete in 12/2027.

The exact inclusion and exclusion criteria for CHAMPION-AF are enumerated in Table 22.2. In summary, this study is designed to evaluate patients who:

- Are adults with non-valvular atrial fibrillation who are at elevated risk of thromboembolism as a cause of stroke (CHA2DS2-VASc score of ≥2 in men or ≥ 3 in women) and AF felt not to be due to a reversible cause such as major surgery or hyperthyroidism.
- Are not at elevated risk of stroke from other causes (i.e., cerebrovascular atherosclerosis or risk of left ventricular thrombus or cardiac tumor).

Table 22.2 Inclusion and exclusion criteria for CHAMPION-AF [10]

Inclusion criteria
The subject is of legal age to participate in the study per the laws of their respective geography.
The subject has documented non-valvular atrial fibrillation (i.e., atrial fibrillation in the absence of moderate or greater mitral stenosis or a mechanical heart valve).
The subject has a calculated CHA2DS2-VASc (congestive heart failure, hypertension, age ≥75 years, diabetes mellitus, stroke or transient ischemic attack (TIA), vascular disease, age 65–74 years, sex category) score of 2 or greater for men and 3 or greater for women.
The subject is deemed to be suitable for the protocol-defined pharmacologic regimens in both the test and control arms.
The subject or legal representative is able to understand and willing to provide written informed consent to participate in the trial.
The subject is able and willing to return for required follow-up visits and examinations.
Exclusion criteria
Subjects who are currently enrolled in another investigational study, except when the subject is participating in a mandatory governmental registry, or a purely observational registry with no associated treatments.
The subject requires long-term anticoagulation therapy for reasons other than AF-related stroke risk reduction, for example, due to an underlying hypercoagulable state (i.e., even if the device is implanted, the subjects would not be eligible to discontinue OAC due to other medical conditions requiring chronic OAC therapy).
The subject is contraindicated or allergic to oral anticoagulation medication and/or aspirin.
The subject is indicated for chronic P2Y12 platelet inhibitor therapy.
The subject had or is planning to have any cardiac or non-cardiac intervention or surgical procedure within 30 days prior to or 60 days after implant (including, but not limited to, cardioversion, percutaneous coronary intervention (PCI), cardiac ablation, cataract surgery, etc.).
The subject had a prior stroke (of any cause, whether ischemic or hemorrhagic) or transient ischemic attack (TIA) within the 30 days prior to enrollment.
The subject had a prior major bleeding event per ISTH definition within the 30 days prior to randomization. Lack of resolution of related clinical sequelae or planned and pending interventions to resolve bleeding/bleeding source are a further exclusion regardless of timing of the bleeding event.
The subject has an active bleed.
The subject has a reversible cause of AF or transient AF.
The subject is absent of a left atrial appendage (LAA) or the LAA is surgically ligated.
The subject has had a myocardial infarction (MI) documented in the clinical record as either a non-ST elevation MI (NSTEMI) or as an ST-elevation MI (STEMI), with or without intervention, within 30 days prior to enrollment.
The subject has a history of atrial septal repair or has an atrial septal device (ASD)/patent foramen ovale (PFO) device.
The subject has an implanted mechanical valve prosthesis in any position.
The subject has a known contraindication to percutaneous catheterization procedure.
The subject has a known contraindication to transesophageal echo (TEE).
The subject has a cardiac tumor.
The subject has signs/symptoms of acute or chronic pericarditis.
The subject has an active infection.
There is evidence of tamponade physiology.

(continued)

Table 22.2 (continued)

The subject has New York Heart Association Class IV Congestive Heart Failure at the time of enrollment.
The subject is of childbearing potential and is, or plans to become, pregnant during the time of the study (method of assessment upon study physician's discretion).
The subject has a documented life expectancy of less than 3 years.
Transthoracic echo exclusion criteria:
The subject has left ventricular ejection fraction (LVEF) < 30%.
The subject has an existing pericardial effusion with a circumferential echo-free space >5 mm.
The subject has a high-risk PFO with an atrial septal aneurysm excursion >15 mm or length > 15 mm.
The subject has a significant mitral valve (MV) stenosis (i.e., MV area < 1.5 cm^2).

- Would typically be treated with DOAC in the current treatment paradigm and are expected to be able to adhere to long-term DOAC therapy (in the control arm) or antiplatelet regimen (in the intervention arm).
- Do not have another indication for long-term anticoagulation or P2Y12 inhibitor.
- Have technically feasible anatomy for the procedure (no ASD or PFO repair or closure, no IVC filter, no contraindication to transesophageal echocardiogram, no hypersensitivity to components of the LAA occlude device, i.e., nickel allergy, LAA is obliterated or surgically ligated).
- Do not have a competing life-limiting comorbidity that would significantly change the risk/benefit ratio of the procedure.
- Do not have significant mitral stenosis (i.e., valve area < 1.5 cm^2).
- Without active or recent major bleed within the past 30 days.

The post-implant drug regimen in CHAMPION-AF includes DOAC + aspirin, DOAC alone, or DAPT with 75 mg clopidogrel and 75–100 mg aspirin. The preferred DOAC is apixaban or rivaroxaban at standard AF dosing. If technical success was achieved at the time of implant (leak 5 mm or less), then the treatment regimen is de-escalated to monotherapy with either aspirin or a P2Y12 inhibitor (if tolerated better than aspirin) for at least 12 months post-implant. If there is a leak greater than 5 mm, then DOAC is continued with aspirin until the leak is 5 mm or less on LAA imaging. If a device-related thrombus is detected at 4 months, then the patient is recommended to be restarted on anticoagulation therapy with aspirin [11].

The primary pre-specified outcomes of CHAMPION-AF are the following:

- Non-inferiority for the composite of stroke, cardiovascular death, and systemic embolism at 36 months.
- Superiority for non-procedural bleeding at 36 months (ISTH major bleeding and clinically relevant non-major bleeding).
- Non-inferiority for the composite outcome of ischemic stroke and systemic embolism at 60 months.

The secondary outcome measures are the following:

- Superiority of ISTH major bleeding at 60 months.

- Superiority of the composite outcome of cardiovascular death, all stroke, systemic embolism, and non-procedural bleeding (ISTH major bleeding and clinically relevant non-major bleeding) at 60 months.

Conclusion

Taken together, these trials will help address the role of LAAO in a contemporary setting where DOAC is the current standard anticoagulation treatment for atrial fibrillation. These trials will build upon the findings of PRAGUE-17, where 402 high-risk AF patients were randomized to LAAO vs. DOAC with non-inferiority of LAAC to DOAC in preventing major AF-related cardiovascular, neurological, and bleeding events [12]. Moreover, these large trials will allow for a better estimate of procedural risk and long-term effects of LAAO given longer follow-up and larger sample size than the initial LAAO trials. Once these results are available, physicians will be better equipped to discuss the risks and benefits of LAAO with more patients with AF and potentially lower the risk of hemorrhagic stroke while still protecting them from thromboembolism.

References

1. January CT, Wann LS, Calkins H, Chen LY, Cigarroa JE, Cleveland JC Jr, Ellinor PT, Ezekowitz MD, Field ME, Furie KL, Heidenreich PA, Murray KT, Shea JB, Tracy CM, Yancy CW. AHA/ACC/HRS focused update of the 2014 AHA/ACC/HRS guideline for the management of patients with atrial fibrillation: a report of the American College of Cardiology/American Heart Association Task Force on Clinical Practice Guidelines and the Heart Rhythm Society. J Am Coll Cardiol. 2019;74(1):104–32. https://doi.org/10.1016/j.jacc.2019.01.011. Epub 2019 Jan 28. Erratum in: J Am Coll Cardiol. 2019 Jul 30;74(4):599.
2. Hindricks G, Potpara T, Dagres N, Arbelo E, Bax JJ, Blomström-Lundqvist C, Boriani G, Castella M, Dan GA, Dilaveris PE, Fauchier L, Filippatos G, Kalman JM, La Meir M, Lane DA, Lebeau JP, Lettino M, Lip GYH, Pinto FJ, Thomas GN, Valgimigli M, Van Gelder IC, Van Putte BP, Watkins CL, ESC Scientific Document Group. 2020 ESC guidelines for the diagnosis and management of atrial fibrillation developed in collaboration with the European Association for Cardio-Thoracic Surgery (EACTS): The Task Force for the diagnosis and management of atrial fibrillation of the European Society of Cardiology (ESC) Developed with the special contribution of the European Heart Rhythm Association (EHRA) of the ESC. Eur Heart J. 2021;42(5):373–498. https://doi.org/10.1093/eurheartj/ehaa612. Erratum in: Eur Heart J. 2021 Feb 1;42(5):507. Erratum in: Eur Heart J. 2021 Feb 1;42(5):546–547. Erratum in: Eur Heart J. 2021 Oct 21;42(40):4194.
3. Hindricks G, Potpara T, Dagres N, Arbelo E, Bax JJ, Blomström-Lundqvist C, Boriani G, Castella M, Dan GA, Dilaveris PE, Fauchier L, Filippatos G, Kalman JM, La Meir M, Lane DA, Lebeau JP, Lettino M, Lip GYH, Pinto FJ, Thomas GN, Valgimigli M, Van Gelder IC, Van Putte BP, Watkins CL, ESC Scientific Document Group. 2020 ESC Guidelines for the diagnosis and management of atrial fibrillation developed in collaboration with the European Association for Cardio-Thoracic Surgery (EACTS): The Task Force for the diagnosis and management of atrial fibrillation of the European Society of Cardiology (ESC) Developed with

the special contribution of the European Heart Rhythm Association (EHRA) of the ESC. Eur Heart J. 2021;42(5):373–498. https://doi.org/10.1093/eurheartj/ehaa612. Erratum in: Eur Heart J. 2021 Feb 1;42(5):507. Erratum in: Eur Heart J. 2021 Feb 1;42(5):546–547. Erratum in: Eur Heart J. 2021 Oct 21;42(40):4194.

4. Joglar JA, Chung MK, Armbruster AL, Benjamin EJ, Chyou JY, Cronin EM, Deswal A, Eckhardt L, Goldberger ZD, Gopinathannair R, Gorenek B, Hess PL, Hlatky M, Hogan G, Ibeh C, Indik JH, Kido K, Kusumoto F, Link MS, Linta KT, Marcus GM, McCarthy PM, Patel N, Patton KK, Perez MV, Piccini JP, Russo AM, Sanders P, Streur MM, Thomas KL, Times S, Tisdale JE, Valente AM, Van Wagoner DR. 2023 ACC/AHA/ACCP/HRS guideline for the diagnosis and management of atrial fibrillation: a report of the American College of Cardiology/American Heart Association Joint Committee on Clinical Practice Guidelines. Circulation. 2024;149:e1–e156. https://doi.org/10.1161/CIR.0000000000001193.
5. Reddy VY, Sievert H, Halperin J, Doshi SK, Buchbinder M, Neuzil P, Huber K, Whisenant B, Kar S, Swarup V, Gordon N, Holmes D. PROTECT AF Steering Committee and Investigators. Percutaneous left atrial appendage closure vs warfarin for atrial fibrillation: a randomized clinical trial. JAMA. 2014;312(19):1988–98. https://doi.org/10.1001/jama.2014.15192. Erratum in: JAMA 2015 Mar 10;313(10):1061.
6. Holmes DR Jr, Kar S, Price MJ, Whisenant B, Sievert H, Doshi SK, Huber K, Reddy VY. Prospective randomized evaluation of the Watchman Left Atrial Appendage Closure device in patients with atrial fibrillation versus long-term warfarin therapy: the PREVAIL trial. J Am Coll Cardiol. 2014;64(1):1–12. https://doi.org/10.1016/j.jacc.2014.04.029. Erratum in: J Am Coll Cardiol 2014 Sep 16;64(11):1186.
7. Holmes DR Jr, Doshi SK, Kar S, Price MJ, Sanchez JM, Sievert H, Valderrabano M, Reddy VY. Left atrial appendage closure as an alternative to warfarin for stroke prevention in atrial fibrillation: a patient-level meta-analysis. J Am Coll Cardiol. 2015;65(24):2614–23. https://doi.org/10.1016/j.jacc.2015.04.025.
8. ClinicalTrials.gov [Internet]. Bethesda (MD): National Library of Medicine (US). 2000 Feb 29 - . Identifier NCT04226547, Amplatzer Amulet LAAO vs. NOAC (CATALYST); first posted 2020 Jan 13, last updated 2023 Sep 13 [cited 2023 Nov 29]; [about 6 screens]. Available from: https://clinicaltrials.gov/study/NCT04226547.
9. CATALYST study protocol.
10. ClinicalTrials.gov [Internet]. Bethesda (MD): National Library of Medicine (US). 2000 Feb 29. Identifier NCT04394546, CHAMPION-AF Clinical Trial (CHAMPION-AF); first posted 2020 May 19, last updated 2023 Nov 21 [cited 2023 Nov 29]; [about 6 screens]. Available from: https://www.clinicaltrials.gov/study/NCT04394546.
11. Kar S, Doshi SK, Alkhouli M, Camm AJ, Coylewright M, Gibson MC, Granger CB, Gurol ME, Huber K, Mansour M, Nair DG, Natale A, Pocock SJ, Reddy VR, Saliba W, Christen T, Allocco DJ, Ellenbogen KA, Leon MB. Rationale and design of a randomized study comparing the Watchman FLX device to DOACs in patients with atrial fibrillation. Am Heart J. 2023;264:123–32. https://doi.org/10.1016/j.ahj.2023.05.022. Epub 2023 Jun 4.
12. Osmancik P, Herman D, Neuzil P, Hala P, Taborsky M, Kala P, Poloczek M, Stasek J, Haman L, Branny M, Chovancik J, Cervinka P, Holy J, Kovarnik T, Zemanek D, Havranek S, Vancura V, Opatrny J, Peichl P, Tousek P, Lekesova V, Jarkovsky J, Novackova M, Benesova K, Widimsky P, Reddy VY, PRAGUE-17 Trial Investigators. Left atrial appendage closure versus direct oral anticoagulants in high-risk patients with atrial fibrillation. J Am Coll Cardiol. 2020;75(25):3122–35. https://doi.org/10.1016/j.jacc.2020.04.067.

Index

S. J. Filby et al. (eds.), *A Contemporary Manual of Left Atrial Appendage Closure*, https://doi.org/10.1007/978-3-031-68441-8

MIX
Papier aus verantwortungsvollen Quellen
Paper from responsible sources
FSC® C105338
FSC
www.fsc.org

If you have any concerns about our products,
you can contact us on
ProductSafety@springernature.com

In case Publisher is established outside the EU,
the EU authorized representative is:
Springer Nature Customer Service Center GmbH
Europaplatz 3, 69115 Heidelberg, Germany

Printed by Libri Plureos GmbH
in Hamburg, Germany